Microbial Biofilms
Omics Biology, Antimicrobials and Clinical Implications

Microbial Biofilms
Omics Biology, Antimicrobials and Clinical Implications

Edited by
Chaminda Jayampath Seneviratne

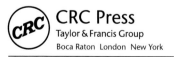

CRC Press
Taylor & Francis Group
Boca Raton London New York

CRC Press is an imprint of the
Taylor & Francis Group, an **informa** business

CRC Press
Taylor & Francis Group
6000 Broken Sound Parkway NW, Suite 300
Boca Raton, FL 33487-2742

First issued in paperback 2020

© 2017 by Taylor & Francis Group, LLC
CRC Press is an imprint of Taylor & Francis Group, an Informa business

No claim to original U.S. Government works

ISBN-13: 978-1-4987-2219-3 (hbk)
ISBN-13: 978-0-367-65799-4 (pbk)

Library of Congress Cataloging-in-Publication Data

Names: Seneviratne, Chaminda Jayampath, editor.
Title: Microbial biofilms : omics biology, antimicrobials and clinical
implications / [edited by] Chaminda Jayampath Seneviratne.
Description: Boca Raton, FL : CRC Press, 2017.
Identifiers: LCCN 2016050540 | ISBN 9781498722193 (hardback : alk. paper)
Subjects: | MESH: Biofilms | Anti-Infective Agents
Classification: LCC RM410 | NLM QW 90 | DDC 615.7/92--dc23
LC record available at https://lccn.loc.gov/2016050540

Visit the Taylor & Francis Web site at
http://www.taylorandfrancis.com

and the CRC Press Web site at
http://www.crcpress.com

To my loving mother and father

ආදරණීය අම්මා සහ තාත්තා වෙත බැතින්

Contents

Foreword

The new textbook *Microbial Biofilms: Omics Biology Antimicrobials and Clinical Implications* authored by renowned world experts and edited by Dr. Chaminda Jayampath Seneviratne is most welcome and relevant. Concepts of microbiome and 'omics' in general have changed the paradigm in infectious diseases and microbial ecology in many areas, including the mouth. The earlier concept where one infectious agent was thought to cause a certain disease seems outdated in many cases, being now replaced by the better understanding of complex microbial communities. There, individual microbes work together and also communicate with each other. Modern research techniques have enabled scrutinising the mysteries of the microbial communities, and we have learnt a lot about their genetics, metabolism and behaviour. These aspects are thoroughly covered in this new textbook.

In many regards, research on oral microbiota has been pioneering in investigating 'dental plaque' and understanding indeed that only seldom can one micro-organism be pointed out as the culprit of a certain condition. Similarly it has been important to realise that most micro-organisms harbouring the human being are not pathogens but, on the contrary, needed and beneficial to health. The homeostasis between the microbiome and the host is prerequisite for healthy life as we understand it. Taken into consideration the fact that micro-organisms have been there millions of years before man, research in this co-existence cannot be over-emphasised. The new textbook elegantly summarises current knowledge of microbial biofilms in the perspective of oral health and clinical implications. The book is going to be an invaluable tool in the hands of students and researchers interested in this highly relevant topic.

Jukka H. Meurman
MD, PhD, Dr. Odont, Dr. hc. (multi), FDSRCSEd.
Professor
Department of Oral and Maxillofacial Diseases
University of Helsinki and Helsinki University Hospital
Helsinki, Finland

Preface

The field of microbiology has indeed come a long way from the very first observation of microbes by Antonie van Leeuwenhoek in 1663 to the science of the twenty-first century. The study of 'microbial biofilms' is, however, a relatively new discipline in the field of microbiology, consolidated in the 1980s. Consequently, there are only a handful of books on the topic. Moreover, as the field of microbial biofilms encompasses both clinical and environmental microbiology, the spectrum of topics that can be covered in this area is very diverse. A closer look at the available resources shows that books on clinical implications of microbial biofilms, keeping in mind a target audience of medical, dental and pharmacology students and researchers, are relatively sparse. This book attempts to fill this resource gap for the educators, researchers and clinicians working on biofilms.

One of the most promising vistas of our book is the ready information available on exploratory omics of microbial biofilms. The chapters dedicated to metagenomics, proteomics and metabolomics analysis of microbial biofilms are intended to provide a simple and holistic view of current knowledge, examples and applications of these cutting-edge technologies in the field of microbial biofilms. The next-generation and futuristic omics approaches that could be applied in biofilm research are also briefly discussed at the conclusion of these chapters. The book starts with two introductory chapters on microbial biofilms and their clinical implications, subsequently expanding into the topics of oral biofilms and their compositional and diversity mapping using metagenomics, drug resistance mechanisms observed in microbial biofilms and their characterisation using proteomics approaches, metabolomics characterisation of microbial biofilms, molecular mechanisms and strategies for tackling persister cells, host–microbial interactions at mucosal surfaces and finally concluding with a chapter on the application of novel therapeutic approaches such as synbiotics and biogenics against biofilms. Both bacterial and fungal biofilms have been discussed in this book along with their clinical implications. An overview of the cutting-edge technologies in metagenomics, proteomics and metabolomics characterisation of biofilms has been provided for readers to appreciate the value of these approaches in future research. An insight into the higher drug resistance of microbial biofilms as well as a discussion of 'persisters', which are highly drug-resistant populations found in microbial biofilms, will shed light on the clinical problems associated with biofilm infections. The diversity of microbial communities associated with different mucosal surfaces and their interplay with the host can provide an idea of the multitude of possibilities that can arise from host–microbial interactions. Finally, some very interesting therapeutic options including prebiotics, probiotics and synbiotics are described to give an idea of the direction towards which the future treatment of biofilms is heading. Overall, the book has been tailored in a way such as to have an equal appeal to both researchers and clinicians.

Publishing a tome of this proportion involves teamwork that encompasses editor, contributors and publisher. I was fortunate to have thoughtful and enthusiastic contributors for the chapters, to whom I am earnestly grateful. I would like to convey my sincere thanks to the team at CRC Press/Taylor & Francis Group, particularly Chuck Crumly and Jennifer Blaise, for providing me with excellent support during this entire process. I am thankful to my research team at the Faculty of Dentistry, National University of Singapore and to Tanujaa, Thuyen, Kassapa, Preethi, Nitya and Neha for their wonderful suggestions and support throughout this period. Academic and research work always comes with the certain price of losing good family time. I am indebted to my wonderful family, Thanuja, Desadu and Thalya, for their love and kindness in patiently allowing me to complete this work.

The book promises to provide a foundational knowledge on microbial biofilms to its readers. However, researchers and clinicians should keep abreast of this evolving, dynamic field of microbial biofilms. We hope that readers will find the chapters informative and that the information presented in the book may provide a stimulus to them to venture into devising new solutions for the clinical problems associated with microbial biofilms, ultimately benefitting patients' health.

Chaminda Jayampath Seneviratne
Singapore

Contributors

Finbarr Allen
Discipline of Endodontics, Operative
 Dentistry & Prosthodontics
Faculty of Dentistry
National University of Singapore
Singapore

Preethi Balan
Discipline of Oral Sciences
Faculty of Dentistry
National University of Singapore
Singapore

Georgios N. Belibasakis
Department of Dental Medicine
Karolinska Institute
Stockholm, Sweden

Nagihan Bostanci
Division of Periodontology
Department of Dental Medicine
Karolinska Institute
Stockholm, Sweden

Wim Crielaard
Department of Preventive Dentistry
Academic Centre for Dentistry
 Amsterdam (ACTA)
University of Amsterdam and
 VU University
Amsterdam, the Netherlands

Kassapa Ellepola
Discipline of Oral Sciences
Faculty of Dentistry
National University of Singapore
Singapore

Kelvin Foong
Discipline of Orthodontics and
 Paediatric Dentistry
Faculty of Dentistry
National University of Singapore
Singapore

Intekhab Islam
Discipline of Oral & Maxillofacial
 Surgery
Faculty of Dentistry
National University of Singapore
Singapore

Lijian Jin
Faculty of Dentistry
The University of Hong Kong
Pok Fu Lam, Hong Kong

Tomomi Kawai
Department of Oral Microbiology
School of Dental Medicine
Tsurumi University
Kanagawa, Japan

Ryan Kean
Oral Sciences Research Group
Glasgow Dental School
School of Medicine
College of Medical, Veterinary and Life
 Sciences
University of Glasgow
Glasgow, United Kingdom

Yukako Kojima
Department of Oral Microbiology
School of Dental Medicine
Tsurumi University
Kanagawa, Japan

Yuan Kun Lee
Department of Microbiology
Yong Loo Lin School of Medicine
National University of Singapore
Singapore

Peng Li
Faculty of Dentistry
The University of Hong Kong
Pok Fu Lam, Hong Kong

Nobuko Maeda
Department of Oral Microbiology
School of Dental Medicine
Tsurumi University
Kanagawa, Japan

Wei Ling Ng
Metabolites Biology Lab
Department of Biological Sciences
National University of Singapore
Singapore

Lindsay E. O'Donnell
Oral Sciences Research Group
Glasgow Dental School
School of Medicine
College of Medical, Veterinary and Life
    Sciences
University of Glasgow
Glasgow, United Kingdom

Tomoko Ohshima
Department of Oral Microbiology
School of Dental Medicine
Tsurumi University
Kanagawa, Japan

Shruti Pavagadhi
Singapore Centre on Environmental
    Life Sciences Engineering
    (SCELSE)
National University of Singapore,
    Centre for Life Sciences
Singapore

Kia Joo Puan
Singapore Immunology Network (SIgN)
Agency for Science, Technology and
    Research (A*STAR)
Singapore

Lin Qingsong
Department of Biological Sciences
National University of Singapore
Singapore

Ranjith Rajendran
Oral Sciences Research Group
Glasgow Dental School
School of Medicine
College of Medical, Veterinary and Life
    Sciences
University of Glasgow
Glasgow, United Kingdom

Gordon Ramage
Oral Sciences Research Group
Glasgow Dental School
School of Medicine
College of Medical, Veterinary and Life
    Sciences
University of Glasgow
Glasgow, United Kingdom

Chaminda Jayampath Seneviratne
Discipline of Oral Sciences
Faculty of Dentistry
National University of Singapore
Singapore

Neha Srivastava
Discipline of Oral Sciences
Faculty of Dentistry
National University of Singapore
Singapore

Tanujaa Suriyanarayanan
Discipline of Oral Sciences
Faculty of Dentistry
National University of Singapore
Singapore

Sanjay Swarup
Metabolites Biology Lab
Department of Biological Sciences
   (DBS)
Singapore Centre on Environmental
   Life Sciences Engineering
   (SCELSE)
NUS Environmental Research Institute
   (NERI)
Synthetic Biology for Clinical and
   Technological Innovation (SynCTI)
National University of Singapore
Singapore

Eleanor Townsend
Oral Sciences Research Group
Glasgow Dental School
School of Medicine
College of Medical, Veterinary and Life
   Sciences
University of Glasgow
Glasgow, United Kingdom

Thuyen Truong
Discipline of Oral Sciences
Faculty of Dentistry
National University of Singapore
Singapore

Nityasri Venkiteswaran
Discipline of Oral Sciences
Faculty of Dentistry
National University of Singapore
Singapore

Juan Antonio Vizcaíno
European Molecular Biology Laboratory,
   European Bioinformatics Institute
   (EMBL-EBI)
Wellcome Trust Genome Campus
Cambridge, United Kingdom

Yue Wang
Institute of Cellular and Molecular
   Biology
Agency for Science, Technology and
   Research
Department of Biochemistry
Yong Loo Lin School of Medicine
National University of Singapore
Singapore

Siew Cheng Wong
Singapore Immunology Network (SIgN)
Agency for Science, Technology and
   Research (A*STAR)
Singapore

1 Microbial Biofilms

An Introduction to Their Development, Properties and Clinical Implications

Chaminda Jayampath Seneviratne, Neha Srivastava,
Intekhab Islam, Kelvin Foong and Finbarr Allen

CONTENTS

My work, which I've done for a long time, was not pursued in order to gain the praise I now enjoy, but chiefly from a craving after knowledge, which I notice resides in me more than in most other men.

And therewithal, whenever I found out anything remarkable, I have thought it my duty to put down my discovery on paper, so that all ingenious people might be informed thereof.

Antonie van Leeuwenhoek (1632–1723), Letter of 12th June 1716

HISTORICAL PERSPECTIVES

The existence of microorganisms – living beings invisible to the naked eye – had always been an intriguing concept in the history of mankind, popular among both religious and scientific communities. Jain scriptures described submicroscopic creatures living in clusters which are present universally. Similarly, certain factions of the scientific community held the view that epidemic diseases such as tuberculosis are caused by the transfer of seed-like materials. However, most of these reports were insubstantial as they were based either on suppositions or indirect observations. The first solid proof for the existence of microorganisms came in 1663 from the work of the Dutch scientist Antonie van Leeuwenhoek, who is regarded as the father of microbiology. Van Leeuwenhoek developed a series of lenses through which he was able to observe the presence of microorganisms [1]. Dental plaque was one of the first specimens he observed under the microscope, where he found the presence of 'animalcules' [i.e. bacteria] in the 'white little matter' between his teeth, which he described as 'a living of animalcules swimming nimbly than any I have ever seen… the biggest short bending their body into curves in going forward' in his correspondence to the Royal Society of London.

Van Leeuwenhoek's microscopic observations paved the foundation for modern microbiology. He performed a number of studies on dental plaque and was the first to observe the resistance phenomena of microorganisms in biofilms. On the basis of these experiments, he reported that the treatment of dental plaque by gargling with vinegar was able to kill only those 'little animals' present on the outside of the plaque and could not penetrate the inside of the plaque. These and several other of van Leeuwenhoek's studies raised the possibility that 'there are more little animals living on the teeth than men in a whole kingdom' as well as the community existence of microorganisms referred to in modern terms as biofilms. A number of microscopic observations of bacteria were also made by Leeuwenhoek's contemporary Robert Hooke, who first coined the term 'cell' to describe these microorganisms.

Van Leeuwenhoek's reports, although establishing the ubiquitous occurrence of microorganisms, did not focus on the causal relationship between microorganisms and disease. The work of Robert Koch was instrumental in developing the aetiological basis of the 'germ theory of disease'. In 1876 Koch described *Bacillus anthracis*, a rod-shaped bacterium, as the causative agent of anthrax. In 1878, he developed several methods to obtain pathogenic microorganisms in pure culture, with his work providing the first clue that specific microorganisms could be causative agents of specific diseases in animals and humans. Later studies based on Koch's postulates successfully established the causal relationship between an infectious agent and a disease [2].

Some of the most significant breakthroughs in the field of microbiology were made in the eighteenth, nineteenth and early twentieth centuries, with the pioneering development of vaccines by Edward Jenner in 1796, pasteurisation by Louis Pasteur in 1864, disinfection by Joseph Lister in 1883, and antibiotics by Paul Ehrlich in 1912. The discovery of penicillin by Alexander Fleming in 1929 ushered in the 'antibiotics era'. While working with *Staphylococcus* cultures, Fleming observed that the plates contaminated with a large mould exhibited lysis of the bacterial colonies. Subsequently, the mould was identified as *Penicillium* and the antibacterial component in the broth of the mould was named *penicillin*. The discovery of viruses and prions led to further understanding of the pathogenicity of microorganisms. Development of DNA sequencing methods by Walter Gilbert and Fred Sanger in 1977 and the polymerase chain reaction (PCR) by Kary Mullis in 1986 provided methodological tools to identify uncultivable microorganisms using PCR-based technology.

The community-style existence of microorganisms was reported by several groups following the initial observations of van Leeuwenhoek. In the 1930s, marine biologists found that fouling of submerged surfaces in ships is caused by clumps consisting of marine bacteria. In 1970s Niels Høiby observed cystic fibrosis (CF) was associated with heaps of a mucoid variant of *Pseudomonas aeruginosa* present in the sputum and lung tissues of the patients. However, the concept of 'biofilms' or a community of microorganisms as a major bacterial lifestyle was popularised largely owing to the work of William Costerton. Until the 1970s, most microbiological studies were based on the notion that bacteria live predominantly in a suspension as free-swimming organisms called the 'planktonic mode' of growth. As a result of the pioneering work of William 'Bill' Costerton, it became increasingly evident that biofilm or 'surface-associated community lifestyle' is the preferred growth mode of microorganisms in nature. One of the first reports on 'biofilms' from Costeron's group was on the natural population of bacteria associated with slime on submerged surfaces in a mountain stream [3]. They observed that the slime contained large numbers of bacteria enmeshed within an extensive fibrous matrix promoting microcolony development and anchoring to surface. They proposed that these slime-enmeshed microcolonies constitute functional communities within which most sessile bacteria live [4,5]. The term *biofilm* used to describe these surface-attached bacterial communities was coined by Costerton, who later started the Centre for Biofilm Engineering at Montana State University, Bozeman. Subsequently, extensive studies were performed on microbial biofilms by various research groups to understand their development, properties and implications in human health and disease [6].

Biofilms can be formed on both biotic and abiotic surfaces including animals, plants, the human body, river valleys, volcanoes, pipelines, and rivers. In fact, there are reports suggesting that biofilm communities existed nearly 3.5 billion years ago [7]. It is noteworthy to recall that Earth was formed about 4.5 billion years ago. Therefore, biofilms could possibly be one of the earliest communities that existed on Earth. The concept of 'biofilm' is an important landmark in the field of microbiology that influenced many other associated scientific areas. According to the Centers for Disease Control and Prevention (CDC) in the United States, at least 65–80% of infectious diseases are related to the biofilm mode of growth [8]. In addition, microorganisms undergoing the biofilm mode of growth exhibit a higher level of drug resistance which is associated with therapeutic failure. An understanding of microbial biofilms and their formation mechanisms therefore goes a long way towards the advancement of the field of medicine and drug development.

STAGES OF BIOFILM DEVELOPMENT

Over the past few decades, much research has been expended on exploring the various properties of biofilms to understand microbial behavior better [9,10]. Biofilms are formed only under specific environmental and flow conditions. Mere surface contact of microorganisms or sedimentation does not necessarily lead to biofilm formation, as biofilms are more than just a continuous collection of microbial cells [11,12]. The development of biofilm on any surface involves a well-organised series of five sequential events: (1) initial reversible attachment of the planktonic microorganisms to the surface, (2) irreversible attachment of the organisms to the surface, (3) development of microcolonies by the adhered microorganisms, (4) secretion of extracellular polymeric substances (EPS) and development of a three-dimensional mature biofilm community and (5) dispersal of microorganisms from the biofilm community to seek new surfaces (Figure 1.1) [10,11]. These developmental stages are common to both bacterial and fungal biofilms. The production of EPS is a salient and unique feature of microbial biofilms [13,14]. Microbial cells become embedded in the EPS, which not only acts as a scaffold for the biofilm community but also contributes to antimicrobial resistance. Therefore, microbial biofilms could be defined as surface-attached structured microbial communities that are encased in a matrix of exopolymeric substances displaying features that are different from those

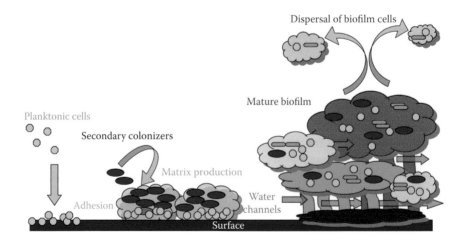

FIGURE 1.1 Sequence of biofilm formation on surfaces. (Reproduced from Seneviratne CJ et al. *Oral Diseases*, 2008. With permission.)

of their free-floating or planktonic counterparts [15]. The critical steps involved in the attachment and maturation of biofilms are described in more detail in the subsections that follow.

EARLY ADHESION PHASE

The successful initiation of biofilm formation on surfaces depends on the firm attachment of the microorganisms to the surfaces. The adhesion of bacteria to surfaces is both an important stage in biofilm development as well as a survival strategy adapted by bacteria over millions of years of evolution on Earth [16]. This trait allows the microorganisms to select a suitable environment to build a biofilm community. Bacterial adhesion occurs in two phases: reversible attachment followed by irreversible attachment. This process is also governed by various environmental factors. A number of theories have been proposed to describe the interactions between the microbe and the surface. However, adhesion is a complex process determined by the properties of the microorganism, attachment surface, and the immediate environment. Therefore, a complete understanding of this process has not yet been achieved.

The critical question that needs to be addressed is the trigger that makes a bacterium adhere to a particular surface, abandoning its free-floating or 'planktonic' mode of growth. Although contact with a surface is a primary requisite, not all bacteria in close proximity to a surface adhere to it. The properties of the surfaces and their interactions with the bacteria play a major role in the initial attachment phase. Microorganisms can come into contact with a given surface by means of Brownian motion, sedimentation, movement with liquid flow, bacterial motility conferred by cell surface appendages or by travelling with other cells as aggregates [17]. A bacterium in liquid without any means of active locomotion will move as a result of random collisions with its surrounding molecules. Random walks describe the trajectory of a particle that steps in any direction in space with equal probability per unit time [18]. These random movements are called diffusion or Brownian motion. Bacterial surface appendages such as type IV pili (TFP) facilitate surface sensing by the bacterium, allowing it to transit from vertical into horizontal cell orientation such as seen in *Pseudomonas aeruginosa* [18]. The net interactions occurring as a result of these motions or surface appendages determine the course of attachment of the microbe to the surface. For example, it is suggested that a low level of TFP production primes planktonic microorganisms to use their pili to 'feel' the surface [19]. Once attached to the surface, TFP helps microbes to 'crawl' when the surface is oriented parallel to the cell and 'walk' when the cell is in upright position [20]. However, adhesion mediated by TFP seems to be unspecific, as it allows the bacterium to adhere to almost all known abiotic and biotic surfaces [18]. The critical proximity distance determining microbial attachment to a surface is less than 1 nm. At this proximity, the net sum of attractive and repulsive forces determines the adhesion process. These include electrostatic and hydrophobic interactions, steric hindrance, van der Waals forces, temperature and hydrodynamic forces. Though bacterial surfaces are negatively charged in general [21], surface charges may become irrelevant in the case of dead cells among floating bacterial communities, as they may change their coadhesion properties. For example, bacteria swimming in close proximity to surfaces experience hydrodynamic forces that both attract them towards the surface and cause them to move in circular trajectories [22].

IRREVERSIBLE ADHESION TO THE SURFACE

The second stage of bacterial adhesion is the irreversible attachment stage or 'locking'. Bacterial surface protein called 'adhesins' and appendages such as pili are important players in this adhesion stage. In addition, receptor-specific ligands located on pili and fimbriae may lock the microorganism to the surface, especially in the case of biotic surfaces. Interactions between microbial adhesins and host cell receptors are discussed in detail in Chapter 9. In general, the microorganisms attached to a particular surface exist as a mixture of multiple species rather than belonging to any single species. In such cases, competition or synergism among the multispecific community may occur. For instance, some bacteria tend to stick to each other, forming bacterial aggregates on the surface. *Fusobacterium nucleatum*, a bacterium found in dental plaque biofilm, is known to carry multiple binding sites for various other bacteria such as *Streptococcus* and is known as a 'bridging' organism [23].

Apart from the properties of the microbe and its proximity to the attachment surface, the nature of the attachment surface also has an important role in the process of adhesion. Some of the important surface properties that determine microbial attachment include surface charge, surface free energy, roughness, hydrophobicity, configuration topography and stiffness [17,24]. For example, surface hydrophobicity can either promote or inhibit bacterial adhesion. In oral environments, especially in supragingival regions (above the gum margin), less biofilm is formed on hydrophobic surfaces than on hydrophilic ones, whereas no such difference is observed for subgingival biofilms [17].

MICROCOLONY FORMATION AND EARLY DEVELOPMENT STAGES OF BIOFILMS

Once microorganisms irreversibly adhere to a surface, the next step in biofilm development is community growth, intercellular communication and networking of microorganisms which ultimately leads to a well-organised, three-dimensional biofilm structure. This stage is characterised by the development of microcolonies that are enmeshed in the extracellular matrix. At this stage, coadhesion and coaggregation occur, resulting in localised microcolonies. Generally, the motility appendages of microorganisms are suppressed on attachment. For example, the synthesis of the flagella is repressed in motile bacteria after attachment. However, it is unclear whether the flagellum is functional, or lost and degraded, or if it is a structural component in the biofilm on surface attachment [22]. Mutations in the flagellar structural gene, flagellin A (*flaA*), resulted in increased exopolysaccharide production which suggested that the lack of flagellum may serve as a signal for biofilm formation. Moreover, studies on *Bacillus subtilis* have shown motility and matrix formation are linked by SinR, a protein that up-regulates expression of flagellar genes and down-regulates expression of matrix-forming genes [25]. *B. subtilis* developed enhanced biofilm formation ability when the *sinR* gene is deleted.

Once the microbes are attached to a surface, other cell wall components or adhesions of the microbial surface may also undergo expression changes or be instrumental in subsequent development steps. Bacteria such as *Staphylococcus* have a cell wall exopolysaccharide named polysaccharide intercellular adhesin (PIA) [26]. The importance of PIA for biofilm formation has been demonstrated in numerous *in vitro* and *in vivo* studies. Lipoteichoic acid (LTA), a cell wall component of Gram-positive bacteria, has also been shown to be important for biofilm formation, possibly because of its interaction with other surface polymers via electrostatic forces. However, there are also reports showing that the impact of LTA in bacteria such as *Staphylococcus aureus* and *Staphylococcus epidermidis* is not directly related to the attachment, but indirect via alteration of surface hydrophobicity [27]. In several Gram-negative bacteria, attachment is reinforced by specific adhesins located on the bacterial cell surface or on cellular appendages such as pili and flagella [28]. Extracellular DNA (eDNA) secreted by the bacteria is also important as it provides a negative charge to interact with positively charged surface molecules [29,30]. However, it must be noted that the adhesion to a biotic surface such as human skin or gut mucosa may be considerably different from the adhesion to an abiotic surface [26]. *In vivo* attachment is governed by the interaction of microorganisms with human matrix proteins [27]. For instance, bacteria such as *Staphylococcus* express a large variety of surface-anchored proteins, collectively called MSCRAMMs (microbial surface components recognising adhesive matrix molecules), that bind to host matrix proteins such as fibronectin. The mechanism of host–microbial interaction is discussed in detail in Chapter 9.

BIOFILM MATURATION

The development of microcolonies is followed by the maturation of the biofilm into a spatially organised three-dimensional community. Though the demarcations between young and mature biofilms are not always clear, certain hallmark features such as the formation of extracellular matrix encasing the microbial community help in distinguishing the mature from the young biofilms [27]. The exopolymeric matrix surrounding the biofilms has also been termed a 'slime layer' in the past [16]. This layer of extracellular polymeric substances (EPS) provides various advantages to the biofilm community such as facilitating adhesion to surfaces, enabling the development of multilayered biofilm and serving as a barrier to influx of drugs and other toxic substances. The EPS layer comprises various components with different chemical natures such as exopolysaccharides, proteins, eDNA and other polymers [30]. While the EPS confer the mature architecture of the biofilms, the shape of mature biofilms is determined by various environmental factors, particularly the flow conditions in the immediate environment. Depending on the fluid flow rates, bacteria such as *P. aeruginosa* and *V. cholerae* have been shown to develop mushroom stalk architecture biofilms indicating the onset of maturation [31,32]. Development of EPS observed *in vivo* using labeling strategies in *V. cholerae* biofilms has shown distinct levels of spatial organisation [33]. In general, the EPS may act as a physical barrier that prevents the access of antimicrobials to cells embedded in the biofilm community, in turn contributing to enhanced drug resistance. This hindrance is thought to depend largely on the amount and nature of the EPS, as well as the physicochemical properties of the drug.

Mature biofilms have several layers of cells embedded within the matrix and are therefore composed of heterogeneous cell populations with differing levels of metabolic activities depending on their spatio-temporal location. This gradation of metabolic activities has been observed in *Candida* biofilms and *P. aeruginosa* by several groups [34–36]. According to these studies, within a multilayered biofilm structure, the bottom layers are usually in a state of quiescence, while the middle and top layers exhibit higher levels of metabolic activities. Furthermore, as maturation of the biofilm progresses, quiescence of certain cell populations seems to occur along with a concomitant reduction in metabolic activity and cellular viability. These subpopulations of cells are termed 'persisters', and have been observed in bacterial biofilms such as *P. aeruginosa*, *E. coli* and *S. aureus* and in fungal biofilms such as *C. albicans* [35,37]. Persister cells demonstrate exceeding levels of higher resistance to antimicrobial agents [36,38]. The properties of persister cells and their implications in biofilm biology are discussed later in Chapter 8.

BIOFILM DISPERSAL

The final stage in a biofilm life cycle is called the dispersal stage and involves the detachment of cells from mature biofilms followed by colonisation of a different surface. Detachment is considered a passive process caused by shear stress [39]. Some suggest that the detachment occurs only in biofilms grown under laminar shear forces and biofilm cells are more likely to detach when shear forces become more turbulent [40]. Dispersal, on the other hand, is considered an active process, which is usually triggered by several environmental factors and quorum sensing mechanisms [26]. It is important for the expansion of biofilm communities and has serious clinical consequences in the context of *in vivo* biofilm infections [39]. Detached cells from biofilms usually establish secondary biofilm infections elsewhere, possibly with increased severity, such as in the case of endocarditis. In addition, the detached cells may also cause acute infections which are not associated with biofilms per se [30].

Dispersal is the least understood and perhaps the most complicated process in both fungal and bacterial biofilm development. The trigger for the dispersal process to occur and the biological pathways modulating dispersal may vary considerably among different microorganisms [41]. Cells from the biofilm may detach singly or as a group and move through a fluid phase to seed new sites. Numerous research groups have put forth efforts to understand this mechanism in pathogenic organisms such as *P. aeruginosa* and *C. albicans*. Bacterial secondary messengers such as cyclic di-GMP have been shown to provide critical signals for biofilm formation as well as dispersal [42]. The factors which signal dispersion can vary, ranging from environmental stimuli, nutrients, certain chemicals such as *cis*-2-decenoic acid or nitric oxide or proteins such as BdlA, a chemotaxis regulator [43–45]. It has also been shown recently that phosphorylation status of diguanylate cyclase NIcD can affect the dispersal of biofilms in *P. aeruginosa* [46]. The aforementioned study demonstrated dispersal inducing environmental cues are sensed by the diguanylate cyclase NicD belonging to a seven transmembrane receptor family. The sensing of dispersal cues by NicD results in NicD dephosphorylation, followed by activation of a chemotaxis regulator BdlA, which in turn activates DipA, a phosphodiesterase molecule. This leads to altered levels of second messenger cyclic-di-GMP molecules signalling dispersion. Studies on *C. albicans* biofilms have found Set3–NRG1 complex as possible regulators of biofilm dispersal. Set3, an NAD-dependent histone deacetylation complex, modulates NRG, a transcriptional regulator of biofilm dispersal and a repressor of filamentation [47]. The typical dispersal of *C. albicans* from biofilms is in the yeast form [48]. Moreover, it was shown that deletion of *Nrg1* gene in *C. albicans* attenuates *in vivo* virulence of the fungus in systemic candidiasis [49]. Therefore, with proper understanding of the dispersal process, alternative therapeutic strategies may be devised for controlling the spread of these pathogenic organisms.

MIXED-SPECIES BIOFILMS

Most of the research on microbial biofilms has focused entirely on understanding the nature of monospecific biofilms. However, in the natural environment and in most infections, biofilms exist as part of a multispecific community (Figure 1.2) [50,51]. The various interactions among the different microbial species in the biofilm community such as quorum sensing, metabolic relationships and competitions can influence each other's properties and virulence [52,53]. Whereas some species exhibit synergism, some may exhibit antagonistic effects. Some examples of synergism between microorganisms include the promotion of biofilm formation by coaggregation; metabolic cooperation, where one species utilises a metabolite produced by a neighbouring species; and increased resistance to antibiotics and clinical implications. A synergistic effect has been observed in mixed-species biofilms of *C. albicans* and *P. aeruginosa*, which are more virulent in CF patients than their respective monospecific biofilms [54]. Interspecific interactions of bacterial–bacterial as well as bacterial–fungal mixed-species biofilms and their implications in polymicrobial diseases are discussed in subsequent chapters.

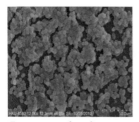
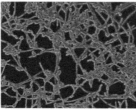
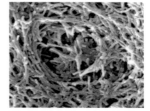

Enterococcus faecalis monospecies bacterial biofilm

Candida albicans monospecies fungal biofilm

Mixed-species bacterial biofilms *Actinomyces naelundii, Lactobacillus acidophilus, Lactobacillus rhamnosus, Streptococcus mutans* and *Streptococcus sobrinus* species

FIGURE 1.2 Scanning electron microscopic images of microbial biofilms. (Reproduced from Seneviratne CJ et al. *Proteomics*, 2012. With permission.)

PROPERTIES OF MICROBIAL BIOFILMS

The properties and behavior of microbial biofilms differ considerably from those of their planktonic counterparts. The existence of microorganisms in the biofilm mode confers numerous survival advantages, mainly owing to the nature and composition of biofilms. One of the most important distinguishing traits of biofilms is their exceedingly high level of drug resistance, which is a major concern in clinical settings [55,56]. The clinical relevance of the biofilm-associated drug resistance is discussed comprehensively in subsequent chapters. Only a brief overview of the biofilm properties is given in the text that follows.

Antimicrobial resistance in the biofilm mode of growth could be as high as a thousand-fold over the planktonic mode, rendering the use of antimicrobial therapy ineffective under such conditions. For instance, common antimicrobials such as penicillin and metronidazole, which are used for Gram-positive and Gram-negative bacterial infections, respectively, may not be active against the biofilm infections of these pathogens [57]. Similarly, chlorhexidine, a widely used chemical antibacterial agent in mouth rinses, is reported to be ineffective at a 0.2% concentration for some oral biofilms [58,59]. Therefore, considerable efforts have been made by various research groups worldwide to understand the reasons for the high drug resistance observed in the biofilm mode of growth. Based on these studies, researchers have proposed several hypotheses to explain this phenomenon: (1) altered metabolic activity, (2) presence of extracellular polymeric substance, (3) presence of highly drug-resistant populations called persisters, (4) higher antioxidative capacities and (5) differential gene/protein expression (Figure 1.3) [56]. These concepts and their implications are comprehensively discussed in other chapters.

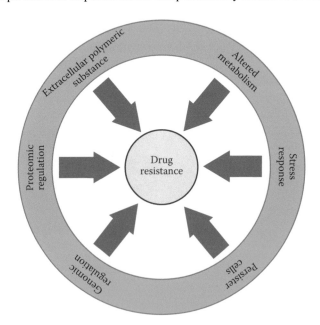

FIGURE 1.3   Factors that may contribute to the higher drug resistance in microbial biofilms. (Reproduced from Seneviratne CJ et al. *Proteomics*, 2012. With permission.)

CLINICAL IMPLICATIONS OF MICROBIAL BIOFILMS

At this juncture of this chapter, we have established that biofilms are the predominant mode of microbial existence. We have discussed the formation of microbial biofilms on both abiotic and biotic surfaces and their life cycle stages in the previous sections of this chapter. The rest of the chapter focuses on the clinical implication of microbial biofilms, in particular, biofilm-associated infections (BAIs). The pathogenic role of microbial biofilms formed on medical devices and human tissues is well established [60]. Even under healthy conditions, human body surfaces such as skin, teeth, oral mucosa and gut harbour millions of commensal microorganisms, which reside predominantly in the biofilm mode of growth. However, under certain circumstances, breakdown of the harmonious host–microbial relationship, may lead to serious consequences to the host. As mentioned previously, according to the CDC at least 65–80% of human infections are associated with the biofilm mode of growth of microorganisms [8]. Hence, approximately two-thirds of nosocomial infections are BAIs [60].

BAIs are broadly categorised as medical device–associated infections and tissue-associated infections [61]. In some cases, hosts may suffer from both types of infections, as a consequence of the other. The primary difference between two types is that tissue biofilm–associated infections do not involve a foreign body surface. Common examples include biofilm infections associated with teeth, gastrointestinal tract, vagina and skin. Moreover, biofilm in wound infections and infected lungs of CF patients are also considered as tissue biofilms. BAIs in medical devices such as catheters, various surgical implants, prosthetic heart valves, contact lenses and others are discussed in the text that follows. Although the main pathogenic agents responsible for biofilm infections are well characterised, it should be noted that with advanced technology such as next-generation sequencing, the list continues to grow. The new information on biofilm microbiome derived from novel gene sequencing technologies is discussed in Chapter 4. A brief overview of the clinical implications of BAIs is given in the text that follows. It should be noted that the following discussion is not an exhaustive list of BAIs, as there are too many to cover under this topic. The clinical implications of microbial biofilms are also comprehensively discussed in subsequent chapters.

MEDICAL DEVICE–ASSOCIATED BIOFILM INFECTIONS

Medical device–associated biofilm infections occur when microorganisms adhere to the indwelling or implanted medical prosthesis. If favorable conditions prevail, microbial adherence leads to biofilm formation on these surfaces. These biofilms, if not eradicated, can be a prelude to both infection and malfunction of the device, giving dire consequences to the host [62]. Biofilm formation has been reported on virtually all medical devices which are being used currently – central venous, urinary and peritoneal dialysis catheters and prosthetic heart valves, cardiac pacemakers, artificial voice prostheses, replacement joints, cerebrospinal fluid shunts, endotracheal tubes, contact lenses and implanted prosthetic devices for erectile dysfunction [61,63]. Hence, medical devices are responsible for a large portion of nosocomial infections, particularly in critically ill patients [64]. Although the predominant species on medical device biofilms may vary depending on the properties of the medical device, they are colonised primarily by a single bacterial species. It is reconstituted as a multispecific community as the biofilm development progresses [40].

The formation of biofilms on indwelling medical devices is influenced by factors related to the microorganisms, device properties and host microenvironment. These include irreversible attachment of microorganisms to the exposed surfaces of the device, the number and types of cells in the liquid to which the device is exposed, the flow rate of liquid through the device and the physicochemical characteristics of the surface [63,65]. For instance, it has been shown that adhesion of *S. epidermidis* and *P. aeruginosa* are dependent on pyrolytic carbon surface, free energy and roughness. On the contrary, adhesion of *S. aureus* is independent of the foregoing factors [66]. When the indwelling medical devices are inserted, a conditioning film from the organic matter present in the surrounding fluid is deposited on it. The source of this film could be host-derived proteins such as fibrinogen, fibronectin and collagen which influence the subsequent adherence of microorganisms. Thus, an *in vitro* model cannot mimic the composition and structure of biofilms formed *in vivo*. For this reason, the results derived from *in vitro* biofilm models should be interpreted with caution and *in vitro* studies should be complemented with *ex vivo* or *in vivo* models for more clinically relevant results. Some common medical device–associated biofilm infections are discussed in the following subsections.

CATHETER-ASSOCIATED BIOFILM INFECTIONS

Catheters are medical devices which are inserted into the body to deliver or drain medications, fluids or gasses. These catheters provide a binding surface for microorganisms to adhere. Under favourable conditions, adhered microorganisms may develop biofilms on catheters, leading to chronic BAI. The catheter invades through the skin insertion site and invariably comes in contact with the patient's endogenous skin microflora. However, the first contact of microorganisms with the catheter surface does not lead to biofilm formation. The chances of biofilm formation become higher when the catheter is placed for an extended period of time. Biofilms can be formed on the extraluminal as well as the interluminal surfaces of the catheter, which have considerable differences in terms of source and composition. Some common examples of catheter-associated biofilm infections are discussed in the paragraphs that follow.

Central venous catheters (CVCs) and urinary catheters associated biofilm infections are a common occurrence in hospital settings. A CVC is a special type of catheter that is placed into a large vein such as internal jugular, subclavian, axillary or femoral veins. A CVC provides an alternative route of administration of medications or nutrients to patients who are unable to take them orally. As CVCs are commonly used for critically ill patients, they might require placement for a considerable period of time. Hence, they become prone to develop biofilms, which eventually leads to catheter-related bloodstream infections [67,68]. An alarming number of catheter-related bloodstream infections (250,000–400,000) occur every year in the United States at a rate of 1.5 per 1,000 CVC days and with an associated mortality rate of 12–25% [67]. Biofilm formed on catheters often necessitates its removal, although the procedure itself carries a relatively high risk of mechanical complications. Moreover, infections in CVCs result in significant healthcare cost, prolonged hospitalisation and patient morbidity [69,70]. The major organisms implicated in CVC biofilms are *S. epidermidis*, *S. aureus*, *C. albicans*, *P. aeruginosa*, *Klebsiella pneumoniae* and *Enterococcus faecalis* [60,63]. These microorganisms may gain access either exogenously through the patient, healthcare workers or hospital environment or endogenously via hematogenous spread from a distant site of infection [69]. In addition to the microorganisms, the CVC biofilm matrix may integrate the host products such as fibrin, fibronectin, fibrinogen, collagen and elastin. This forms a protective barrier for the biofilm community from antimicrobials and host immune defenses [70]. Subsequently, embolization of cells or cell aggregates from the mature biofilm can occur, causing distant infections in the body. CVC biofilms colonised with *S. aureus* have been implicated as a source of infection, with 25% of patients developing endocarditis and 31% developing metastatic infections [71].

Biofilms are also known to develop readily on the inner and outer surfaces of urinary catheters [72]. The pathogenic microorganisms may originate exogenously from personnel and the environment or endogenously through the gastrointestinal tract. The pathogens common in catheter-related infections are bacteria such as *E. faecalis*, *P. aeruginosa*, *E. coli*, *P. mirabilis* and *S. aureus* and fungi such as *Candida* species. Once the biofilm develops on the urinary catheters, it becomes a cause of persistent urinary tract infections [73]. The situation becomes critical particularly when biofilms involve urease-producing bacteria such as *P. mirabilis* [72]. The urease produced by *P. mirabilis* generates ammonia by hydrolyzing urea, which raises the pH of the urine. As the urine becomes alkaline, biofilms become crystalline by precipitation of calcium phosphate and magnesium phosphate crystals obstructing the catheter lumen. This can lead to serious complications such as pyelonephritis and septicemia. *Candida* biofilms have also been implicated in urinary catheter infections [69].

SURGICAL IMPLANT–ASSOCIATED BIOFILM INFECTIONS

Surgical implants are medical devices that help to restore a missing body structure or enhance a compromised part of the body. Over the years, various types of surgical implants have developed depending on the area of the human body in which they are used. To name a few, they include artificial heart valves, cardiac pacemakers, orthopedic implants, intraocular lenses, breast implants and dental implants. Unlike catheters, implants are permanent or semi-permanent medical devices which remain in the body for a considerable period of time. Therefore, infections associated with surgical implants are generally more difficult to manage because they require a longer period of antibiotic therapy and repeated surgical procedures [74]. Biofilm infection is a major risk factor leading to implant failure and creating a life-threatening condition in the host. Some of the common BAIs in surgical implants are discussed in brief.

Cardiac surgical implants such as prosthetic heart valves, pacemakers and cardiac defibrillators are prone to biofilm formation which may subsequently lead to endocarditis [75–77]. Following surgical implantation, circulating platelets and plasma proteins form a 'conditioning' film on the mechanical heart valves, which provides bindings sites for the circulating microorganisms. The most common pathogens associated with heart valve endocarditis are *S. aureus* and coagulase-negative staphylococcus (ConS) such as *S. epidermidis* derived from the normal microflora of the patient [75,78]. In addition, studies have suggested the implication of other bacterial pathogens such as streptococci, enterococci and HACEK bacteria (*Haemophilus*, *Aggregatibacter*, *Cardiobacterium*, *Eikenella*, *Kingella*) [75,79]. *Candida* species may also be accountable for the biofilm infections in prosthetic heart valves. *Propionibacterium*, a bacterium with a good biofilm-forming ability, has also been involved in infective endocarditis [80]. Because endocarditis is associated with continuous bacteraemia arising from daily life activities, it may be possible to isolate the causative organism by routine culture of blood of patients. However, the results of blood cultures may be negative if the patient has recently received antibiotics or if the organism is fastidious. Clinical practice dictates surgical replacement of almost all prosthetic valves infected by *S. aureus* or *Candida* species [81]. Surgical intervention may not be required in patients infected by ConS who have already responded to antibiotic therapy. Regardless of the causative pathogen, cardiac complications [e.g. congestive heart failure, conduction abnormalities, paravalvular abscesses, valve dehiscence, and serious peripheral embolisation] necessitate the surgical replacement of the infected prosthesis. Although relatively uncommon, prosthetic-valve endocarditis is life threatening, with mortality exceeding 30% [78].

Orthopaedic implants are designed to restore the functionality of hip, knee, ankle, shoulder and elbow joints. However, biofilm-associated infection is a devastating complication in orthopaedic joint replacement surgeries [82]. Hence, biofilm infections may result in implant failure and in extreme cases may lead to amputation or mortality [83]. A patient can develop infections from the immediate environment of the surgery room, surgical equipment and medical staff, or from bacteria from the patient's body itself. Similar to prosthetic heart values, orthopaedic implants are also covered with a conditioning film of extracellular matrix proteins such as fibronectin, fibrinogen, albumin, vitronectin and collagen after insertion [84]. Bacteria reaching the orthopaedic implants by a haematogenous route bind to these extracellular matrix surfaces on the surface of the material. Subsequently a multilayered biofilm develops which protects the bacteria from phagocytosis and antibiotics, resulting in chronic osteomyelitis [85]. Most of the orthopaedic implant–associated infections are caused by Gram-positive staphylococci, particularly *S. aureus* and *S. epidermidis*. The treatment of orthopaedic implants often becomes complex when methicillin-resistant *Staphylococcus aureus* [MRSA] is involved in the biofilm formation [86,87]. Therefore, therapeutic strategies that target anti-adhesion, anti-bacterial, anti-biofilm properties and modification of orthopaedic implants are being developed to minimise the risk of BAI after orthopaedic surgeries [88].

Bacterial biofilms have been demonstrated on materials relevant to the eye such as contact lenses, scleral buckles, suture material and intraocular lenses. Many ocular infections often occur when such prosthetic devices come in contact with or are implanted in the eye. Approximately 56% of corneal ulcers in the United States are associated with contact lens wear [89]. Because of their proximity to the cornea, contact lenses may modify and compromise the corneal epithelium and make it easier for microorganisms in the vicinity to adhere to the ocular surfaces [90]. Continuous contact of the eye with the biofilm-infested lens may lead to serious ocular conditions such as endophthalmitis and keratitis [91,92]. The physical properties and surface chemistry of contact lenses can influence the variation in adherence of organism onto it. For instance, *in vitro* studies have shown that silicone hydrogel lenses have a greater propensity to biofilm formation than hydroxyethyl methacrylate–based soft lenses [93]. In particular, more hydrophobic surfaces of silicone hydrogel facilitate *P. aeruginosa* biofilm formation. In addition, during contact lens wear, a protein-rich coating or conditioning film derived from host products forms on the contact lens surface. Such conditioning films have been found to influence the microbial adherence [93].

Culture-dependent methodologies have identified *P. aeruginosa* as the most common pathogen in contact lens–related infections, followed by *Serratia marcescens*, *S. aureus*, *Acanthamoeba*, and *Fusarium* [90]. Bacterial composition based on 16S ribosomal RNA gene sequencing has revealed that *Achromobacter*, *Stenotrophomonas*, and *Delftia* as the predominant bacteria, showing their role in contact lens–related disease [90]. Moreover, bacterial biofilms may provide binding sites for protozoa such as *Acanthamoeba*, predisposing lens wearers at increased risk for *Acanthamoeba* infection if lenses had been previously contaminated with bacterial biofilm [94]. Fungal keratitis is commonly caused by filamentous fungi *Fusarium* and *Aspergillus* species and less commonly by yeast-like fungi *Candida* species [95]. *Fusarium* adhere to contact lenses and form penetration pegs, which are hyphae of the fungi that traverse into the matrix of lenses. Biofilm on contact lenses can also be mixed species in nature.

Microbial biofilm established on lenses or within the lens case becomes much more resistant to the biocide properties of lens care products [96]. Multidrug-resistant, biofilm-forming *P. aeruginosa* isolates have been identified in contact lens–associated infections [97]. *Serratia marcescens* biofilm on the surface of etafilcon A lenses become resistant to phagocytosis by polymorphonuclear leukocytes [98]. Fungal biofilms can be less susceptible to the disinfectant agents. Therefore, proper postoperative eye care and sanitisation procedures are required to reduce the BAI in contact lenses.

OTHER MEDICAL DEVICE–ASSOCIATED BIOFILM INFECTION

Medical devices which temporarily come into contact with human body surfaces may also develop microbial biofilms on their surfaces. Some common examples are discussed in the text that follows. Endotracheal tubes are placed in the lower airways to assist breathing in critically ill patients who are unable to breathe normally [99]. However, this provides an opportunity for microorganisms to adhere and form biofilms on endotracheal tubes, leading to ventilator-associated pneumonia (VAP) [100]. VAP is a major nosocomial infection associated with significant morbidity and mortality in critically ill patients. Bacterial colonisation occurs within hours of endotracheal intubation [60]. Subsequently, biofilm microorganisms may gain access to the sterile lung tissues leading to pneumonia [99]. To support this association, studies have observed identical bacterial populations between endotracheal biofilms and the infected lungs of 70% of VAP patients [101]. These bacteria may come from oropharyngeal and enteric flora and are usually mixed-species in nature. Various bacterial groups of oral origin have been associated with VAP [99]. In addition, the ESKAPE group of bacteria – *Enterococcus faecium, Staphylococcus aureus, Klebsiella pneumoniae, Acinetobacter baumannii, Pseudomonas aeruginosa* and *Enterobacter* spp.–has also been frequently recovered from endotracheal tube biofilms [60,99]. In addition, fungal species such as *Candida* can also be accountable for VAP [102].

Voice prostheses are widely used as a part of voice rehabilitation after laryngectomy, particularly in management of laryngeal cancer [103]. Voice prostheses are prone to microbial adhesion and biofilm formation, commonly by organisms that are part of oropharyngeal microflora. These are usually mixed-species biofilms composed of bacterial and fungal species such as *Staphylococcus, Streptococcus, Escherichia, Enterobacter, Proteus, Pseudomonas* and *Candida*. Voice prostheses are highly subjected to *Candida* biofilms, as the fungus can easily gain access to the surface of the prosthesis, from the oral microbiota, where it resides in most human oral cavities [104]. Intrauterine devices (IUDs) are a common contraceptive procedure used by women throughout the world. However, in certain cases their use becomes limited because of increased risk of pelvic inflammatory diseases (PIDs) and subsequent complications, such as infertility and ectopic pregnancy. Bacteriological investigations have revealed that an IUD may become contaminated by the indigenous vaginal microbiome and predisposes a woman to BAI [105]. The commonly involved microorganisms in IUD biofilms are *S. aureus, S. epidermidis, P. aeruginosa, E. coli, Neisseria gonorrhoeae* and *Candida* species [106]. *Candida* biofilms in IUDs are a common cause of recurrent vulvovaginal candidiasis (Figure 1.4) [107,108].

Microorganisms adhere to the surfaces of reusable medical devices when they are in use [109]. If the medical device is not properly cleaned after usage, these adhered

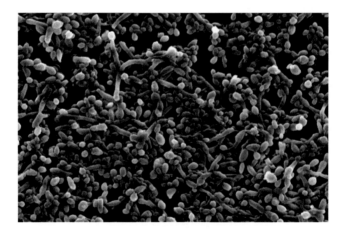

FIGURE 1.4 *Candida* biofilms formed on vaginal ring pessary.

organisms may progress to form biofilms, which can be a potential problem in clinical settings. For example, endoscopes that examine the interior of body organs are reusable medical devices on which biofilm formation will readily occur if reprocessing protocols are not strictly followed [40,109]. The moist, nutrient-rich conditions inside the lumens of an endoscope provide an ideal biofilm-forming environment for common pathogens such as *Legionella* and *Mycobacteria* species. However, some studies have reported that viable microorganisms could still be detected even after a complete disinfection procedure, highlighting the significant clinical problem in BAIs [110].

Biomaterials widely used to restore oral functions are invariably associated with microbial adhesion and biofilm formation [111]. These include restorative materials – composite resins, dental primers and dental adhesives; endodontic materials; and orthodontic and implanted materials such as ceramics, resin composites and metallic alloys [17]. Oral biomaterials readily come in contact with saliva, which helps formation of a conditioning film composed of salivary proteins. Acrylic dentures are particularly prone to biofilm formation by the fungal pathogen, *Candida* spp. If not properly controlled, these biofilms can lead to denture stomatitis, which is the most common form of oral candidiasis (Figure 1.5a). In addition, tooth restorative materials such as amalgam, ceramic, resin composites and glass–ionomer cements can become colonised with oral bacterial biofilms, predominantly of streptococcal origin, leading to secondary caries [111]. In particular, this can occur at the interface between tooth tissue and the restorative material because of microleakage. Periodontitis or biofilm-associated inflammatory disease of the tooth supporting tissues is a major cause of tooth loss worldwide [112]. It is caused by the pathological dental plaque biofilm that accumulates on teeth adjacent to the gingiva which is colonised predominantly by the 'red-complex bacteria' viz., *P. gingivalis*, *Tannerella forsythia* and *Treponema denticola* [113]. Similarly to natural dentition, biofilms can form on dental implants. This may subsequently trigger infection and cause inflammatory destruction of the peri-implant tissue or peri-implantitis (Figure 1.5b) [114]. Studies have shown that microbiota colonising clinically healthy implants consists mainly of Gram-positive cocci and non-motile bacilli and a limited number of Gram-negative anaerobic species, that resembles healthy periodontal sites of healthy subjects [114,115]. The transition to peri-implantitis is accompanied by emergence of Gram-negative, anaerobic species such as *Porphyromonas gingivalis*, *Tannerella forsythia* and *Treponema denticola* that are commonly found in periodontitis. Significantly higher counts of *S. aureus* and *Staphylococcus anaerobius* have been detected in implants with peri-implantitis compared to those of healthy peri-implant pockets. Newer gene sequencing studies have revealed biofilms associated with peri-implantitis are different from biofilms in periodontitis [115]. Biofilm-associated peri-implantitis is discussed further in Chapters 3 and 4. In addition, orthodontic patients with fixed appliances often show increased dental plaque biofilm formation and elevated levels of cariogenic pathogens such as *Streptococcus mutans* (Figure 1.5b) [116]. Biofilms formed on fixed appliances may lead to decalcification of the enamel surfaces, resulting in white spot lesions [117].

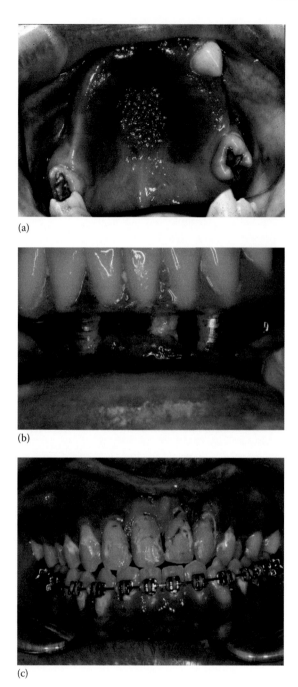

(a)

(b)

(c)

FIGURE 1.5 (a) Denture biofilm–associated denture stomatitis. (b) Biofilms formed on dental implants. (Courtesy of Prof. Finbarr Allen, Faculty of Dentistry, National University of Singapore.) (c) Biofilms on orthodontic biomaterials. (Courtesy of Prof. Kelvin Foong, Faculty of Dentistry, National University of Singapore.)

Biofilms in Hospital Water Systems

Biofilms formed in hospital water systems can be a major source of nosocomial infections, as the biofilm cells can disperse to healthcare personnel and to medical devices. Hence, biofilm organisms have been reported in common water sources in the hospital setting including water used in taps, showers and storage tanks; humidifiers and air-conditioning water systems; water used for washing medical devices; water for dialysis; and waterlines in dental clinics [40,118]. Drinking water used in hospitals is commonly disinfected. However, biofilms formed on water systems may resist disinfection strategies and survive [119]. The common microorganisms associated with such biofilms include *Legionella* spp., *P. aeruginosa*, *Mycobacteria* spp., *Acinetobacter* spp., *Aeromonas* spp. and *Aspergillus* spp. [40,120]. Species belonging to the non-tuberculous mycobacteria (NTM) are common microorganisms found in the biofilms in hospital water systems [121]. The environmental nature of NTM and their ability to form biofilms on different surfaces are key in their pathogenesis in pulmonary infections, which are becoming increasingly common in immuno-compromised individuals and elderly patients [122]. Biofilms of NTM are highly tolerant to disinfectant chlorine, thus posing a significant public health challenge [123]. A recent study which used next-generation sequencing technology identified novel '*Mycobacterium*-like' species closely related to *Mycobacterium rhodesiae* and *Mycobacterium tusciae* as responsible for the biofilms on hospital shower hoses [119]. The biofilm communities harboured genes related to disinfectant tolerance.

Dental chair units have a complex network of interconnected waterline systems to cool and irrigate instruments and tooth surfaces and provide rinse water during various dental treatment procedures [124]. Dental units, particularly the waterline tubes that supply water to the dental instruments, inevitably harbour a wide variety of microorganisms including bacteria, fungi and protozoans. The microorganisms adhering to the waterlines inevitably lead to biofilm formation on these surfaces. However, dental water unit biofilms are not harmful unless colonised with pathogenic bacteria or exceeding certain microbiological levels [40]. Current CDC guidelines for infection control in dental healthcare settings recommend that output water from dental units should not exceed 500 colony-forming units (CFU)/mL of aerobic heterotrophic bacteria [124]. Hence, mostly saprophites, such as *Moraxella* spp., *Flavobacterium* spp., *Micrococcus* spp. and *Actinomyces* spp. and yeast species can be present in the dental waterline output in harmless concentrations. Under certain circumstances, pathogenic species such as *P. aeruginosa*, *Legionella* spp. and *Mycobacteria* spp. have also been isolated from these biofilms [125]. A further concern of colonised dental unit waterlines is the potential for cross-contamination of patients with infectious microorganisms Therefore, if proper infection control of dental units is not followed, it can be a serious source of cross-contamination.

TISSUE-ASSOCIATED BIOFILM INFECTIONS

The human body carries approximately 10 times more microbial than human cells [126,127]. In brief, microorganisms reside on all body surfaces and cavities open to the exterior environment. The oral cavity, gastrointestinal tract, respiratory tract, genital organs and conjunctiva are colonised by niche-specific microbiota which fluctuates between planktonic and biofilm modes. Biofilms on these surfaces under healthy conditions are discussed in detail in Chapters 4 and 9. Tissue-associated biofilm infections can occur as a result of either opportunistic infections such as oral candidiasis or of invasion of pathogenic organisms, as in the case of CF. These infections pervade the hospitals and are a major burden to healthcare systems. Treatment of tissue-associated biofilm infections can be challenging and varies depending on the type of tissue colonised and the severity of infection. Some of the classical examples of tissue-associated biofilm infections are discussed in brief in the text that follows.

BIOFILMS ASSOCIATED WITH CF LUNG INFECTIONS

Persistent lung infection in CF patients is a classic example of tissue-related biofilm infections. CF is an autosomal recessive disease occurring as a result of the mutation of the gene for CF transmembrane conductance regulator (CFTR) protein. This defect in the gene alters the consistency of mucosal secretions, which may result in impaired resistance to pathogenic infections [128,129]. Bacterial biofilms have been recognised as contributing factors in the pathogenesis of CF. *P. aeruginosa* and *Burkholderia cepacia* are the two major Gram-negative rods that infect the lungs of patients with CF [130]. The major organism responsible for patient morbidity and mortality in CF is *P. aeruginosa*. The presence of *P. aeruginosa* biofilms in the lower respiratory tract results in refractory treatment and chronic inflammation, subsequently leading to pulmonary damage and decreased lung function [131]. *P. aeruginosa* biofilms can be prevented by early aggressive antibiotic prophylaxis or therapy [132]. In infants and children with CF, the most commonly implicated bacterial pathogens are *S. aureus* and *H. influenzae* while *B. cepacia*, *Achromobacter xylosoxidans*, *Stenotrophomonas maltophilia* and NTM are commonly isolated in adult cases [133]. In certain extreme cases, anaerobic bacteria such as *Prevotella intermedia* may be found in patients [134,135]. Gene sequencing techniques have revealed a 'cystic fibrosis microbiome' which is implicated in the pathogenesis of this disease [136]. Taken together, these pulmonary infections are a major cause of mortality in CF patients.

WOUND INFECTIONS

Wound-related infections occur because of colonizing bacteria that exist as biofilm communities (Figure 1.6) [137]. Hence, studies have shown that bacteria colonising chronic human wounds exist as biofilm communities [138]. Wound-associated biofilms are often initiated by Gram-positive bacteria such as coagulase-negative staphylococci, as their optimum pH for growth is around 7 [139]. Subsequently, microbes such as *P. aeruginosa* and *E. faecalis* that are able to grow in a wider range of pH begin to colonise the wound biofilm, resulting in further complications. As the wound becomes chronic and more alkaline, anaerobic infections due to organisms such as *Peptostreptococci* may follow. In addition, methicillin-resistant *S. aureus*, *Klebsiella* spp., *E. coli* and *Acinetobacter* spp. are particularly linked as a causative

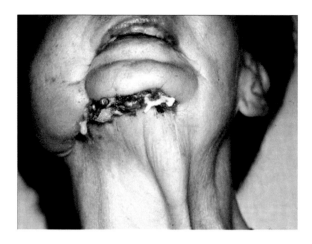

FIGURE 1.6 Biofilm on wound infections. (Courtesy of Dr. Intekhab Islam, Faculty of Dentistry, National University of Singapore.)

factor in the burn wound infections [40]. Anaerobic bacteria may grow as a biofilm in the deep layers of the wounds, which may not be present in the swab samples. Therefore, where possible, it is advisable to take biopsy samples for the determination of appropriate antibiotics [61].

ORAL BIOFILM INFECTIONS

Oral microbiota exists both on the hard surfaces of the oral cavity such as teeth and soft tissue surfaces such as mucosa [23]. In addition, saliva contains millions of planktonic microbiota. Transient colonisers may also appear in the oral cavity during daily activities. Hence, dental plaque is a fine example of complex biofilm lifestyle of microorganisms [140]. All common oral infectious diseases such as dental caries, periodontal diseases, oral candidiasis and peri-implantitis are associated with biofilm mode of growth (Figures 1.7 and 1.8). The microbial composition and pathogenesis of oral biofilm infections will be elaborated by Chapters 3 and 4, which will provide a comprehensive understanding of this topic to readers.

BIOFILM INFECTIONS OF THE GASTROINTESTINAL TRACT

Cholera is an acute waterborne diarrhoeal disease caused by the Gram-negative bacterium *Vibrio cholerae*. *V. cholerae* can effectively colonise ecological niches such as the nutrient-rich human small intestine or aquatic environments. There is plentiful evidence suggesting that the capacity of *V. cholerae* to develop biofilms is critical to intestinal colonisation [141]. It is likely that all these factors, at least indirectly, influence virulence and biofilm formation. *Helicobacter pylori* is another bacterial pathogen that has biofilm-forming ability on human gastric mucosal epithelium. *H. pylori* infection often persists throughout life and the biofilms make them less susceptible to antibiotics [142]. *H. pylori* infection can lead to chronic active gastritis,

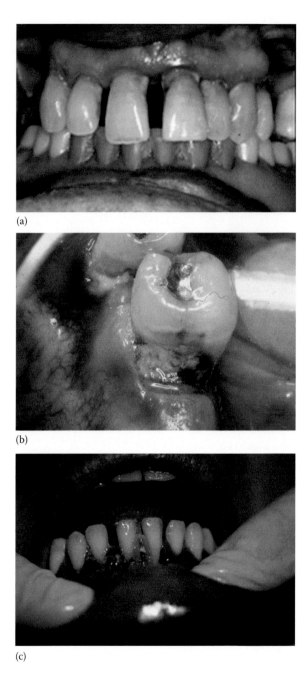

(a)

(b)

(c)

FIGURE 1.7 Dental plaque biofilm-associated dental caries (a, b) and periodontal disease (c). (Courtesy of Prof. Finbarr Allen, Faculty of Dentistry, National University of Singapore.)

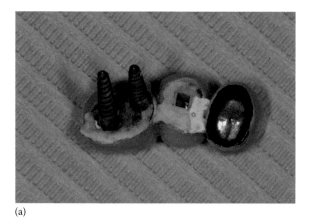

(a)

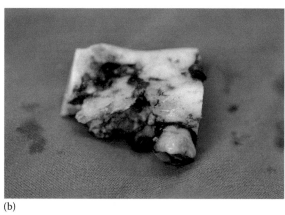

(b)

FIGURE 1.8 (a) Explanted failed mini-implants from the mandible due to biofilm infection associated with dental implants. (b) Resection of necrotic bone and tooth with infected oral biofilms in a patient with osteoradionecrosis.

peptic ulcer disease, gastric adenocarcinoma and mucosa-associated lymphoid tissue lymphoma.

BIOFILM INFECTIONS IN THE VAGINA

Biofilms are implicated in vaginal infections such as bacterial vaginosis and vulvo-vaginal candidiasis [143]. Bacterial vaginosis is the most common genital tract infection in women during their reproductive years. It is associated with serious health complications such as preterm delivery and sexually transmitted diseases [144]. Bacterial vaginosis is characterised by a reduction of beneficial lactobacilli and a significant increase in the number of anaerobic bacteria, including *Gardnerella vaginalis*, *Atopobium vaginae*, *Mobiluncus* spp., *Bacteroides* spp. and *Prevotella* spp., resulting in a thick multispecific vaginal biofilm, with *G. vaginalis* as the dominant player. *Candida* species are common inhabitants of the vagina, which can form biofilms leading to vulvovaginal candidiasis. *C. albicans* is the most commonly isolated species of *Candida*, followed by *C. glabrata*, from cervicovaginal swabs in vulvovaginal candidiasis [145].

PROSTATE INFECTIONS

Bacterial infection of the prostate gland is the most frequent cause of recurrent urinary tract infections in young and middle-aged men. Chronic bacterial prostatitis is also associated with bacterial species that are able to form biofilms and infect prostate cells [146]. *E. coli* is the most commonly isolated organism from these infections, but other Gram-negative organisms belonging to the genera *Klebsiella*, *Proteus* and *Pseudomonas* are also common. Studies suggest that the *E. coli* strains often seen in chronic bacterial prostatitis have a high virulence factor and great degree of biofilm formation. The pathogenesis of chronic bacterial prostatitis has not yet been scientifically proven, but it is assumed that the infection moves from the distal urethra to the prostate. Although haemolysin is the main virulence factor by which *E. coli* causes acute prostatitis, the association between haemolysin and biofilm formation may result in increased ability of *E. coli* strains to persist in the prostate [147].

NAIL INFECTIONS

Fungi form complex sessile biofilm communities which can irreversibly attach to epithelial surfaces such as nails. These fungal biofilms can lead to onychomycosis, or fungal infection of the nails. *Trichophyton rubrum* and *T. mentagrophytes* are the most commonly involved fungal species in onychomycosis [148]. Fungal biofilms in the nails may act as a persistent source of infection and account for antifungal resistance. Severe or persistent fungal nail infections demand surgical removal of the nail.

CONCLUSIONS AND PERSPECTIVES

The path from the discovery of microorganisms to the understanding of their prevalence and significance in modern settings has been a long and interesting one marked by several landmark discoveries. However, with every new breakthrough, there arises a potential landscape of information yet to be uncovered, complicating our understanding of microbes and microbial biofilms. The aim of this introductory chapter was to provide a brief overview of the historical perspectives about microorganisms, biofilm lifestyle of microbes, nature of biofilm formation and development, properties of microbial biofilms and their implications in clinical settings. An insight into the inherent complexity of biofilms, their multispecific existence in nature and interactions with their hosts are some of the aspects that will be covered in the next few chapters of this book. A detailed discussion on the multidrug-resistant properties of microbial biofilms and their characterisation by different omics approaches such as genomics, transcriptomics, proteomics and metabolomics will be the focus of the latter half of the book.

CORRESPONDING AUTHOR

Chaminda Jayampath Seneviratne
Discipline of Oral Sciences
Faculty of Dentistry
National University of Singapore
Singapore
jaya@nus.edu.sg

REFERENCES

1. Toledo-Pereyra LH. The strange little animals of Antony van Leeuwenhoek surgical revolution. *J Invest Surg.* 2009;22(1):4–8.
2. Williams JV. Déjà vu all over again: Koch's postulates and virology in the 21st century. *J Infect Dis.* 2010;201(11):1611–4.
3. Geesey GG, Richardson WT, Yeomans HG, Irvin RT, Costerton JW. Microscopic examination of natural sessile bacterial populations from an alpine stream. *Can J Microbiol.* 1977;23(12):1733–6.
4. Costerton JW, Geesey GG, Cheng K-J. How Bacteria Stick. *Sci Am.* 1978;238(1):86–95.
5. Costerton JW. Bacterial biofilms in nature and disease. *Ann Rev Microbiol.* 1987;41:435–64.
6. Potera C. Biofilms invade microbiology. *Science.* 1996;273(5283):1795–7.
7. Bontognali TR, Sessions AL, Allwood AC, Fischer WW, Grotzinger JP, Summons RE et al. Sulfur isotopes of organic matter preserved in 3.45-billion-year-old stromatolites reveal microbial metabolism. *Proc Natl Acad Sci U S A.* 2012;109(38):15146–51.
8. Potera C. Forging a Link Between Biofilms and Disease. *Science.* 1999;283(5409):1837–9.
9. Lopez D, Vlamakis H, Kolter R. Biofilms. *Cold Spring Harb Perspect Biol.* 2(7): a000398.
10. Hall-Stoodley L, Costerton JW, Stoodley P. Bacterial biofilms: From the natural environment to infectious diseases. *Nat Rev Microbiol.* 2004;2(2):95–108.
11. Donlan RM, Costerton JW. Biofilms: Survival mechanisms of clinically relevant microorganisms. *Clin Microbiol Rev.* 2002;15(2):167–93.
12. Seneviratne CJ, Jin L, Samaranayake LP. Biofilm lifestyle of *Candida*: A mini review. *Oral Dis.* 2008;14(7):582–90.
13. Flemming HC, Wingender J. The biofilm matrix. *Nat Rev Microbiol.* 8(9):623–33.
14. Kolter R, Greenberg EP. Microbial sciences: The superficial life of microbes. *Nature.* 2006;441(7091):300–2.
15. Costerton JW, Lewandowski Z, Caldwell DE, Korber DR, Lappin-Scott HM. Microbial biofilms. *Annu Rev Microbiol.* 1995;49:711–45.
16. Dunne WM, Jr. Bacterial adhesion: Seen any good biofilms lately? *Clin Microbiol Rev.* 2002;15(2):155–66.
17. Song F, Koo H, Ren D. Effects of material properties on bacterial adhesion and biofilm formation. *J Dent Res.* 2015;94(8):1027–34.
18. Maier B, Wong GC. How bacteria use type IV pili machinery on surfaces. *Trends Microbiol.* 2015;23(12):775–88.
19. O'Toole GA, Wong GC. Sensational biofilms: Surface sensing in bacteria. *Curr Opin Microbiol.* 2016;30:139–46.
20. Gibiansky ML, Conrad JC, Jin F, Gordon VD, Motto DA, Mathewson MA et al. Bacteria use type IV pili to walk upright and detach from surfaces. *Science.* 2010;330(6001):197.

21. Dickson JS, Koohmaraie M. Cell surface charge characteristics and their relationship to bacterial attachment to meat surfaces. *Appl Environ Microbiol.* 1989;55(4):832–6.

22. Teschler JK, Zamorano-Sanchez D, Utada AS, Warner CJ, Wong GC, Linington RG et al. Living in the matrix: Assembly and control of *Vibrio cholerae* biofilms. *Nat Rev Microbiol.* 2015;13(5):255–68.

23. Seneviratne CJ, Zhang CF, Samaranayake LP. Dental plaque biofilm in oral health and disease. *Chin J Dent Res.* 2011;14(2):87–94.

24. Low B, Lee W, Seneviratne CJ, Samaranayake LP, Hagg U. Ultrastructure and morphology of biofilms on thermoplastic orthodontic appliances in 'fast' and 'slow' plaque formers. *Eur J Orthod.* 2011;33(5):577–83.

25. Berry RM, Armitage JP. Microbiology. How bacteria change gear. *Science.* 2008; 320(5883):1599–600.

26. Otto M. Staphylococcal infections: Mechanisms of biofilm maturation and detachment as critical determinants of pathogenicity. *Annu Rev Med.* 2013;64:175–88.

27. Joo HS, Otto M. Molecular basis of in vivo biofilm formation by bacterial pathogens. *Chem Biol.* 2012;19(12):1503–13.

28. Kostakioti M, Hadjifrangiskou M, Hultgren SJ. Bacterial biofilms: Development, dispersal, and therapeutic strategies in the dawn of the postantibiotic era. *Cold Spring Harb Perspect Med.* 2013;3(4):a010306.

29. Okshevsky M, Regina VR, Meyer RL. Extracellular DNA as a target for biofilm control. *Curr Opin Biotechnol.* 2015;33:73–80.

30. Whitchurch CB, Tolker-Nielsen T, Ragas PC, Mattick JS. Extracellular DNA required for bacterial biofilm formation. *Science.* 2002;295(5559):1487.

31. Greenberg EP. Bacterial communication: Tiny teamwork. *Nature.* 2003;424(6945):134.

32. Klausen M, Aaes-Jorgensen A, Molin S, Tolker-Nielsen T. Involvement of bacterial migration in the development of complex multicellular structures in *Pseudomonas aeruginosa* biofilms. *Mol Microbiol.* 2003;50(1):61–8.

33. Berk V, Fong JC, Dempsey GT, Develioglu ON, Zhuang X, Liphardt J et al. Molecular architecture and assembly principles of *Vibrio cholerae* biofilms. *Science.* 2012;337(6091): 236–9.

34. Uppuluri P, Sarmah B, Chaffin WL. *Candida albicans* SNO1 and SNZ1 expressed in stationary-phase planktonic yeast cells and base of biofilm. *Microbiology.* 2006;152(Pt 7): 2031–8.

35. LaFleur MD, Kumamoto CA, Lewis K. *Candida albicans* biofilms produce antifungal-tolerant persister cells. *Antimicrob Agents Chemother.* 2006;50(11):3839–46.

36. Li P, Seneviratne CJ, Alpi E, Vizcaino JA, Jin L. Delicate metabolic control and coordinated stress response critically determine antifungal tolerance of *Candida albicans* biofilm persisters. *Antimicrob Agents Chemother.* 2015;59(10):6101–12.

37. Dawson CC, Intapa C, Jabra-Rizk MA. 'Persisters': Survival at the cellular level. *PLoS Pathog.* 2011;7(7):e1002121.

38. Lewis K. Persister cells. *Annu Rev Microbiol.* 2010;64:357–72.

39. Hall-Stoodley L, Stoodley P. Biofilm formation and dispersal and the transmission of human pathogens. *Trends Microbiol.* 2005;13(1):7–10.

40. Lindsay D, von Holy A. Bacterial biofilms within the clinical setting: What healthcare professionals should know. *J Hosp Infect.* 2006;64(4):313–25.

41. Kaplan JB. Biofilm dispersal: Mechanisms, clinical implications, and potential therapeutic uses. *J Dent Res.* 2010;89(3):205–18.

42. Wood TK, Hong SH, Ma Q. Engineering biofilm formation and dispersal. *Trends Biotechnol.* 2011;29(2):87–94.

43. Sauer K, Cullen MC, Rickard AH, Zeef LA, Davies DG, Gilbert P. Characterization of nutrient-induced dispersion in *Pseudomonas aeruginosa* PAO1 biofilm. *J Bacteriol.* 2004;186(21):7312-26.

44. Barraud N, Hassett DJ, Hwang S-H, Rice SA, Kjelleberg S, Webb JS. Involvement of nitric oxide in biofilm dispersal of *Pseudomonas aeruginosa. J Bacteriol.* 2006 Nov 1; 188(21):7344–53.
45. Morgan R, Kohn S, Hwang SH, Hassett DJ, Sauer K. BdlA, a chemotaxis regulator essential for biofilm dispersion in *Pseudomonas aeruginosa. J Bacteriol.* 2006;188(21):7335-43.
46. Basu Roy A, Sauer K. Diguanylate cyclase NicD-based signalling mechanism of nutrient-induced dispersion by *Pseudomonas aeruginosa. Mol Microbiol.* 2014;94(4): 771–93.
47. Hnisz D, Majer O, Frohner IE, Komnenovic V, Kuchler K. The Set3/Hos2 histone deacetylase complex attenuates cAMP/PKA signaling to regulate morphogenesis and virulence of *Candida albicans. PLoS Pathog.* 2010;6(5):e1000889.
48. Uppuluri P, Chaturvedi AK, Srinivasan A, Banerjee M, Ramasubramaniam AK, Kohler JR et al. Dispersion as an important step in the *Candida albicans* biofilm developmental cycle. *PLoS Pathog.* 2010;6(3):e1000828.
49. Murad AM, Leng P, Straffon M, Wishart J, Macaskill S, MacCallum D et al. NRG1 represses yeast-hypha morphogenesis and hypha-specific gene expression in *Candida albicans. EMBO J.* 2001;20(17):4742–52.
50. Elias S, Banin E. Multi-species biofilms: Living with friendly neighbors. *FEMS Microbiol Rev.* 2012;36(5):990–1004.
51. Thein ZM, Seneviratne CJ, Samaranayake YH, Samaranayake LP. Community lifestyle of *Candida* in mixed biofilms: A mini review. *Mycoses.* 2009;52(6):467–75.
52. Hansen SK, Rainey PB, Haagensen JA, Molin S. Evolution of species interactions in a biofilm community. *Nature.* 2007;445(7127):533–6.
53. Roder HL, Sorensen SJ, Burmolle M. Studying bacterial multispecies biofilms: Where to start? *Trends Microbiol.* 2016;24(6):503–13.
54. Mear JB, Kipnis E, Faure E, Dessein R, Schurtz G, Faure K et al. *Candida albicans* and *Pseudomonas aeruginosa* interactions: More than an opportunistic criminal association? *Med Malad Infect.* 2013;43(4):146–51.
55. Høiby N, Bjarnsholt T, Givskov M, Molin S, Ciofu O. Antibiotic resistance of bacterial biofilms. *Int J Antimicrob Agents.* 2010;35(4):322–32.
56. Seneviratne CJ, Wang Y, Jin L, Wong SSW, Herath TDK, Samaranayake LP. Unraveling the resistance of microbial biofilms: Has proteomics been helpful? *Proteomics.* 2012;12(4–5):651–65.
57. Lewis K. Riddle of Biofilm Resistance. Antimicrob Agents Chemother. 2001;45(4): 999–1007.
58. Leung CY, Chan YC, Samaranayake LP, Seneviratne CJ. Biocide resistance of *Candida* and *Escherichia coli* biofilms is associated with higher antioxidative capacities. *J Hosp Infect.* 2012;81(2):79–86.
59. Smith K, Robertson DP, Lappin DF, Ramage G. Commercial mouthwashes are ineffective against oral MRSA biofilms. *Oral Surg Oral Med Oral Pathol Oral Radiol.* 2013;115(5):624–9.
60. Boisvert AA, Cheng MP, Sheppard DC, Nguyen D. Microbial biofilms in pulmonary and critical care diseases. *Ann Am Thorac Soc.* 2016.
61. Hoiby N, Bjarnsholt T, Moser C, Bassi GL, Coenye T, Donelli G et al. ESCMID guideline for the diagnosis and treatment of biofilm infections 2014. *Clin Microbiol Infect.* 2015;21(Suppl 1):S1–25.
62. Costerton JW, Stewart PS, Greenberg EP. Bacterial biofilms: A common cause of persistent infections. *Science.* 1999;284(5418):1318–22.
63. Donlan RM. Biofilms and device-associated infections. *Emerg Infect Dis.* 2001; 7(2):277–81.

64. Darouiche RO. Device-associated infections: A macroproblem that starts with micro-adherence. *Clin Infect Dis.* 2001;33(9):1567–72.
65. Estivill D, Arias A, Torres-Lana A, Carrillo-Munoz AJ, Arevalo MP. Biofilm formation by five species of *Candida* on three clinical materials. *J Microb Methods.* 2011;86(2):238–42.
66. Litzler PY, Benard L, Barbier-Frebourg N, Vilain S, Jouenne T, Beucher E et al. Biofilm formation on pyrolytic carbon heart valves: Influence of surface free energy, roughness, and bacterial species. *J Thorac Cardiovasc Surg.* 2007;134(4):1025–32.
67. Yousif A, Jamal MA, Raad I. Biofilm-based central line-associated bloodstream infections. *Adv Exp Med Biol.* 2015;830:157–79.
68. Sousa C, Henriques M, Oliveira R. Mini-review: Antimicrobial central venous catheters – Recent advances and strategies. *Biofouling.* 2011;27(6):609–20.
69. Ramage G, Martinez JP, Lopez-Ribot JL. *Candida* biofilms on implanted biomaterials: A clinically significant problem. *FEMS Yeast Res.* 2006;6(7):979–86.
70. Walz JM, Memtsoudis SG, Heard SO. Prevention of central venous catheter blood-stream infections. *J Intens Care Med.* 2010;25(3):131–8.
71. Ryder MA. Catheter-related infections: It's all about biofilm. *Top Adv Pract Nurs.* 2005.
72. Tenke P, Koves B, Nagy K, Hultgren SJ, Mendling W, Wullt B et al. Update on biofilm infections in the urinary tract. *World J Urol.* 2012;30(1):51–7.
73. Stickler DJ. Bacterial biofilms in patients with indwelling urinary catheters. *Nat Clin Pract Urol.* 2008;5(11):598–608.
74. Darouiche RO. Treatment of infections associated with surgical implants. *N Engl J Med.* 2004;350(14):1422–9.
75. Cahill TJ, Prendergast BD. Infective endocarditis. *Lancet.* 2016;387(10021):882–93.
76. Inacio RC, Klautau GB, Murca MA, da Silva CB, Nigro S, Rivetti LA et al. Microbial diagnosis of infection and colonization of cardiac implantable electronic devices by use of sonication. *Int J Infect Dis.* 2015;38:54–9.
77. Padera RF. Infection in ventricular assist devices: The role of biofilm. *Cardiovasc Pathol.* 2006;15(5):264–70.
78. Vongpatanasin W, Hillis LD, Lange RA. Prosthetic heart valves. *N Engl J Med.* 1996; 335(6):407–16.
79. Chifiriuc MC, Banu O, Bleotu C, Lazar V. Interaction of bacteria isolated from clini-cal biofilms with cardiovascular prosthetic devices and eukaryotic cells. *Anaerobe.* 2011;17(6):419–21.
80. Braun DL, Hasse BK, Stricker J, Fehr JS. Prosthetic valve endocarditis caused by Propionibacterium species successfully treated with coadministered rifampin: Report of two cases. *BMJ Case Rep.* 2013;2013.
81. Darouiche RO. Treatment of infections associated with surgical implants. *N Engl J Med.* 2004;350:1422–9.
82. Mauffrey C, Herbert B, Young H, Wilson ML, Hake M, Stahel PF. The role of biofilm on orthopaedic implants: The 'Holy Grail' of post-traumatic infection management? *Eur J Trauma Emerg Surg.* 2016.
83. Ercan B, Kummer KM, Tarquinio KM, Webster TJ. Decreased *Staphylococcus aureus* biofilm growth on anodized nanotubular titanium and the effect of electrical stimula-tion. *Acta Biomaterial.* 2011;7(7):3003–12.
84. Brady RA, Leid JG, Calhoun JH, Costerton JW, Shirtliff ME. Osteomyelitis and the role of biofilms in chronic infection. *FEMS Immunol Med Microbiol.* 2008;52(1):13–22.
85. Gristina AG, Oga M, Webb LX, Hobgood CD. Adherent bacterial colonization in the pathogenesis of osteomyelitis. *Science.* 1985;228(4702):990–3.
86. Kawamura H, Nishi J, Imuta N, Tokuda K, Miyanohara H, Hashiguchi T et al. Quanti-tative analysis of biofilm formation of methicillin-resistant *Staphylococcus aureus* (MRSA) strains from patients with orthopaedic device-related infections. *FEMS Immunol Med Microbiol.* 2011;63(1):10–5.

87. Lauderdale KJ, Malone CL, Boles BR, Morcuende J, Horswill AR. Biofilm dispersal of community-associated methicillin-resistant *Staphylococcus aureus* on orthopedic implant material. *J Orthopaed Res.* 2010;28(1):55–61.
88. Nana A, Nelson SB, McLaren A, Chen AF. What's new in musculoskeletal infection: Update on biofilms. *J Bone Joint Surg Am.* 2016;98(14):1226–34.
89. Zegans ME, Becker HI, Budzik J, O'Toole G. The role of bacterial biofilms in ocular infections. *DNA Cell Biol.* 2002;21(5–6):415–20.
90. Wiley L, Bridge DR, Wiley LA, Odom JV, Elliott T, Olson JC. Bacterial biofilm diversity in contact lens-related disease: Emerging role of *Achromobacter, Stenotrophomonas,* and *Delftia. Invest Ophthalmol Vis Sci.* 2012;53(7):3896–905.
91. Bispo PJ, Haas W, Gilmore MS. Biofilms in infections of the eye. *Pathogens.* 2015; 4(1):111–36.
92. McLaughlin-Borlace L, Stapleton F, Matheson M, Dart JK. Bacterial biofilm on contact lenses and lens storage cases in wearers with microbial keratitis. *J Appl Microbiol.* 1998;84(5):827–38.
93. Willcox MD. Microbial adhesion to silicone hydrogel lenses: A review. *Eye Contact Lens.* 2013;39(1):61–6.
94. Simmons PA, Tomlinson A, Seal DV. The role of *Pseudomonas aeruginosa* biofilm in the attachment of *Acanthamoeba* to four types of hydrogel contact lens materials. *Optom Vis Sci.* 1998;75(12):860–6.
95. Imamura Y, Chandra J, Mukherjee PK, Lattif AA, Szczotka-Flynn LB, Pearlman E et al. *Fusarium* and *Candida albicans* biofilms on soft contact lenses: Model development, influence of lens type, and susceptibility to lens care solutions. *Antimicrob Agents Chemother.* 2008;52(1):171–82.
96. Szczotka-Flynn LB, Pearlman E, Ghannoum M. Microbial contamination of contact lenses, lens care solutions, and their accessories: A literature review. *Eye Contact Lens.* 2010;36(2):116–29.
97. Abidi SH, Sherwani SK, Siddiqui TR, Bashir A, Kazmi SU. Drug resistance profile and biofilm forming potential of *Pseudomonas aeruginosa* isolated from contact lenses in Karachi-Pakistan. *BMC Ophthalmol.* 2013;13:57.
98. Hume EB, Stapleton F, Willcox MD. Evasion of cellular ocular defenses by contact lens isolates of *Serratia marcescens. Eye Contact Lens.* 2003;29(2):108–12.
99. Vandecandelaere I, Coenye T. Microbial composition and antibiotic resistance of biofilms recovered from endotracheal tubes of mechanically ventilated patients. *Adv Exp Med Biol.* 2015;830:137–55.
100. Gil-Perotin S, Ramirez P, Marti V, Sahuquillo JM, Gonzalez E, Calleja I et al. Implications of endotracheal tube biofilm in ventilator-associated pneumonia response: A state of concept. *Crit Care.* 2012;16(3):R93.
101. Adair CG, Gorman SP, Feron BM, Byers LM, Jones DS, Goldsmith CE et al. Implications of endotracheal tube biofilm for ventilator-associated pneumonia. *Intens Care Med.* 1999;25(10):1072–6.
102. Danin PE, Girou E, Legrand P, Louis B, Fodil R, Christov C et al. Description and microbiology of endotracheal tube biofilm in mechanically ventilated subjects. *Respir Care.* 2015;60(1):21–9.
103. Leonhard M, Schneider-Stickler B. Voice prostheses, microbial colonization and biofilm formation. *Adv Exp Med Biol.* 2015;830:123–36.
104. Talpaert MJ, Balfour A, Stevens S, Baker M, Muhlschlegel FA, Gourlay CW. *Candida* biofilm formation on voice prostheses. *J Med Microbiol.* 2015;64(Pt 3):199–208.
105. Pal Z, Urban E, Dosa E, Pal A, Nagy E. Biofilm formation on intrauterine devices in relation to duration of use. *J Med Microbiol.* 2005;54(Pt 12):1199–203.
106. Pruthi V, Al-Janabi A, Pereira BM. Characterization of biofilm formed on intrauterine devices. *Indian J Med Microbiol.* 2003;21(3):161–5.

107. Chassot F, Negri MF, Svidzinski AE, Donatti L, Peralta RM, Svidzinski TI et al. Can intrauterine contraceptive devices be a *Candida albicans* reservoir? *Contraception.* 2008;77(5):355–9.
108. Auler ME, Morreira D, Rodrigues FF, Abr Ao MS, Margarido PF, Matsumoto FE et al. Biofilm formation on intrauterine devices in patients with recurrent vulvovaginal candidiasis. *Med Mycol.* 2010;48(1):211–6.
109. Roberts CG. The role of biofilms in reprocessing medical devices. *Am J Infect Control.* 2013;41(5 Suppl):S77–80.
110. Neves MS, da Silva MG, Ventura GM, Cortes PB, Duarte RS, de Souza HS. Effectiveness of current disinfection procedures against biofilm on contaminated GI endoscopes. *Gastrointest Endosc.* 2016;83(5):944–53.
111. Busscher HJ, Rinastiti M, Siswomihardjo W, van der Mei HC. Biofilm formation on dental restorative and implant materials. *J Dent Res.* 2010;89(7):657–65.
112. Berezow AB, Darveau RP. Microbial shift and periodontitis. *Periodontology.* 2000. 2011;55(1):36–47.
113. Pihlstrom BL, Michalowicz BS, Johnson NW. Periodontal diseases. *Lancet.* 2005; 366(9499):1809–20.
114. Belibasakis GN, Charalampakis G, Bostanci N, Stadlinger B. Peri-implant infections of oral biofilm etiology. *Adv Exp Med Biol.* 2015;830:69–84.
115. Faveri M, Figueiredo LC, Shibli JA, Perez-Chaparro PJ, Feres M. Microbiological diversity of peri-implantitis biofilms. *Adv Exp Med Biol.* 2015;830:85–96.
116. Ren Y, Jongsma MA, Mei L, van der Mei HC, Busscher HJ. Orthodontic treatment with fixed appliances and biofilm formation – A potential public health threat? *Clin Oral Invest.* 2014;18(7):1711–8.
117. Morrier JJ. (White spot lesions and orthodontic treatment. Prevention and treatment). *Orthodont Fr.* 2014;85(3):235–44.
118. Capelletti RV, Moraes AM. Waterborne microorganisms and biofilms related to hospital infections: Strategies for prevention and control in healthcare facilities. *J Water Health.* 2016;14(1):52–67.
119. Soto-Giron MJ, Rodriguez RL, Luo C, Elk M, Ryu H, Hoelle J et al. Biofilms on hospital shower hoses: Characterization and implications for nosocomial infections. *Appl Environ Microbiol.* 2016;82(9):2872–83.
120. Exner M, Kramer A, Lajoie L, Gebel J, Engelhart S, Hartemann P. Prevention and control of health care-associated waterborne infections in health care facilities. *Am J Infect Control.* 2005;33(5 Suppl 1):S26–40.
121. Vaerewijck MJ, Huys G, Palomino JC, Swings J, Portaels F. Mycobacteria in drinking water distribution systems: Ecology and significance for human health. *FEMS Microbiol Rev.* 2005;29(5):911–34.
122. Halstrom S, Price P, Thomson R. Review: Environmental mycobacteria as a cause of human infection. *Int J Mycobacteriol.* 2015;4(2):81–91.
123. Faria S, Joao I, Jordao L. General Overview on Nontuberculous Mycobacteria, Biofilms, and Human Infection. *J Pathog.* 2015;2015:1–10.
124. O'Donnell MJ, Boyle MA, Russell RJ, Coleman DC. Management of dental unit waterline biofilms in the 21st century. *Fut Microbiol.* 2011;6(10):1209–26.
125. Coleman DC, O'Donnell MJ, Shore AC, Russell RJ. Biofilm problems in dental unit water systems and its practical control. *J Appl Microbiol.* 2009;106(5):1424–37.
126. Morgan XC, Huttenhower C. Human microbiome analysis. *PLoS Comput Biol.* 2012; 8(12):e1002808.
127. Pflughoeft KJ, Versalovic J. Human microbiome in health and disease. *Annu Rev Pathol.* 2012;7:99–122.
128. Elborn JS. Cystic fibrosis. *Lancet.* 2016;388(10059):2519–31.

129. Filkins LM, O'Toole GA. Cystic Fibrosis Lung Infections: Polymicrobial, Complex, and Hard to Treat. *PLoS Pathog.* 2015;11(12):e1005258.

130. George AM, Jones PM, Middleton PG. Cystic fibrosis infections: Treatment strategies and prospects. *FEMS Microbiol Lett.* 2009;300(2):153–64.

131. Hoiby N, Ciofu O, Bjarnsholt T. *Pseudomonas aeruginosa* biofilms in cystic fibrosis. *Future Microbiol.* 2010;5(11):1663–74.

132. Döring G, Flume P, Heijerman H, Elborn JS. Treatment of lung infection in patients with cystic fibrosis: Current and future strategies. *J Cyst Fibros.* European Cystic Fibrosis Society, 2012;11(6):461–79.

133. Davies JC, Bilton D. Bugs, biofilms, and resistance in cystic fibrosis. *Respir Care.* 2009;54(5):628–40.

134. Ulrich M, Beer I, Braitmaier P, Dierkes M, Kummer F, Krismer B, Schumacher U, Gräpler-Mainka U, Riethmüller J, Jensen PO, Bjarnsholt T, Høiby N, Bellon G, Doring G. Relative contribution of Prevotella intermedia and *Pseudomonas aeruginosa* to lung pathology in airways of patients with cystic fibrosis. *Thorax.* 2010;65(11):978–84.

135. Tunney MM, Field TR, Moriarty TF, Patrick S, Doering G, Muhlebach MS et al. Detection of anaerobic bacteria in high numbers in sputum from patients with cystic fibrosis. *Am J Respir Crit Care Med.* 2008;177(9):995–1001.

136. Caverly LJ, Zhao J, LiPuma JJ. Cystic fibrosis lung microbiome: Opportunities to reconsider management of airway infection. *Pediatr Pulmonol.* 2015;50(Suppl 40):S31–8.

137. Clinton A, Carter T. Chronic wound biofilms: Pathogenesis and potential therapies. *Lab Med.* 2015;46(4):277–84.

138. Hurlow J, Couch K, Laforet K, Bolton L, Metcalf D, Bowler P. Clinical biofilms: A challenging frontier in wound care. *Adv Wound Care* (New Rochelle). 2015;4(5):295–301.

139. Scalise A, Bianchi A, Tartaglione C, Bolletta E, Pierangeli M, Torresetti M et al. Microenvironment and microbiology of skin wounds: The role of bacterial biofilms and related factors. *Semin Vasc Surg.* 2015;28(3–4):151–9.

140. Marsh PD, Moter A, Devine DA. Dental plaque biofilms: Communities, conflict and control. *Periodontology.* 2000. 2011;55(1):16–35.

141. Silva AJ, Benitez JA. *Vibrio cholerae* biofilms and cholera pathogenesis. *PLoS Negl Trop Dis.* 2016;10(2):e0004330.

142. Yonezawa H, Osaki T, Kamiya S. Biofilm formation by *Helicobacter pylori* and its involvement for antibiotic resistance. *Biomed Res Int.* 2015;2015:914791.

143. Muzny CA, Schwebke JR. Biofilms: An underappreciated mechanism of treatment failure and recurrence in vaginal infections. *Clin Infect Dis.* 2015;61(4):601–6.

144. Machado D, Castro J, Palmeira-de Oliveira A, Martinez-de Oliveira J, Cerca N. Bacterial vaginosis biofilms: Challenges to current therapies and emerging solutions. *Front Microbiol.* 2015;6:1528.

145. Vermitsky JP, Self MJ, Chadwick SG, Trama JP, Adelson ME, Mordechai E et al. Survey of vaginal-flora *Candida* species isolates from women of different age groups by use of species-specific PCR detection. *J Clin Microbiol.* 2008;46(4):1501–3.

146. Mazzoli S. Biofilms in chronic bacterial prostatitis (NIH-II) and in prostatic calcifications. *FEMS Immunol Med Microbiol.* 2010;59(3):337–44.

147. Soto SM, Smithson A, Martinez JA, Horcajada JP, Mensa J, Vila J. Biofilm formation in uropathogenic *Escherichia coli* strains: Relationship with prostatitis, urovirulence factors and antimicrobial resistance. *J Urol.* 2007;177(1):365–8.

148. Gupta AK, Daigle D, Carviel JL. The role of biofilms in onychomycosis. *J Am Acad Dermatol.* 2016;74(6):1241–6.

2 Clinical Implications of Interkingdom Fungal and Bacterial Biofilms

Gordon Ramage, Lindsay E. O'Donnell, Ryan Kean, Eleanor Townsend and Ranjith Rajendran

CONTENTS

INTRODUCTION

Fungal biofilms, in particular *Candida albicans*, remain an important healthcare issue as a consequence of ineffectual clinical management strategies [1]. Over the past several decades, we have learned a great deal about their mechanistic and clinical importance, particularly in relation to resisting the challenge of host and antimicrobial molecules [2,3]. However, it is generally acknowledged that *Candida* rarely exist within a monospecies environment, and that mixed-species biofilm populations consisting of aggregates of other fungi and bacteria are ubiquitous, and as such are a clinically important entity exemplified by an increasing volume of literature [4–7]. Traditional microbiology approaches invested time and effort in unravelling the importance of specific bacterial–bacterial interactions, which has been to the relative detriment of the study of polymicrobial interactions. This has led to a knowledge gap on the significance of fungal–bacterial interactions, which is pertinent given the growing evidence from the literature that polymicrobial interactions may synergise the pathogenic potential of one or other microorganism [8,9]. Moreover, these coinfections may resist antimicrobial treatment strategies, which collectively serve to highlight the importance of a dual approach to microbial analysis [10]. This chapter aims to critically evaluate the available evidence as a means of appraising the clinical importance of fungi in polymicrobial environments, using key biofilm diseases and groups of microorganisms to illustrate these points.

POLYMICROBIALITY ON THE MUCOSA AND BEYOND: CLINICAL CONSIDERATIONS

Within the human host, mucosal surfaces including the oral cavity, nasopharynx, respiratory tract, gastrointestinal tract and genitourinary tract support the growth and colonisation of a diverse microbiome, a microbial consortia of both bacterial and fungal species [4]. Moreover, breaches of the skin and development of wounds resultant from systemic disease (e.g. diabetic ulcers), or insertion of biomaterials, can create environments for the development of polymicrobial biofilm infections from endogenous and exogenous microbes. The potential for this is explained by the human mycobiome, which includes almost 400 fungal species detected in the oral cavity, skin, vagina and digestive tract [11].

ORAL CAVITY AND SINUSES

The oral cavity is a primary route of entry for pathogens, and is home to this rich and diverse microbial flora. Data suggest that up to 10^8 microbes per millilitre of saliva are present, but these data are based on bacterial estimates [12]. Regardless of this diverse bacterial microbiome, the oral cavity represents an optimal environment for biofilm growth of a variety of fungal species. The first fungal mycobiome analysis of the oral cavity identified 74 culturable and 11 non-culturable fungal genera from a basal healthy population of 20 individuals using a pyrosequencing approach [13]. In fact, 101 genera in total were identified, which individually ranged from 9 to 23 different species. *Candida* spp. were shown to be the most prominent genera from patients (75%), followed by *Cladosporium* (65%), *Aureobasidium* (50%), *Saccharomycetales* (50%), *Aspergillus* (35%), *Fusarium* (30%) and *Cryptococcus* (20%). Although several of these genera are known to be pathogenic to humans, these data must be reviewed with caution, as these organisms were not cultured and their ecological role in the oral cavity is unknown. *Candida* spp. are the best characterised in the context of the oral cavity. Next-generation sequencing (NGS) technology is beginning to reveal the importance of *Candida* spp. within these complex communities [14]. For example, NGS analysis of elderly Dutch patients demonstrated that an increased candidal load was associated with an altered bacterial flora, which favoured coexistence with oral streptococci [15]. Fungi such as *Candida* spp. are involved in a number of oral diseases and have been identified in numerous sites within the oral cavity. The sites from which *C. albicans* has been isolated include periodontal pockets, root canals, orthodontic appliances, enamel, dentures and mucosal surfaces [16–21]. Such polymicrobial biofilms are able to flourish in these environments because of the moisture, nutrients, hyphal growth and presence of commensal bacteria, all of which are required to form strong, virulent biofilms [22].

There is a growing appreciation that chronic rhinosinusitis, an inflammation of the mucous membrane that lines the paranasal sinuses, is typified by biofilm growth [23–25]. NGS revealed that 244 strains of microorganisms representing more than 50 families were identified in the maxillary sinus and middle nasal meatus (164 and 80, respectively). *Streptococcus* and *Prevotella* species, two key oral bacteria, were shown to predominate [26]. Though there is substantial evidence for the role of bacterial biofilms in sinus infection, the role of fungi is less well defined [27]. Given the anatomical location of the sinuses it is difficult to ascertain whether they form defined biofilms per se, though paranasal sinus fungus balls have been described [28,29], and these have been likened to fungal biofilms [30,31]. Of 118 patients studied over a 14-year period, 23.7% had a sphenoid fungus ball, of which *Aspergillus fumigatus* and *Aspergillus nidulans* hyphae were observed microscopically [29]. Other fungi are associated with these infections, including *Schizophyllum commune* [32,33], *Trichosporon inkin* [34], *Mucorales* [35], and *Fusarium* [36]. Infection with *A. fumigatus* within the maxillary sinus associated with a zygomatic implant has also been reported [37]. Therefore, the sinus is clearly a host environment for polymicrobial interactions [38].

RESPIRATORY TRACT

The close proximity of the trachea and bronchioles to the oral cavity and its warm moist environment makes for an attractive biofilm niche. The lung mycobiome has been suggested to have a significant impact on clinical outcome of chronic respiratory diseases (CRD) such as asthma, chronic obstructive pulmonary disease, cystic fibrosis (CF), and bronchiectasis [39]. Ventilator-associated pneumonia (VAP) is of particular interest, as the oral microbiota are known to form biofilms. Studies have shown that *Candida* spp. isolated alone or in combination from respiratory secretions in individuals with suspected VAP were shown to be associated with increased mortality compared to those in whom bacteria were isolated, with an unadjusted odds ratio of 2.9 [40]. Moreover, *Candida* colonisation has been associated with an increased risk of isolation of multidrug-resistant bacteria [41]. It is unknown whether *Candida* spp. represent a cause of disease or are a marker of disease. A study of VAP following cardiac surgery revealed that 30.19% of patients were culture positive for fungi, including *C. albicans* (16.97%); *Pneumocystis jirovecii* (3.77%); and *C. glabrata*, *C. sake*, *C. krusei*, *Geotrichum capitatum* and *Cryptococcus humicola* (1.89%) each] [42]. It is possible that the incidence of fungi within these VAP samples may be due to broad-spectrum antibiotics. Methods to prevent these biofilm infections include care bundles that include infection control measures, such as oral decontamination with chlorhexidine, which have dramatically cut the rates of VAP in the intensive care setting [43,44].

The lower respiratory tract is also associated with biofilm infection, of which *Pseudomonas aeruginosa* is a primary causative agent [45], though it is increasingly recognised that the fungal biofilms can persist in the lung and contribute towards infection. Filamentous moulds such as *A. fumigatus* can cause a spectrum of respiratory disease, including allergic bronchopulmonary aspergillosis (ABPA), an aspergilloma and invasive aspergillosis (IA) [46]. Bronchopulmonary lavage (BAL) of these individuals often reveals the presence of numerous intertwined hyphae forming complex multicellular structures indicative of a biofilm phenotype when examined histologically [47]. Aspergillary bronchitis is also a problematic biofilm-associated disease, characterised by bronchial casts containing mycelia forming compact masses [48]. Collectively, this evidence shows that *Aspergillus* species form medically important biofilms [49,50], so understanding their clinical role in the respiratory tract and how they interact with bacterial species is crucial, as these structures are highly resistant to antifungal therapy [51,52].

CF is an autosomal recessive disease caused by a mutation in the CF transmembrane conductance regulator [CFTR] protein, which is responsible for maintaining airway homeostasis and mucociliary clearance [53]. The morbidity and mortality associated with CF are linked to the irreversible decline in lung function caused by microbial colonisation of the airways and the resulting overactive neutrophilic immunological response [15]. The most commonly isolated pathogen is *P. aeruginosa*, which has been reported to colonise the airways of up to 75% of adult patients with CF [6]. This is the most prevalent and persistent microbe found in the CF lung [54], and is associated with a more rapid decline in lung function, increased hospitalisation and a decreased life expectancy [55,56]. Infection in CF patients is also commonly associated with *Staphylococcus aureus* and *Haemophilus influenzae*, and recent advances in culture-independent, NGS technologies have revealed that the microbiome of the CF lung is much richer than previously appreciated, comprising a diverse range of bacterial and fungal pathogens, of which *Aspergillus fumigatus* is the most prevalent filamentous fungus [50]. *A. fumigatus* has a prevalence rate of between 10% and 57% [57,58], though other fungi have been isolated from the lungs including *Scedosporium* species, *A. niger*, *A. flavus*, *A. nidulans* and *A. terrus* [59,60], as well as several yeasts such as *C. albicans*, *C. glabrata*, *C. krusei* and *C. parapsilosis*. Lungs of persons with CF are lined with a thick viscous mucus layer susceptible to polymicrobial infections, leading to recurrent infections and continuous inflammation [53]. The interplay between the pathogens residing in the lung may be responsible for the acute exacerbations associated with CF, where the balance is tipped towards an environment with excess inflammatory, oxidative and proteolytic activity [22]. Several studies have identified an association between *A. fumigatus* and *P. aeruginosa*, where decreased pulmonary function was seen in coinfection in comparison to a mono-infection [61], a phenomenon also reported with *Candida* spp. and *P. aeruginosa* [62]. Evidence is therefore increasing for the improved clinical management of these patients [63]. Indeed, interkingdom interactions of the CF lung, and elsewhere, may lead to adverse clinical outcomes [64]. The ability of these microbes to form strong mixed-species biofilms likely contributes towards their persistence, making it extremely difficult to eradicate the infection [52,65].

GASTROINTESTINAL TRACT

The mucosa of the gastrointestinal (GI) tract is heavily laden with bacterial microbiota, growing as healthy biofilm communities [66]. The GI tract is composed predominately of bacterial microflora, with estimates suggesting that its total metagenome comprises some 150 times more genetic material than the human genome. Review of 36 mycology-focussed studies found that at least 267 distinct fungal taxa have been reported from the human gut, a list that is ever expanding [67]. If we examine this more closely, however, there is a small number of commonly detected yeast species and a long tail of taxa that have been reported only once, suggesting transient colonisation. Other studies suggest that the GI mycobiome includes 335 species and 158 genera. Use of 454 pyrosequencing, targeting the internal transcribed spacer (ITS) region of the rRNA genes in faecal samples, demonstrated that fungi were detected in at least 46 distinct fungal operational taxonomic units (OTUs) from two phyla (Ascomycota and Basidiomycota). *Fusarium* was the most abundant genus, followed by *Malassezia, Penicillium, Aspergillus* and *Candida*, although these are presumed to be transient owing to their abundance in the environment or dietary associations [68].

Clinically polymicrobial biofilms present a problem, for example, when they are located in the stomach of those with percutaneous endoscopy gastronomy (PEG) feeding tubes for enteral nutrition, or in the large intestines in diseases such as ulcerative colitis [69]. *C. albicans* and *C. tropicalis* have been shown to colonise these PEG tubes and contribute to degradation of the polyurethane [70,71]. Clinically this may lead to diarrhoea, or possibly cause translocation of microbes across the epithelial barrier, leading to sepsis. *Candida* spp. colonisation of the GI tract is common, accounting for 30% to 80% in normal healthy adults [72]. Chronic colonisation may lead to GI candidiasis, which in immunocompromised individuals may lead to systemic candidiasis. Although little direct work has focussed on fungal biofilm in the GI tract per se, this environment is largely a polymicrobial biofilm, and interactions between yeasts and bacteria are likely to exist and play a role in health and disease, particularly *Escherichia coli* and various anaerobic Gram-negative microorganisms. In fact, it has been suggested that *Candida* colonisation may enhance inflammation in the GI tract [73].

URINARY TRACT

The urinary tract is also a polymicrobial environment, with a diverse metagenome present that is capable of preventing bacterial vaginosis, yeast infections, sexually transmitted disease and urinary tract infections (UTIs) [74]. It has been estimated that up to a third of UTIs in the elderly are polymicrobial and that with both increasing age and recurrent use of antimicrobials, fungal UTIs become more frequent [75]. Several studies have shown that *E. coli* and *C. albicans* are the most prevalent bacterial and fungal urinary pathogens, respectively [76–78]. It is therefore increasingly realised that polymicrobial infections are important in the urinary tract. High acidity from lactic acid bacterial metabolism is a key mediator of selective inhibition of other species [79]. Therefore, control of candidal biofilms may be best achieved through competitive inhibition by bacterial flora, such as lactobacilli, though no definitive studies have focussed in this area yet [80]. Nonetheless, it is suggested that 75% of woman experience vulvovaginal candidiasis at some point in their lives, suggesting that *Candida* spp. are important at this body site. *Candida* spp. have been associated with pyelonephritis, cystitis and prostatitis [81,82]. *Candida* biofilms have been detected on ureteral stents and have been shown to grow in this lifestyle experimentally on vaginal mucosa [83,84]. Urinary catheters are also a significant risk factor in intensive care units for healthcare-associated fungal infections [85]. Moreover, they are commonly detected on intrauterine contraceptive devices [86]. Although relatively rare, reports of an aspergilloma within the urinary tract are also possible [87,88].

WOUNDS

The skin microbiome is composed primarily of *Staphylococcus epidermidis* and other coagulase-negative staphylococci (CoNS), alongside *Corynebacterium, Propionibacterium, Brevibacterium* and *Micrococcus*, from the phylum Actinobacteria [89]. The most common fungi in the skin microbiome are *Malassezia* spp.; they are more prevalent in sebaceous areas and are thought to contribute to as much as 80% of the total fungal skin population [89,90]. Studies show that *Candida* spp. rarely colonise healthy intact skin, but are commonly implicated in infections in patients with immunodeficiency, diabetes and post-antibiotic use [5]. The skin is also thought to be colonised by *Debaryomyces* and *Cryptococcus* spp., although this has not been confirmed by molecular analysis [89].

Chronic wounds, associated with diabetic patients, vascular disease and immobility, are increasing as obesity, cardiovascular disease and urbanised sedentary lifestyles are becoming more common. Chronic wounds are an example of commensal skin organisms, including bacteria and fungi, invading and becoming pathogens on breach of the skin barrier when they form a diverse polymicrobial biofilm [89,91–93]. Biofilms have been observed in soft tissue samples from diabetic foot ulcers, pressure ulcers and venous leg ulcers by means of confocal microscopy, and at higher rates than acute wounds, using scanning electron microscopy and molecular techniques [94,95], and these represent a significant clinical burden to patients [96]. *S. aureus* and *P. aeruginosa* are the most significant pathogenic determinants of this process, which are often isolated together and have been shown to have a non-random association within the wound site [97]. A number of recent studies have investigated the diversity of chronic wounds, focussing on bacterial 16S ribosomal sequencing [98–101]. Evidence is emerging that pathogenic fungal species also play a role in these infections [102], and although generally uncommon various factors have led to an increased awareness, and even the development of novel diagnostics [103]. In a survey of 915 chronic wounds, 23% were identified as containing fungi as determined by quantitative real-time polymerase chain reaction (qPCR). There was a large diversity, with 34 genera, including 48 unique species, represented in at least five wounds. The most abundant fungi identified were from the genus *Candida*. Quantification of the relative abundance of bacteria versus fungus revealed that 67% wounds positive for fungi had fungal ratios accounting for more than half the microbial component. In this subset, 24 wounds were composed of more than 90% fungal component [104]. These data suggest that ignoring the fungal component of chronic wounds will result in 23% of wounds not being adequately treated. This estimate of the prevalence of fungi is reinforced by a culture study in which 25% of the diabetic foot wounds surveyed contained fungi, either alone or in conjunction with bacteria [105]. The presence of fungi was also found to be associated with poor glycaemic control [105]. In a study of US military personnel injured during combat who had persistent evidence of wound necrosis and evidence of fungal infection by microbiology and/or histopathology, mould isolates were recovered in 83% of cases (*Mucorales*, $n = 16$; *Aspergillus* spp., $n = 16$; *Fusarium* spp., $n = 9$), commonly with multiple mould species among infected wounds (28%). Clinical outcomes included three related deaths (8.1%), frequent debridements (median, 11 cases), and amputation revisions (58%) [106], thus highlighting the clinical importance of these infections. Sophisticated NGS approaches of samples from venous leg ulcers have shown that *C. albicans*, *C. glabrata* and *Aspergillus* species are present, but most intriguingly the authors report that individuals have unique microbial profiles, suggesting that a personalised approach to treating these infections is required alongside current biofilm-based wound care therapeutics [107]. This becomes apparent when a recent retrospective molecular analysis of 915 chronic wound infections is considered; in 208 (23%) of these, pathogenic fungi were isolated from pressure ulcers, diabetic foot ulcers, non-healing surgical wounds and venous leg ulcers [108]. Yeasts were the most abundant fungi (*Candida* spp.), but *Aureobasidium*, *Cladosporium*, *Curvularia*, *Engodontium*, *Malessezia*, *Trichtophyton* and *Ulocladium* were also found to be prevalent amongst polymicrobial infections. Overall, fungal species represented more than 50% of the microbial burden in the majority of specimens examined, prompting empiric antifungal treatment.

MEDICAL DEVICES

The hospital represents a significant burden of fungal and bacterial biofilm infection to the patient population with temporary and permanent biomaterials (Table 2.1). Moreover, broad-spectrum antibiotics, parenteral nutrition and immunosuppression due to chemotherapy and radiotherapy, and disruption of mucosal barriers due to surgery, are among the most important predisposing factors for invasive fungal infection [109]. Prominent pathogens associated with indwelling medical devices are either commensal flora that have migrated from around the skin onto the device, or of nosocomial origin [110,111]. Prevalent Gram-positive organisms include CoNS, partially because of their widespread presence on the skin [89], but also because of their ability to adhere to surfaces including host tissue, fibronectin and the indwelling medical device itself [110]. *S. aureus* is also commonly implicated; it is commonly carried in the nares and is a well-documented nosocomial pathogen [112]. *S. aureus* is a highly virulent organism, with the ability to produce multiple toxins, leading to tissue damage that incites a vigorous immune response, leading to an acute infection [113]. *S. aureus* device-related infections often lead to the patient developing a bacteraemia, which itself leads to further complications such as endocarditis and increased mortality [114]. Estimates suggest that around 27% of candidaemias are

TABLE 2.1
Medical Devices Commonly Associated with Biofilm Infections

Devices	Fungi	Bacteria	References
Pacemakers	*C. albicans*	*S. epidermidis*	[115,116]
Artificial heart valves	*Candida* spp. *Aspergillus* spp.	*Staphylococcus aureus* Coagulase-negative *Staphylococcus* Viridans *Streptococci* *Enterococcus* spp.	[117–119]
Ventilators	*Candida* spp. *Aspergillus* spp.	*Staphylococcus* spp. *Pseudomonas* spp. *Acinetobacter* spp. *Enterobacteriaceae*	[5,120]
Vascular catheters	*Candida* spp.	*Staphylococcus* spp. Viridans *Streptococci* *Escherichia coli* *Klebsiella* spp.	[5,121–124]
Urinary catheters	*C. albicans*	*E. coli*	[5,125–127]
Dentures	*Candida* spp.	*Lactobacillus* spp.	[128]
Breast implants	*C. albicans* *Aspergillus niger* *Curvularia* spp.	*Staphylococcus* spp. *Streptococcus* spp. *Klebsiella* spp. *Bacillus* spp. *Propionibacterium* spp.	[129,130]
Prosthetic joints	*Candida* spp.	*Staphylococcus* spp. *Streptococcus* spp. *Propionibacterium* spp.	[131,132]
Intragastric balloons	*Candida* spp.	*Enterobacter cloacae*	[133]
Neurosurgical shunts	*Candida* spp.	*Staphylococcus* spp. *Streptococcus* spp. *Enterococcus faecium* *Corynebacteria* sp. Gram-negative rods	[134,135]
Voice prosthesis	*Candida* spp.	*Rothia dentocariosa* *Staphylococcus* spp. *Streptococcus* spp. *Lactobacillus* spp.	[136,137]

polymicrobial, with a large proportion of this mixed with *S. aureus*, which is the third most commonly isolated pathogen [138].

Candida spp. are important nosocomial bloodstream infections, and are the fourth most common infectious agent in the intensive care unit, and are the most common aetiologic agent of fungal-related biofilm infection. Alongside these infections are the more common CoNS, which are the most common biomaterial-related bacteria. CoNS follow a more low-grade chronic disease progression [139]. Although bacteria are commonly implicated as the source of device-related infection, as alluded to earlier, fungi such as *Candida* are important and their involvement often leads to lower patient survival rates [140,141]. *S. epidermidis*, a CoNS, has been found in coinfections with *Candida* in pacemaker infective endocarditis [115] and on central venous catheters (CVCs) [142]. Scanning electron microscopy of *S. epidermidis* and *Candida* biofilm growing within vascular catheter material shows that the bacteria attach to both morphological forms of the fungus [116]. These types of infection are inherently difficult to resolve and may require both long-term antimicrobial therapy and/or physical removal of the implant to control the infection. Indwelling medical devices, such as intravascular catheters, can become colonised with *Candida* spp., allowing the development of adherent biofilm structures from which cells can then detach and cause an acute fungaemia and/or disseminated infection. It was shown that *Candida* bloodstream infections caused by biofilm forming isolates could be independently predicted by the presence of central venous catheters, urinary catheters, total parenteral nutrition and diabetes mellitus [143], and that high levels of biofilm formation significantly impacted mortality [144]. Studies of this nature highlight the clinical importance of biofilm forming isolates of *C. albicans*, particularly those associated with indwelling catheters, and the likelihood of these being of a polymicrobial interkingdom nature.

Other biofilm-related yeast and filamentous fungi infections have also been increasingly described, including *Aspergillus*, *Cryptococcus*, *Coccidioides*, *Zygomycetes*, *Blastoschizomyces* and *Malassezia*. *Aspergillus* species have been reported to cause serious biomaterial-related biofilm infections, involving catheters, joint replacements, cardiac pacemakers, heart valves and breast augmentation implants. *C. neoformans* has been shown to colonise and subsequently form biofilms on cardiac valves, peritoneal dialysis fistulas, ventricular shunts, and prosthetic hip joints [1]. This list of biomaterial-associated fungal species is by no means exhaustive, but does provide a vivid picture of the true extent of clinically important fungal biofilms associated directly with the human host [145]. Given our knowledge of how bacterial pathogens interact with these same materials, it highlights how important polymicrobial interkingdom biofilm infections can be in this arena.

CROSS-KINGDOM INTERACTIONS

Staphylococcal Interactions

Angular cheilitis is an inflammation of one, or more commonly both, corners of the mouth. Although not particularly common per se, this condition is of interest as it is often associated with the co-isolation of *Candida* spp. with *Staphylococcus aureus*, microorganisms not unaccustomed to one another within the human host [146–148]. Both species are leading pathogens in blood-borne and systemic infections, a major cause of morbidity and mortality in hospitalised patients. These species are of significant interest because of the escalating development of antimicrobial resistance and their increasing involvement in chronic and systemic polymicrobial biofilm infections [149], and have been shown to coaggregate together and exist within a dynamic and interactive state [6,150,151]. The relationship between these two has been described as mutualistic, synergistic and antagonistic, yet most of the evidence indicates synergy, as the majority of their interactions are associated with enhanced pathogenicity and disease severity [152,153].

The interaction between *C. albicans* and *S. aureus* has been associated with enhanced pathogenic behaviour, disease severity and morbidity [154]. They form mixed polymicrobial biofilms in which *S. aureus* cells are found attached to *C. albicans* hyphal filaments [155,156]. Their colocalisation within biofilms is still unclear, as some describe them interspersed throughout the biofilm three-dimensional structure [155], whereas others describe them as only found attached within the upper layers of the biofilm [157]. This disparity could be explained by different experimental conditions (e.g. growth medium). The initial colonising species plays a key role in dictating their interaction, as it has been shown that *C. albicans* biofilm formation was delayed when *S. aureus* colonised first, yet when added simultaneously biofilms formed rapidly [156]. The reason for this inhibition is unknown; perhaps *S. aureus* secretes an inhibitory molecule preventing *Candida* adhesion.

It has also been shown that *S. aureus* preferentially adhere to hyphal filaments (Figure 2.1) by relying on the adhesion to the *C. albicans* agglutinin-like sequence 3 protein (Als3p) [151,155], though it is likely that other proteins are involved. *S. epidermidis* have also been shown to adhere preferentially to hyphae (Figure 2.1), with large adhesion forces (~5 nN) evident between single bacterial and fungal germ tubes [158]. Studies have shown that *S. aureus* binding to *C. albicans* hyphae was significantly stronger than that of all other bacteria tested, including *P. aeruginosa* [155]. Interestingly, it was reported that none of the members of the ALS family of adhesins, (*ALS1–7* and *ALS9*), including *ALS3*, are involved in interspecies adhesion [159]. Thus further insight is required before we can fully understand the mechanisms responsible for adherence, yet it is likely that this is a complex process in which a multitude of proteins are involved. Nevertheless, it is thought that adhesion to hyphae may assist *S. aureus* in penetrating into the host [153], in a manner analogous to injection from a needle-stick injury (Figure 2.2). This has been demonstrated

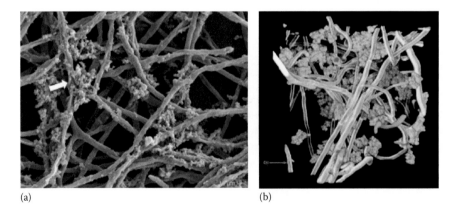

(a)   (b)

FIGURE 2.1   Mixed polymicrobial biofilm. (a) Scanning electron micrograph and (b) confocal micrograph illustrate the adhesion of *S. aureus* (denoted by arrow or yellow colour) to *Candida* hyphal filaments forming a complex polymicrobial biofilm.

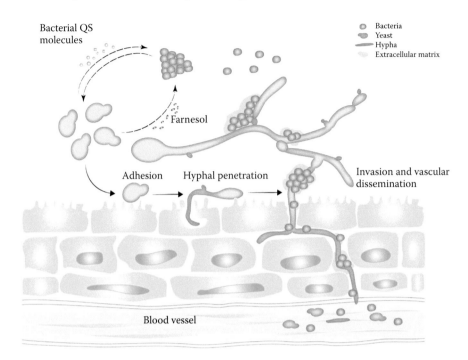

FIGURE 2.2 Cross-kingdom interactions. Bacteria and fungi interact with each other in a variety of forms including physical associations and molecular exchanges (e.g. farnesol and QS molecules). The hyphal growth of fungi acts as a niche for bacterial biofilm formation and potentially assists them in penetrating into the host.

in mice studies, in which mixed infections with *C. albicans als3Δ* strains together with *S. aureus* were unable to invade the tongue, whereas the wild-type infections demonstrated coinfection [151]. The ramifications of this enhanced invasive capacity have been shown historically to impact mortality, where synergism between the coinfected species administered intraperitoneally in a mouse model led to 100% mortality, whereas monospecies infections caused no mortality whatsoever [160]. Whether or not the relationship between the two organisms is physical or chemical remains to be determined, although there is evidence that growth-related synergy is an important factor in their cohabitation of micro-niches [161]. Indeed, the physical relationship between the organisms is important, but not fundamental. Recent studies indicated that morphogenesis, that is, the presence of hyphae, is not critical for their pathogenic potential, as demonstrated in some intricate murine studies using *C. albicans* genetically locked into the yeast state [162]. This suggests that physical cellular interactions are not solely responsible.

Metabolic signalling between *C. albicans* and *S. aureus* may play an important role in orchestrating this relationship. Chemically mediated signalling in the form of quorum sensing (QS) could potentiate both positive and negative interactions between these two microorganisms, which may inadvertently impact clinical outcomes. *C. albicans* secretion of farnesol, a QS molecule, decreases *S. aureus* biofilm formation, as well as increasing its susceptibility to antibiotics [163–165]. Moreover, it was shown to competitively inhibit *S. aureus* lipase activity [166]. However, it was found that *S. aureus* conditioned media had a striking impact on *C. albicans* biofilm growth rate, indicating that *S. aureus* secretes a reciprocal QS molecule that stimulates *C. albicans* growth [167]. Nonetheless, whether *C. albicans* secretes sufficient farnesol *in vivo* to have an effect on *S. aureus* remains unknown. Yet despite these conflicting results, the majority of studies support the idea of a synergistic relationship between the two.

Indeed, affinity panning of an *S. aureus* phage display library against *C. albicans* biofilms demonstrated that *S. aureus* released extracellular fibrinogen binding protein (Efb) during the interaction. This was shown to coat *C. albicans* yeast cells and reduce phagocytosis by granulocytes [168]. To gain a better understanding of the molecular interaction between C. *albicans* and *S. aureus*, Peters and colleagues undertook a proteomics approach to identify proteins up-regulated during their interaction [155]. The majority of the 27 proteins that were up-regulated were involved in processes including stress and growth responses and metabolism. *S. aureus* up-regulated stress-related genes in response to both yeast and hyphae, yet, interestingly most of these genes were up-regulated in response to yeast rather than hyphal biofilms. As for *C. albicans*, yeast cells increased a number of stress-related proteins such as Tsa1p and aconitate hydratase, yet *C. albicans* in hyphal formation showed minimal changes in gene expression in response to *S. aureus*. These results suggest that both organisms induce a stress response on their initial encounter with one another, particularly while *Candida* exists in yeast form. However, as they mature and develop into a hyphal biofilm, they may down-regulate these genes as a survival strategy, facilitating survival within the host.

Clearly, these two pathogens have the ability to influence one another's behaviour, so care must be taken in their clinical management. Broad-spectrum antimicrobial activity is crucial, accounting for both prokaryotes and eukaryotes. The use of ethanol has been shown to be effective at preventing both mono- and polymicrobial biofilms [169]. However, the successful use of miconazole in angular cheilitis is interesting given no precise mechanism of action for this azole to *S. aureus* [170]. It could therefore be hypothesised that given the polymicrobiality of the disease miconazole acts by inhibiting *C. albicans* activity, thereby destabilising *S. aureus* colonisation, which is physically supported by the hyphal biofilm meshwork. Studies in *S. epidermidis* have shown that extracellular DNA (eDNA) release through autolysis is an important entity in supporting mixed biofilm growth [171], and is a feature also critical for *C. albicans* biofilm extracellular matrix (ECM) integrity [172,173]. Therefore, it is not surprising that eDNA and the ECM from both *C. albicans* and *S. aureus* biofilms are both involved in affecting the action of antibacterial agents. In fact, it has been shown that *S. aureus* is protected against vancomycin treatment using concentrations as high as 1600 mg/mL within the mixed biofilm environment, through *C. albicans* ECM preventing diffusion and access to *S. aureus* [157]. There are, however, other adaptive resistance mechanisms that play a role in this resistance phenotype [159]. In a study on the effects of fluconazole and vancomycin on coculture biofilms, increased drug resistance was shown in the coculture compared to the single species [116]. This supports the hypothesis that slime production by *S. epidermidis* contributes to drug resistance. It also suggests that resistance can be enhanced by the presence of *Candida* [116]. Mixed biofilms have also been shown to cause increased catheter infection with increased dissemination of the *S. epidermidis* in a mouse model, which could provide an explanation for adverse clinical outcomes [174].

STREPTOCOCCAL INTERACTIONS

Dental caries is one of the most common conditions worldwide, impacting 36% of the entire global population [approx. 2.43 billion] [175]. Dental plaque biofilms play a key role in the development of dental caries, through carbohydrate metabolism (predominantly sucrose) that leads to the production of large quantities of lactic acid and ultimately the dissolution of tooth surfaces. *Streptococcus mutans* and *Lactobacillus* species are most commonly associated with caries [176,177], however, recent oral microbiome studies have highlighted the polymicrobial aetiology of carious lesions [178,179]. Candidal yeasts have been isolated in patients with caries [180,181], though the evidence for their direct role has not yet been shown directly. There is now growing evidence that *C. albicans* actively participates in cariogenic biofilms, through synergistic interaction with *S. mutans* [181,182]. Evidence of enhanced exopolymeric matrix production, facilitated by the increased surface area associated with hyphal networks, supports mixed biofilm growth of dense communities cemented to tooth enamel. There are a range of streptococci amongst the primary colonisers of the oral cavity that comprise a large proportion of the overall flora [183,184]. Oral streptococcal species are often termed the mitis group streptococci (MGS), which include *S. gordonii*, *S. oralis*, *S. mitis*, *S. sanguinis* and *S. parasanguinis* species [185]. MGS are thought to comprise approximately 60–80% of the flora [186], although use of NGS technology has revealed them to also be predominant colonisers of oral mucosal surfaces [186].

The relationship between *Candida* and streptococci is generally considered to be synergistic, with advanced microscopy showing streptococcal interactions with the hyphal filaments of *Candida* [187]. Streptococci provide *Candida* with nutrients from the salivary pellicle, such as lactate and glucose, which *Candida* utilises as a source of carbon [188]. Furthermore, streptococci are aciduric and thus create an acidic environment through the fermentation of carbohydrates [189]. At low pH *Candida* grows in its yeast form, though when cocolonised with streptococci it can grow and survive at a lower pH (<4.5), and the H_2O_2 produced by streptococci can induce hyphal growth by inducing oxidative stress [190,191]. This interaction is bidirectional, as *C. albicans* can promote the survival of streptococci by lowering oxygen tension levels to those more acceptable for streptococcal growth, as well as providing nutrients to stimulate bacterial growth [192]. This synergistic relationship can prove detrimental for the host. Studies have shown that streptococci augment the persistence of *Candida* spp. It was demonstrated that coinfection with *C. albicans* and *S. oralis* resulted in a more pathogenic inflammatory response compared with infection with either microorganism alone, as illustrated through an exaggerated upregulation of TLR2-dependent inflammatory genes [187,193].

Adherence to mucosal surfaces occurs through binding interactions with components of the salivary pellicle, but there are a limited number of niches for *C. albicans* to inhabit, and *C. albicans* has to compete [194]. To overcome this, it has evolved a mechanism allowing it to bind directly to MGS species [190]. This interaction is mutually beneficial, as *C. albicans* can support the outgrowth of streptococci by enabling them to form robust biofilms [193]. Adherence between these two species occurs via interactions of the *C. albicans* hyphal cell wall protein Als3 and the streptococcal cell surface adhesins SspA and SspB [195], proteins that belong to the antigen I/II polypeptide family [196]. Als3p is one of eight Als protein family members, and direct binding of SspB to Als3p is required for bacterial–fungal attachment. Interaction between these molecules is associated with the N-terminal domain of Als3 [197], as deletions at the N-terminus abrogate binding to *S. gordonii*. This interaction may be more complex than originally thought, as the peptide-binding domain (PBD) of *C. albicans* is essential for *C. albicans*–*S. gordonii* adherence. The PBD functions by binding to the free C-terminus; however, in *S. gordonii* the SspB C-terminus is covalently linked to peptidoglycan and is thus unavailable to bind. Recent studies suggest that the early stage of cell wall *O*-mannosylation may be important in the development of these polymicrobial communities [187].

An important component of biofilms is the ECM [193]. Streptococcal biofilm ECM is composed of α-glucans [198], whereas *Candida* biofilm ECM is composed primarily of β-glucans [199,200]. *S. mutans* utilises its ECM components to enhance adhesion to fungal cells by depositing α-glucans on the surface of hyphae [198]. The interaction between *S. mutans* and *C. albicans* is promoted by glucosyltransferase-derived ECM and expression of the *S. mutans* virulence gene *gtfB* [201]. It was also shown that Candida-derived β1,3-glucans contribute to ECM matrix structure, while fungal β-glucan and mannan provide sites for GtfB binding and activity. Furthermore, β-glucans are found on the surface of hyphae as well as in the matrix [18], suggesting that streptococci utilise these proteins to adhere to candidal hyphae. Collectively, this suggests the biofilm ECM contributes to this mutualistic behavior, favouring their coexistence in the oral environment to the detriment of the host.

QS is an important factor in the relationship between *Candida* and streptococci. Farnesol, a tetraprenoid alcohol and a key intermediate in the sterol biosynthetic pathway in eukaryotic cells, represents the primary QS molecule associated with *C. albicans*, its main role being repression of hyphal growth and biofilm formation [202]. It has been suggested that *S. gordonii* is able to suppress farnesol induced inhibition of biofilm formation via autoinducer 2 (AI-2), as *luxS* mutants were less effective at permitting hyphal formation [196]. Farnesol has also been shown to inhibit *S. mutans* biofilm accumulation and ECM production [203], leading to suggestions that it could be used as a chemotherapeutic strategy [204]. AI-2 is the primary QS molecule secreted by bacteria that allows interspecies communication [205]. The *luxS* gene is associated with AI-2 production. Streptococcal *luxS* mutants can form monospecies biofilms, yet, when cocolonised with *C. albicans*, biofilm formation becomes abrogated, suggesting this molecule is involved in cellular communication between both organisms [196,206]. Another important signalling mechanism in streptococci, including *S. gordonii*, is through the comCDE operon, which encodes a sensor-regulator system (ComDE). The latter is activated by the *comC* gene encoded competence stimulating peptide (CSP). In a coculture model, *S. gordonii* Δ*comCDE* or Δ*comC* mutants with *C. albicans* showed increased biofilm biomass compared to wild-type biofilms. Interestingly, more eDNA was observed in the mixed Δ*comCDE* mutant biofilms. Although purified CSP did not affect *C. albicans* hyphal formation, contrary to earlier findings [207], it did inhibit monospecies biofilm formation, suggesting that the *S. gordonii* comCDE QS-system modulates the production of eDNA [208], an important component of candidal ECM [172].

PORPHYROMONAS INTERACTIONS

Periodontal disease (PD) is a complex polymicrobial disease caused by host–pathogen interactions, affecting around half of the US population younger than 30 years old. It exists in mild (gingivitis) and severe (periodontitis) forms. Both forms of disease can be categorised by the development of polymicrobial biofilms, which form initially above the gum line (supragingival plaque), and can subsequently lead to subgingival plaque biofilms. The composition of these biofilms and their clinical outcomes has been well characterised using Socransky's traffic light analogy [209,210]. However, surprisingly, there has been a distinct lack of research into the role of *Candida* spp. in this disease, especially as *Candida* spp. has been found within the subgingival plaque of patients with severe chronic periodontitis, where quantitatively high levels of *C. albicans* were shown to correlate with moderate and severe chronic periodontitis [211]. Evidence for direct causality is lacking, yet studies involving diabetic patients identified a relationship between subgingival candidal colonisation and periodontitis [212,213], though this could purely be a result of elevated blood sugar levels supporting the growth of *Candida* spp. Furthermore, the use of oral contraceptives (OCs) have implicated *Candida* spp. in PD, as evidence shows an increased carriage rate, as well as higher incidences of oral and vaginal candidiasis among OC users [214–216]. Severe periodontitis is also more common among OC users, suggesting that the hormones lead to the development of a dysbiotic biofilm, enabling *Candida* yeast to colonise [217]. Nonetheless, whether or not *Candida* plays a significant role in periodontal biofilms, and the specific interactions involved, remain to be elucidated.

Life in subgingival plaque is highly anaerobic, favouring many obligate PD pathogens such as *Porphyromonas gingivalis*, *Fusobacterium nucleatum* and *P. intermedia*. However, given the undefined relationship between *Candida* spp. and PD, this remains a relatively neglected area of research. Studies regarding *C. albicans* and *P. gingivalis* have produced conflicting results. It was shown that *P. gingivalis* suppressed *Candida* biofilm formation through a reduction in the number of viable yeast cells coincidental with an increasing *P. gingivalis* concentration [218]. Conversely, it was also shown that *P. gingivalis* induces germ-tube formation in *C. albicans*, producing a more invasive phenotype, thus increasing the risk of infection [219]. Furthermore, both microbes appear to have an antagonistic effect on one another in relation to host cell adhesion, as *P. gingivalis* inhibited adhesion of *C. albicans* to buccal epithelial cells [220], whereas the presence of *C. albicans* did not enhance adhesion to gingival epithelial cells or gingival fibroblasts by *P. gingivalis* [221]. Yet, in the same study preexposure of gingival epithelial cells and fibroblasts to *C. albicans* enhanced cell invasion by *P. gingivalis*. Clearly, further studies are required to decipher how these microorganisms interact with one another. As for

F. nucleatum, coaggregation studies have revealed its ability to adhere to *C. albicans* species [222], as well as *C. dubliniensis* [223]. However, the interaction with *C. albicans* may be temperature dependent as *C. albicans* grown at 37°C did not coaggregate with *F. nucleatum*, yet the two species did coaggregate when grown at 25°C and 45°C [223]. The exact mechanistic behind these interactions remain unknown; however, these observations indicate *C. albicans–F. nucleatum* interactions may be an important factor in oral colonisation by yeasts.

PSEUDOMONAS INTERACTIONS

The CF lung is a site of intense interkingdom interaction, where *P. aeruginosa* is a primary participant. It has been shown that *P. aeruginosa* is able to selectively form biofilms on hyphae and kill *C. albicans*, but not the yeast form [224]. Presumably this occurs through the release of a phenazine toxin [225,226]. It has also been shown to inhibit the morphological transition through a 3-oxo-C12 homoserine lactone [227], a phenomenon replicated in studies of *A. fumigatus* biofilm [228]. Recent evidence from a murine model demonstrated that lung tissue injury caused by *P. aeruginosa* infection is alleviated if preceded by a short-term *C. albicans* colonisation [229]. This was a result of *C. albicans* activating interleukin-22 (IL-22) producing innate lymphoid cells, which provided protection from *P. aeruginosa*–induced injury [230]. Given the dynamic relationship between these organisms, it is not surprising that release of the QS molecule farnesol by *C. albicans* impacts *P. aeurginosa* by inhibiting its quinolone signalling, which controls pyocyanin production [231]. These studies highlight the ongoing and dynamic battle within a polymicrobial environment such as the CF lung, which clearly plays a crucial role in the overall pathogenesis of disease [150]. Elegant studies in a *Drosophila* infection model of polymicrobial infection demonstrate this point; they showed that microorganisms of the CF airways were able to influence the outcome of an infection depending on the presence or absence of *P. aeruginosa* [232,233].

    P. aeruginosa has also been shown to inhibit *A. fumigatus* filamentation via the release of molecules involved in intracellular communication [228]. Investigations into the interactions between these two are limited; however, the release of small molecules designed to inhibit fungal growth appear to be the primary form of interaction. One particular group of metabolites known as phenazines have been reported to inhibit *A. fumigatus* biofilm formation; however, it was also found that *A. fumigatus* was able to convert these metabolites released by *P. aeruginosa* to produce fungal siderophores, which may in turn influence CF progression [234]. Furthermore, *P. aeruginosa* releases the metalloprotease elastase, which has been shown to be toxic to host cells [9]. It was found that elastase production was constitutive, but became significantly increased in the presence of *A. fumigatus* during biofilm coculture. Furthermore, elastase was cytotoxic to human lung cells, therefore indicating that the presence of both of these pathogens could synergistically contribute towards enhanced pathogenicity [9]. Thus, in general, evidence suggests that the co-isolation of both of these organisms indicates a poorer prognosis; however, the relationship between the two remains poorly understood and requires further investigation into their polymicrobial interactions.

ESCHERICHIA INTERACTIONS

C. albicans can exhibit both a mutual and antagonistic relationship with *E. coli*. Studies using lipopolysaccharide (LPS) from a variety of Gram-negative strains have shown that hyphal formation is inhibited, as is biofilm formation in a number of *Candida* spp. [235], indicating that physical interaction may be an important factor in defining their subgingival niches. Subsequent work in *E. coli* demonstrated that secreted elements also play an important role in affecting hyphal formation [236]. It has been shown that the non-pathogenic *E. coli* strain 83972 is able to inhibit the attachment of a range of urinary pathogens, including *C. albicans*, to Foley catheters [237]. The precoating of the catheter surface with the bacteria was able to reduce fungal attachment significantly. Although the underlying mechanisms are unknown, it is likely that an amalgamation of the secretion of antifungal molecules and a competition for both surface area and nutrients are the reasons for this inhibition. The ability of *E. coli*, as well as another Gram-negative bacilli, *Pseudomonas aeruginosa*, to inhibit *C. albicans* biofilm formation on Foley catheters has also been shown [238]. They reported that dual species biofilms containing *C. albicans* and either of the Gram-negative organisms or bacterial lipopolysaccharide alone were able to reduce candidal adhesion to the catheter disc significantly. It should be noted that these observed antagonist relationships appear to be very much strain dependent, yet nonetheless might provide a useful insight into possible probiotic therapeutic approaches.

Contrary to this, multiple studies have shown a synergistic *in vivo* relationship between *E. coli* and *C. albicans* [239,240]. Moreover, it has been shown in a murine model that a concomitant infection with both *C. albicans* and *E. coli* demonstrates a synergistic co-operation in which the bacteria strengthens the colonisation of *C. albicans* to the host bladder mucosa. The reason for this disparity observed between *in vitro* and *in vivo* studies remains unclear, though additional factors associated with the animal hosts are likely to change the dynamic relationship between these organisms. This increased attachment then enhances the probability of a fungal UTI [241]. These same organisms are also found as the principal biofilm forming pathogens that colonise urinary catheters. Recent studies showed that in a *C. albicans–E. coli* polymicrobial biofilm model, ofloxacin tolerance of *E. coli* is significantly increased in comparison to that of its own monospecies biofilm [242]. Furthermore, using a *C. albicans* $zap1\Delta/zap1\Delta$ mutant which overexpresses β-1,3-glucan, these biofilms showed a further increase in ofloxacin resistance than the wild-type polymicrobial biofilm, highlighting the role which integral cell wall protein β-1,3-glucan contributes to this resistance. Recently, experimental murine studies have reported that *C. albicans* is able to modulate the bacterial microbiota composition of non-pathogenic species after antibiotic exposure [243], suggesting that in health there is a bidirectional relationship between bacteria and *C. albicans*, rather than simply competitive inhibition by bacteria.

ENTEROCOCCUS INTERACTIONS

Endodontitis is characterised by an infection of the pulp within the dental root canal system, and is classically of biofilm aetiology. Endodontic infections are associated with four key phyla (*Firmicutes*, *Bacteroidetes*, *Actinobacteria* and *Proteobacteria*), yet bacterial pathogens from more than 100 different genera have been implicated, although *Enterococcus faecalis* is considered the primary aetiological agent [244]. The composition of endodontic biofilms is often reflected in their site of origin, that is, those in periapical infections are composed primarily of anaerobic bacteria, whereas those from cariogenic lesions can be compared to supragingival plaque. Evidence for interkingdom interactions within endodontic infection is scarce; however, *Candida* spp. are becoming increasingly isolated [245]. *In vitro* studies have demonstrated that *C. albicans* is able to penetrate dentine tubules [246]. *C. albicans* has been identified within root canal samples, and an association between *C. albicans* and *E. faecalis* has been identified [247,248]. Yet, despite this, there still remains a distinct lack of evidence regarding polymicrobial interactions in the root canal environment. *Candida* spp. and *E. faecalis* have become increasingly noted for their co-isolation within endodontic infections, both of which play an important role in nosocomial infection. Interestingly, data from a longitudinal study conducted over two years at a German teaching hospital found that *Candida*-positive patients (blood, cerebrospinal fluid, skin, faeces or sputum) were twice as likely to be cocolonised by *E. faecalis* [249]. *E. faecalis* has been found to incorporate itself into *Candida* biofilms, and is the third most predominant bacterial species found in mucosal fungal biofilms [18,250]. It was shown to adhere to *Candida* in both hyphal and yeast forms, yet caused a reduction in the overall biofilm biomass [250]. However, Cruz and colleagues demonstrated that *E. faecalis* inhibited hyphal morphogenesis, which was partially dependent on the *Fsr* QS system, a major regulator of *E. faecalis* virulence [251]. Collectively, this effect impacted virulence during coinfection when compared to monospecies infection, suggesting that they both negatively influence one another's virulence and help maintain a commensal relationship [252]. Further work has revealed that *C. albicans* releases a surface protein Msb2, which binds to host antimicrobial peptides as well as antibiotics, thus conferring protection to both organisms [253]. Furthermore, evaluating the influence of *C. albicans* on the dynamics of the bacterial microbiome following antibiotic treatment found that bacterial recolonisation was enhanced in the presence of *C. albicans* [243]. Moreover, *C. albicans* reduced *Lactobacillus* spp. while enhancing the level of *E. faecalis*, which led to the persistence of *E. faecalis* long term. This effect was not apparent in subjects when *C. albicans* was absent. Whether this effect was due to a synergistic relationship with *E. faecalis* or an antagonistic interaction with lactobacilli remains to be elucidated.

LACTOBACILLUS INTERACTIONS

There is a conceived dogma that lactobacilli antagonise candidal colonisation [254], which forms the basis of why they play a key role in probiotics. It is well documented that probiotics reduces candidal levels at several sites, including oral cavity, bloodstream and urinary tract [255,256]. Early observations indicate that levels of *C. albicans* decreased in the presence of lactobacilli through provision of nutrients for lactobacilli that leads to lactic acid production, thus hindering candidal growth through pH-dependent inhibition. This dynamic relationship suggests that there is a close association between the two, but to date this has been observed mainly in vaginal infection. Our own microbiome studies of denture plaque have shown that *C. albicans* and lactobacilli are positively associated in disease (unpublished work). The role of lactobacilli in maintaining homeostasis at the vaginal mucosa initially came to light as a result of the occurrence of vaginal candidiasis during treatment with systemic antibiotics. The mechanisms by which *Lactobacillus* spp. inhibits growth and virulence of *Candida* spp. are not yet fully understood, but perhaps they involve the production of hydrogen peroxide, as it has been shown to cause anti-candidal activity, albeit in some strains of lactobacilli [257]. This suggests that other interactive mechanisms are involved in disease, including the modulation of the host response whereby lactobacilli cells have been shown to up-regulate inflammatory cytokines when cocultured with *C. albicans* [258], potentially assisting in the clearance of candidal infection. Despite the overwhelming evidence of an antagonistic interaction, certain species of oral *Lactobacillus*, namely *L. casei*, have demonstrated a stimulatory effect on hyphal growth of *C. albicans* [259], and in fact it has been demonstrated that candidal hyphae have the capacity to coaggregate and support lactobacilli levels in patients with higher levels of oral disease [260]. Nevertheless, further studies are required to investigate these interactions in detail to determine the true extent of the dynamic relationship; particularly as the conceived antagonism may exist only for *C. albicans*. For example, recent studies have shown that only one of six probiotic *Lactobacillus* spp. had an inhibitory effect on growth of *C. glabrata* [261]. This suggests that the interaction between *Candida* and lactobacilli may be dependent on the particular environment they cohabit.

CANDIDAL INTERACTIONS

Denture stomatitis (DS) refers to inflammation of the oral mucosa and pathological changes associated with the tissue surfaces in direct contact with the prosthesis [262]. Approximately two thirds of denture wearers will experience DS at some point [263]. Dentures support the growth of polymicrobial biofilm communities which contain up to 10^{11} microbes per milligram of denture plaque [264,265]. In general DS is considered to be of yeast aetiology, as the literature is excessively focussed on *Candida* spp. [266–269]. *C. albicans* is the yeast most commonly isolated from dentures and is responsible for most of the DS-associated pathology; however, *C. glabrata*, *C. dubliniensis*, *C. tropicalis*, *C. krusei* and a range of other *Candida* spp. have been commonly isolated [270,271]. *Candida* colonises the oral cavity of 25–50% of the healthy population, but can become pathogenic under optimal conditions or when the immune response is compromised [272]. It is a dimorphic yeast, with the ability to switch to a hyphal phenotype, a prerequisite for biofilm formation [273]. The hyphal form is associated with a more invasive phenotype and with an enhanced capacity to adhere to the denture surface and is commonly found in individuals affected with DS [263,274]. Nonetheless, it is unlikely that *Candida* is solely responsible for the infection given that recent first NGS microbiome analysis of denture plaque identified hundreds of species of bacteria colonising the denture surface. The predominant bacteria included *Actinomyces*, *Streptococcus*, *Rothia*, *Veillonella* and *Lactobacillus* [275]. This particular composition is likely due to the ability of many of these bacteria to coaggregate with *C. albicans* hyphae [260,276]. The specific interactions in a polymicrobial denture biofilm remain to be elucidated; however, what we do understand is that these biofilms actively release proteolytic and lipolytic enzymes leading to inflammation of the palatal surface [277,278], ultimately causing DS.

Hyphae provide *C. albicans* with an advantage over many of its competitors in terms of size and surface area, enabling them to take advantage of more sites for adhesion and occupation of a variety of niches. This is why it is a more successful pathogen than other members of the genus. Nonetheless, there is hypothesis that *Candida* spp., in particular *C. glabrata*, benefit from *C. albicans*. There have been suggestions that DS pathology may be promoted by the synergistic interaction between these species within denture biofilms. Coco and colleagues [270] first reported that *C. glabrata* and *C. albicans* were often co-isolated from patients, particularly those with severe inflammation. The authors hypothesised that pathogenic synergy existed between the two *Candida* spp. *C. glabrata*, devoid of hyphae, forms relatively structurally poor and unstable biofilms, yet is associated with disease. Therefore, it was hypothesised to use *C. albicans* as a structural scaffold to gain entry into the host. Further studies have confirmed this, where *C. albicans* appeared to assist the invasive capacity of *C. glabrata* within an *in vitro* reconstituted epithelial biofilm model [279]. The mechanistics of this interaction are at present unknown; however, we can speculate that tissue destruction through proteolytic and lipolytic enzymes augments the invasive capacity of the hyphae and allows coaggregative *C. glabrata* to enter and contribute to pathogenesis. Further work by this group has shown similar data with work in a reconstituted human vaginal epithelial model, where *C. glabrata* individually caused minimal tissue damage, though there was a significant increase in *C. glabrata* colonisation and invasiveness in combination with *C. albicans* [280]. Damage was dependent primarily on the process of invasion, with key virulence genes upregulated (*HWP1*, *PLD1* and *ALS3*). Further studies using *in vivo* models to investigate the pathogenesis of denture stomatitis would be useful in this context [281], although as described earlier there is mounting evidence that hitchhiking through adhesion to hyphae is not a limited phenomenon and may also be important with respect to *C. glabrata* using *C. albicans* to gain entry to the host [153].

CONCLUSIONS

Interkingdom interactions within biofilms are an important clinical entity. These interactions may be chemical, physical or both, and are dictated by the particular environment they cohabit. The physical presence of hyphae creates scaffolds for coadhesion, and secretion of signalling molecules from the myriad of microorganisms on mucosal surfaces highlight how the interactome, comprising the micro- and myco-biomes, metagenomes, transcriptomes and metabolomes, makes for a complex clinical scenario. If one brings in the host innate and adaptive immune system this paints a picture of limitless interactions to investigate and unravel. Understanding how each of these specific interactions influences pathogenicity will enable us to target these medically important interkingdom infections. Though, we must be cognisant of the negative influences of changing its role within complex oral biofilm communities and the consequences of dysbiosis [282], as this may support unnecessary proliferation and overgrowth, ultimately leading to poor disease outcomes.

CORRESPONDING AUTHOR

Gordon Ramage
Oral Sciences Research Group
Glasgow Dental School
School of Medicine
College of Medical, Veterinary and Life Sciences
University of Glasgow
Glasgow, United Kingdom
Gordon.Ramage@glasgow.ac.uk

REFERENCES

1. Williams C, Ramage G. Fungal biofilms in human disease. *Adv Exp Med Biol.* 2015;831:11–27.
2. Nett JE. Future directions for anti-biofilm therapeutics targeting *Candida*. *Exp Rev Anti-infect Ther.* 2014;12(3):375–82.
3. Ramage G, Robertson SN, Williams C. Strength in numbers: Antifungal strategies against fungal biofilms. *Int J Antimicrob Agents.* 2014;43(2):114–20.
4. O'Donnell LE, Millhouse E, Sherry L, Kean R, Malcolm J, Nile CJ et al. Polymicrobial *Candida* biofilms: Friends and foe in the oral cavity. *FEMS Yeast Res.* 2015;15(7):77–81.
5. Peleg AY, Hogan DA, Mylonakis E. Medically important bacterial–fungal interactions. *Nat Rev Microbiol.* 2010;8(5):340–9.
6. Shirtliff ME, Peters BM, Jabra-Rizk MA. Cross-kingdom interactions: *Candida albicans* and bacteria. *FEMS Microbiol Lett.* 2009;299(1):1–8.
7. Wright CJ, Burns LH, Jack AA, Back CR, Dutton LC, Nobbs AH et al. Microbial interactions in building of communities. *Mol Oral Microbiol.* 2013;28(2):83–101.
8. Stacy A, Everett J, Jorth P, Trivedi U, Rumbaugh KP, Whiteley M. Bacterial fight-and-flight responses enhance virulence in a polymicrobial infection. *Proc Natl Acad Sci U S A.* 2014;111(21):7819–24.
9. Smith K, Rajendran R, Kerr S, Lappin DF, Mackay WG, Williams C et al. *Aspergillus fumigatus* enhances elastase production in *Pseudomonas aeruginosa* co-cultures. *Med Mycol.* 2015;53(7):645–55.
10. Holmes AR, Cannon RD, Jenkinson HF. Interactions of *Candida albicans* with bacteria and salivary molecules in oral biofilms. *J Indust Microbiol.* 1995;15(3):208–13.
11. Cui L, Morris A, Ghedin E. The human mycobiome in health and disease. *Genome Med.* 2013;5(7):63.
12. Guo L, Shi W. Salivary biomarkers for caries risk assessment. *J Calif Dent Assoc.* 2013;41(2):107–9, 12–8.
13. Ghannoum MA, Jurevic RJ, Mukherjee PK, Cui F, Sikaroodi M, Naqvi A et al. Characterization of the oral fungal microbiome (mycobiome) in healthy individuals. *PLoS Pathog.* 2010;6(1):e1000713.
14. Nobbs AH, Jenkinson HF. Interkingdom networking within the oral microbiome. *Microbes Infect.* 2015;17(7):484–92.
15. Kraneveld EA, Buijs MJ, Bonder MJ, Visser M, Keijser BJ, Crielaard W et al. The relation between oral *Candida* load and bacterial microbiome profiles in Dutch older adults. *PLoS ONE.* 2012;7(8):e42770.
16. Arslan SG, Akpolat N, Kama JD, Ozer T, Hamamci O. One-year follow-up of the effect of fixed orthodontic treatment on colonization by oral *Candida*. *J Oral Pathol Med.* 2008;37(1):26–9.

17. de Carvalho FG, Silva DS, Hebling J, Spolidorio LC, Spolidorio DM. Presence of mutans streptococci and *Candida* spp. in dental plaque/dentine of carious teeth and early childhood caries. *Arch Oral Biol.* 2006;51(11):1024–8.

18. Dongari-Bagtzoglou A, Kashleva H, Dwivedi P, Diaz P, Vasilakos J. Characterization of mucosal Candida albicans biofilms. *PloS ONE.* 2009;4(11):e7967.

19. Freitas AO, Marquezan M, Nojima Mda C, Alviano DS, Maia LC. The influence of orthodontic fixed appliances on the oral microbiota: A systematic review. *Dent Press J Orthodont.* 2014;19(2):46–55.

20. Ramage G, Tomsett K, Wickes BL, Lopez-Ribot JL, Redding SW. Denture stomatitis: A role for *Candida* biofilms. *Oral Surg Oral Med Oral Pathol Oral Radiol Endodont.* 2004;98(1):53–9.

21. Sardi JC, Duque C, Mariano FS, Peixoto IT, Hofling JF, Goncalves RB. *Candida* spp. in periodontal disease: A brief review. *J Oral Sci.* 2010;52(2):177–85.

22. Bertolini MM, Xu H, Sobue T, Nobile CJ, Del Bel Cury AA, Dongari-Bagtzoglou A. Candida-streptococcal mucosal biofilms display distinct structural and virulence characteristics depending on growth conditions and hyphal morphotypes. *Mol Oral Microbiol.* 2015;30(4):307–22.

23. Foreman A, Jervis-Bardy J, Wormald PJ. Do biofilms contribute to the initiation and recalcitrance of chronic rhinosinusitis? *Laryngoscope.* 2011;121(5):1085–91.

24. Keir J, Pedelty L, Swift AC. Biofilms in chronic rhinosinusitis: Systematic review and suggestions for future research. *J Laryngol Otol.* 2011;125(4):331–7.

25. Ebbens FA, Georgalas C, Fokkens WJ. Fungus as the cause of chronic rhinosinusitis: The case remains unproven. *Curr Opin Otolaryngol Head Neck Surg.* 2009;17(1):43–9.

26. Ivanchenko OA, Karpishchenko SA, Kozlov RS, Krechikova OI, Otvagin IV, Sopko ON et al. The microbiome of the maxillary sinus and middle nasal meatus in chronic rhinosinusitis. *Rhinology.* 2016;54(1):68–74.

27. Ebbens FA, Georgalas C, Fokkens WJ. The mold conundrum in chronic hyperplastic sinusitis. *Curr Allergy Asthma Rep.* 2009;9(2):114–20.

28. Grosjean P, Weber R. Fungus balls of the paranasal sinuses: A review. *Eur Arch Otorhinolaryngol.* 2007;264(5):461–70.

29. Karkas A, Rtail R, Reyt E, Timi N, Righini CA. Sphenoid sinus fungus ball. *Eur Arch Otorhinolaryngol.* 2013;270(3):893–8.

30. Harding MW, Marques LL, Howard RJ, Olson ME. Can filamentous fungi form biofilms? *Trends Microbiol.* 2009;17(11):475–80.

31. Mowat E, Williams C, Jones B, McChlery S, Ramage G. The characteristics of *Aspergillus fumigatus* mycetoma development: Is this a biofilm? *Med Mycol.* 2008:1–7.

32. Chowdhary A, Randhawa HS, Gaur SN, Agarwal K, Kathuria S, Roy P et al. *Schizophyllum commune* as an emerging fungal pathogen: A review and report of two cases. *Mycoses.* 2013;56(1):1–10.

33. Sa HS, Ko KS, Woo KI, Peck KR, Kim YD. A case of sino-orbital infection caused by the *Schizophyllum commune. Diagn Microbiol Infect Dis.* 2012;73(4):376–7.

34. Janagond A, Krishnan KM, Kindo AJ, Sumathi G. *Trichosporon inkin*, an unusual agent of fungal sinusitis: A report from south India. *Indian J Med Microbiol.* 2012;30(2):229–32.

35. Mignogna MD, Fortuna G, Leuci S, Adamo D, Ruoppo E, Siano M et al. Mucormycosis in immunocompetent patients: A case-series of patients with maxillary sinus involvement and a critical review of the literature. *Int J Infect Dis.* 2011;15(8):e533–40.

36. Rombaux P, Eloy P, Bertrand B, Delos M, Doyen C. Lethal disseminated *Fusarium* infection with sinus involvement in the immunocompromised host: Case report and review of the literature. *Rhinology.* 1996;34(4):237–41.

37. Sato FR, Sawazaki R, Berretta D, Moreira RW, Vargas PA, de Almeida OP. Aspergillosis of the maxillary sinus associated with a zygomatic implant. *J Am Dent Assoc.* 2010;141(10):1231–5.

38. Boase S, Foreman A, Cleland E, Tan L, Melton-Kreft R, Pant H et al. The microbiome of chronic rhinosinusitis: Culture, molecular diagnostics and biofilm detection. *BMC Infect Dis*. 2013;13:210.
39. Nguyen LD, Viscogliosi E, Delhaes L. The lung mycobiome: An emerging field of the human respiratory microbiome. *Front Microbiol*. 2015;6:89.
40. Delisle MS, Williamson DR, Albert M, Perreault MM, Jiang X, Day AG et al. Impact of *Candida* species on clinical outcomes in patients with suspected ventilator-associated pneumonia. *Can Respir J*. 2011;18(3):131–6.
41. Hamet M, Pavon A, Dalle F, Pechinot A, Prin S, Quenot JP et al. *Candida* spp. airway colonization could promote antibiotic-resistant bacteria selection in patients with suspected ventilator-associated pneumonia. *Intens Care Med*. 2012;38(8):1272–9.
42. Serban RI, Dan M, Panzaru CV, Anghel D, Dascalescu D, Ciucu L et al. Fungi as emergent etiologic agents in ventilator-associated pneumonia after cardiac surgery. *Rev Med Chir Soc Med Nat Iasi*. 2010;114(4):1077–82.
43. Stonecypher K. Ventilator-associated pneumonia: The importance of oral care in intubated adults. *Crit Care Nurs Q*. 2010;33(4):339–47.
44. Caserta RA, Marra AR, Durao MS, Silva CV, Pavao Dos Santos OF, Neves HS et al. A program for sustained improvement in preventing ventilator associated pneumonia in an intensive care setting. *BMC Infect Dis*. 2012;12:234.
45. Singh PK, Schaefer AL, Parsek MR, Moninger TO, Welsh MJ, Greenberg EP. Quorum-sensing signals indicate that cystic fibrosis lungs are infected with bacterial biofilms. *Nature*. 2000;407(6805):762–4.
46. Denning DW. Invasive aspergillosis. *Clin Infect Dis*. 1998;26(4):781–803; quiz 4–5.
47. Jayshree RS, Shafiulla M, George J, David JK, Bapsy PP, Chakrabarti A. Microscopic, cultural and molecular evidence of disseminated invasive aspergillosis involving the lungs and the gastrointestinal tract. *J Med Microbiol*. 2006;55(Pt 7):961–4.
48. Young RC, Bennett JE, Vogel CL, Carbone PP, DeVita VT. Aspergillosis: The spectrum of the disease in 98 patients. *Medicine* (Baltimore). 1970;49(2):147–73.
49. Gutierrez-Correa M, Ludena Y, Ramage G, Villena GK. Recent advances on filamentous fungal biofilms for industrial uses. *Appl Biochem Biotechnol*. 2012;167(5):1235–53.
50. Ramage G, Rajendran R, Gutierrez-Correa M, Jones B, Williams C. *Aspergillus* biofilms: Clinical and industrial significance. *FEMS Microbiol Lett*. 2011;324(2):89–97.
51. Mowat E, Lang S, Williams C, McCulloch E, Jones B, Ramage G. Phase-dependent antifungal activity against *Aspergillus fumigatus* developing multicellular filamentous biofilms. *J Antimicrob Chemother*. 2008;62(6):1281–4.
52. Seidler MJ, Salvenmoser S, Muller FM. *Aspergillus fumigatus* forms biofilms with reduced antifungal drug susceptibility on bronchial epithelial cells. *Antimicrob Agents Chemother*. 2008;52(11):4130–6.
53. Rowe SM, Miller S, Sorscher EJ. Mechanisms of disease: Cystic fibrosis. *New Engl J Med*. 2005;352(19):1992–2001.
54. Delhaes L, Monchy S, Frealle E, Hubans C, Salleron J, Leroy S et al. The airway microbiota in cystic fibrosis: A complex fungal and bacterial community – Implications for therapeutic management. *PloS ONE*. 2012;7(4).
55. Emerson J, Rosenfeld M, McNamara S, Ramsey B, Gibson RL. *Pseudomonas aeruginosa* and other predictors of mortality and morbidity in young children with cystic fibrosis. *Pediatr Pulmonol*. 2002;34(2):91–100.
56. Nixon GM, Armstrong DS, Carzino R, Carlin JB, Olinsky A, Robertson CF et al. Clinical outcome after early *Pseudomonas aeruginosa* infection in cystic fibrosis. *J Pediatr*. 2001;138(5):699–704.
57. Pihet M, Carrere J, Cimon B, Chabasse D, Delhaes L, Symoens F et al. Occurrence and relevance of filamentous fungi in respiratory secretions of patients with cystic fibrosis – A review. *Med Mycol*. 2009;47(4):387–97.

58. Bauernfeind A, Bertele RM, Harms K, Horl G, Jungwirth R, Petermuller C et al. Qualitative and quantitative microbiological analysis of sputa of 102 patients with cystic fibrosis. *Infection*. 1987;15(4):270–7.

59. Sudfeld CR, Dasenbrook EC, Merz WG, Carroll KC, Boyle MP. Prevalence and risk factors for recovery of filamentous fungi in individuals with cystic fibrosis. *J Cyst Fibros*. 2010;9(2):110–6.

60. Cimon B, Zouhair R, Symoens F, Carrere J, Chabasse D, Bouchara JP. *Aspergillus terreus* in a cystic fibrosis clinic: Environmental distribution and patient colonization pattern. *J Hospital Infect*. 2003;53(1):81–2.

61. Amin R, Dupuis A, Aaron SD, Ratjen F. The effect of chronic infection with *Aspergillus fumigatus* on lung function and hospitalization in patients with cystic fibrosis. *Chest*. 2010;137(1):171–6.

62. Chotirmall SH, O'Donoghue E, Bennett K, Gunaratnam C, O'Neill SJ, McElvaney NG. Sputum *Candida albicans* presages FEV decline and hospital-treated exacerbations in cystic fibrosis. *Chest*. 2010;138(5):1186–95.

63. Delhaes L, Monchy S, Frealle E, Hubans C, Salleron J, Leroy S et al. The airway microbiota in cystic fibrosis: A complex fungal and bacterial community – Implications for therapeutic management. *PloS ONE*. 2012;7(4):e36313.

64. Leclair LW, Hogan DA. Mixed bacterial-fungal infections in the CF respiratory tract. *Med Mycol*. 2010;48(Suppl 1):S125–32.

65. Lutz L, Pereira DC, Paiva RM, Zavascki AP, Barth AL. Macrolides decrease the minimal inhibitory concentration of anti-pseudomonal agents against *Pseudomonas aeruginosa* from cystic fibrosis patients in biofilm. *BMC Microbiol*. 2012;12:196.

66. Macfarlane S, Dillon JF. Microbial biofilms in the human gastrointestinal tract. *J Appl Microbiol*. 2007;102(5):1187–96.

67. Suhr MJ, Hallen-Adams HE. The human gut mycobiome: Pitfalls and potentials – A mycologist's perspective. *Mycologia*. 2015;107:1057–73.

68. Suhr MJ, Banjara N, Hallen-Adams HE. Sequence-based methods for detecting and evaluating the human gut mycobiome. *Lett Appl Microbiol*. 2016;62(3):209–15.

69. Macfarlane S. Microbial biofilm communities in the gastrointestinal tract. *J Clin Gastroenterol*. 2008;42(Suppl 3 Pt 1):S142–3.

70. Trevisani L, Sartori S, Rossi MR, Bovolenta R, Scoponi M, Gullini S et al. Degradation of polyurethane gastrostomy devices: What is the role of fungal colonization? *Dig Dis Sci*. 2005;50(3):463–9.

71. Gottlieb K, Leya J, Kruss DM, Mobarhan S, Iber FL. Intraluminal fungal colonization of gastrostomy tubes. *Gastrointest Endosc*. 1993;39(3):413–5.

72. Damman CJ, Miller SI, Surawicz CM, Zisman TL. The microbiome and inflammatory bowel disease: Is there a therapeutic role for fecal microbiota transplantation? *Am J Gastroenterol*. 2012;107(10):1452–9.

73. Kumamoto CA. Inflammation and gastrointestinal *Candida* colonization. *Curr Opin Microbiol*. 2011;14(4):386–91.

74. Ma B, Forney LJ, Ravel J. Vaginal microbiome: Rethinking health and disease. *Annu Rev Microbiol*. 2012;66:371–89.

75. MK C-SAA. Management of urinary tract infections in the elderly. *Trends Urol Gynaecol Sexual Health*. 2007;12(4):31–4.

76. Karchmer TB, Giannetta ET, Muto CA, Strain BA, Farr BM. A randomized crossover study of silver-coated urinary catheters in hospitalized patients. *Arch Intern Med*. 2000;160(21):3294–8.

77. Hidron AI, Edwards JR, Patel J, Horan TC, Sievert DM, Pollock DA et al. NHSN annual update: Antimicrobial-resistant pathogens associated with healthcare-associated infections. Annual summary of data reported to the National Healthcare Safety Network

at the Centers for Disease Control and Prevention, 2006–2007. *Infect Control Hosp Epidemiol.* 2008;29(11):996–1011.

78. Maki DG, Tambyah PA. Engineering out the risk for infection with urinary catheters. *Emerg Infect Dis.* 2001;7(2):342–7.

79. Gajer P, Brotman RM, Bai G, Sakamoto J, Schutte UM, Zhong X et al. Temporal dynamics of the human vaginal microbiota. *Sci Transl Med.* 2012;4(132):132ra52.

80. McMillan A, Dell M, Zellar MP, Cribby S, Martz S, Hong E et al. Disruption of urogenital biofilms by lactobacilli. *Colloids Surf B Biointerfaces.* 2011;86(1):58–64.

81. Kauffman CA, Fisher JF, Sobel JD, Newman CA. *Candida* urinary tract infections – Diagnosis. *Clin Infect Dis.* 2011;52 Suppl 6:S452–6.

82. Sobel JD, Fisher JF, Kauffman CA, Newman CA. *Candida* urinary tract infections – Epidemiology. *Clin Infect Dis.* 2011;52(Suppl 6):S433–6.

83. Reid G, Denstedt JD, Kang YS, Lam D, Nause C. Microbial adhesion and biofilm formation on ureteral stents in vitro and in vivo. *J Urol.* 1992;148(5):1592–4.

84. Harriott MM, Lilly EA, Rodriguez TE, Fidel PL, Jr., Noverr MC. *Candida albicans* forms biofilms on the vaginal mucosa. *Microbiology.* 2010;156(Pt 12):3635–44.

85. Yang SP, Chen YY, Hsu HS, Wang FD, Chen LY, Fung CP. A risk factor analysis of healthcare-associated fungal infections in an intensive care unit: A retrospective cohort study. *BMC Infect Dis.* 2013;13:10.

86. Chassot F, Negri MF, Svidzinski AE, Donatti L, Peralta RM, Svidzinski TI et al. Can intrauterine contraceptive devices be a *Candida albicans* reservoir? *Contraception.* 2008;77(5):355–9.

87. Lee SW. An aspergilloma mistaken for a pelviureteral stone on nonenhanced CT: A fungal bezoar causing ureteral obstruction. *Korean J Urol.* 2010;51(3):216–8.

88. Muller FM, Seidler M, Beauvais A. *Aspergillus fumigatus* biofilms in the clinical setting. *Med Mycol.* 2011;49(Suppl 1):S96–S100.

89. Grice EA, Segre JA. The skin microbiome. *Nat Rev Microbiol.* 2011;9(4):244–53.

90. Gao Z, Perez-Perez GI, Chen Y, Blaser MJ. Quantitation of major human cutaneous bacterial and fungal populations. *J Clin Microbiol.* 2010;48(10):3575–81.

91. Wolcott RD, Gontcharova V, Sun Y, Dowd SE. Evaluation of the bacterial diversity among and within individual venous leg ulcers using bacterial tag-encoded FLX and titanium amplicon pyrosequencing and metagenomic approaches. *BMC Microbiol.* 2009;9(1):226.

92. Leung P. Diabetic foot ulcers – A comprehensive review. *Surgeon.* 2007;5(4):219–31.

93. Davis SC, Martinez L, Kirsner R. The diabetic foot: The importance of biofilms and wound bed preparation. *Curr Diabet Rep.* 2006;6(6):439–45.

94. James GA, Swogger E, Wolcott R, Secor P, Sestrich J, Costerton JW et al. Biofilms in chronic wounds. *Wound Repair Regen.* 2008;16(1):37–44.

95. Neut D, Tijdens-Creusen EJ, Bulstra SK, van der Mei HC, Busscher HJ. Biofilms in chronic diabetic foot ulcers – A study of 2 cases. *Acta Orthopaed.* 2011;82(3):383–5.

96. Seth AK, Geringer MR, Hong SJ, Leung KP, Mustoe TA, Galiano RD. In vivo modeling of biofilm-infected wounds: A review. *J Surg Res.* 2012;178(1):330–8.

97. Fazli M, Bjarnsholt T, Kirketerp-Moller K, Jorgensen B, Andersen AS, Krogfelt KA et al. Nonrandom distribution of *Pseudomonas aeruginosa* and *Staphylococcus aureus* in chronic wounds. *J Clin Microbiol.* 2009;47(12):4084–9.

98. Dowd SE, Wolcott RD, Sun Y, McKeehan T, Smith E, Rhoads D. Polymicrobial nature of chronic diabetic foot ulcer biofilm infections determined using bacterial tag encoded FLX amplicon pyrosequencing (bTEFAP). *PLoS ONE.* 2008;3(10):e3326.

99. Dowd SE, Sun Y, Secor PR, Rhoads DD, Wolcott BM, James GA et al. Survey of bacterial diversity in chronic wounds using pyrosequencing, DGGE, and full ribosome shotgun sequencing. *BMC Microbiol.* 2008;8(1):43.

100. Gontcharova V, Youn E, Sun Y, Wolcott RD, Dowd SE. A comparison of bacterial composition in diabetic ulcers and contralateral intact skin. *Open Microbiol J.* 2010;4:8.
101. Gardner SE, Hillis SL, Heilmann K, Segre JA, Grice EA. The neuropathic diabetic foot ulcer microbiome is associated with clinical factors. *Diabetes.* 2013;62(3):923–30.
102. Branski LK, Al-Mousawi A, Rivero H, Jeschke MG, Sanford AP, Herndon DN. Emerging infections in burns. *Surg Infect* (Larchmt). 2009;10(5):389–97.
103. Leake JL, Dowd SE, Wolcott RD, Zischkau AM. Identification of yeast in chronic wounds using new pathogen-detection technologies. *J Wound Care.* 2009;18(3):103–4, 6, 8.
104. Sun Y. Survey of fungi and yeast in polymicrobial infections in chronic wounds. *J Wound Care.* 2010;20(1):40.
105. Chellan G, Shivaprakash S, Ramaiyar SK, Varma AK, Varma N, Sukumaran MT et al. Spectrum and prevalence of fungi infecting deep tissues of lower-limb wounds in patients with type 2 diabetes. *J Clin Microbiol.* 2010;48(6):2097–102.
106. Warkentien T, Rodriguez C, Lloyd B, Wells J, Weintrob A, Dunne JR et al. Invasive mold infections following combat-related injuries. *Clin Infect Dis.* 2012;55(11):1441–9.
107. Wolcott RD, Gontcharova V, Sun Y, Dowd SE. Evaluation of the bacterial diversity among and within individual venous leg ulcers using bacterial tag-encoded FLX and titanium amplicon pyrosequencing and metagenomic approaches. *BMC Microbiol.* 2009;9:226.
108. Dowd SE, Delton Hanson J, Rees E, Wolcott RD, Zischau AM, Sun Y et al. Survey of fungi and yeast in polymicrobial infections in chronic wounds. *J Wound Care.* 2011;20(1):40–7.
109. Odds F. Candida and candidosis, 2nd ed. London: Bailliere Tindall; 1988.
110. Donlan RM, Costerton JW. Biofilms: Survival mechanisms of clinically relevant microorganisms. *Clin Microbiology Rev.* 2002;15(2):167–93.
111. Bjornson H, Colley R, Bower R, Duty V, Schwartz-Fulton J, Fischer J. Association between microorganism growth at the catheter insertion site and colonization of the catheter in patients receiving total parenteral nutrition. *Surgery.* 1982;92(4):720–7.
112. Davis KA, Stewart JJ, Crouch HK, Florez CE, Hospenthal DR. Methicillin-resistant *Staphylococcus aureus* (MRSA) nares colonization at hospital admission and its effect on subsequent MRSA infection. *Clin Infect Dis.* 2004;39(6):776–82.
113. Peacock SJ, Moore CE, Justice A, Kantzanou M, Story L, Mackie K et al. Virulent combinations of adhesin and toxin genes in natural populations of *Staphylococcus aureus.* *Infect Immun.* 2002;70(9):4987–96.
114. Chu VH, Crosslin DR, Friedman JY, Reed SD, Cabell CH, Griffiths RI et al. *Staphylococcus aureus* bacteremia in patients with prosthetic devices: Costs and outcomes. *Am Journal Med.* 2005;118(12):1416. e19–24.
115. Cacoub P, Leprince P, Nataf P, Hausfater P, Dorent R, Wechsler B et al. Pacemaker infective endocarditis. *Am J Cardiol.* 1998;82(4):480–4.
116. Adam B, Baillie GS, Douglas LJ. Mixed species biofilms of *Candida albicans* and *Staphylococcus epidermidis. J Med Microbiol.* 2002;51(4):344–9.
117. Lee JH, Burner KD, Fealey ME, Edwards WD, Tazelaar HD, Orszulak TA et al. Prosthetic valve endocarditis: Clinicopathological correlates in 122 surgical specimens from 116 patients (1985–2004). *Cardiovasc Pathol.* 2011;20(1):26–35.
118. Mylonakis E, Calderwood SB. Infective endocarditis in adults. *N Engl J Med.* 2001;345(18):1318–30.
119. Anguera I, Miro JM, San Roman JA, de Alarcon A, Anguita M, Almirante B et al. Periannular complications in infective endocarditis involving prosthetic aortic valves. *Am J Cardiol.* 2006;98(9):1261–8.
120. Park DR. The microbiology of ventilator-associated pneumonia. *Respir Care.* 2005;50(6):742–65.

121. Adler A, Yaniv I, Steinberg R, Solter E, Samra Z, Stein J et al. Infectious complications of implantable ports and Hickman catheters in paediatric haematology–oncology patients. *J Hosp Infect.* 2006;62(3):358–65.

122. Kim JS, Holtom P, Vigen C. Reduction of catheter-related bloodstream infections through the use of a central venous line bundle: Epidemiologic and economic consequences. *Am J Infect Control.* 2011;39(8):640–6.

123. Downes KJ, Metlay JP, Bell LM, McGowan KL, Elliott MR, Shah SS. Polymicrobial bloodstream infections among children and adolescents with central venous catheters evaluated in ambulatory care. *Clin Infect Dis.* 2008;46(3):387–94.

124. Tchekmedyian NS, Newman K, Moody MR, Costerton JW, Aisner J, Schumpff SC et al. Special studies of the Hickman catheter of a patient with recurrent bacteremia and candidemia. *Am J Med Sci.* 1986;291(6):419–24.

125. Karchmer TB, Giannetta ET, Muto CA, Strain BA, Farr BM. A randomized crossover study of silver-coated urinary catheters in hospitalized patients. *Arch Intern Med.* 2000;160(21):3294–8.

126. Alicia IH, Edwards J, Patel J, Horan Teresa C, Sievert Dawn M. NHSN Annual update: Antimicrobial-resistant pathogens associated with healthcare-associated infections. Annual summary of data reported to the National Healthcare Safety Network at the Centers for Disease Control and Prevention, 2006–2007. *Infect Control Hosp Epidemiol.* 2008;29(1):996–1011.

127. Maki DG, Tambyah PA. Engineering out the risk for infection with urinary catheters. *Emerg Infect Dis.* 2001;7(2):342.

128. O'Donnell LE, Robertson D, Nile CJ, Cross LJ, Riggio M, Sherriff A et al. The oral microbiome of denture wearers is influenced by levels of natural dentition. *PloS ONE.* 2015;10(9):e0137717.

129. Gravante G, Caruso R, Araco A, Cervelli V. Infections after plastic procedures: Incidences, etiologies, risk factors, and antibiotic prophylaxis. *Aesthet Plast Surg.* 2008;32(2):243–51.

130. Ramage G, Martínez JP, López-Ribot JL. *Candida* biofilms on implanted biomaterials: A clinically significant problem. *FEMS Yeast Res.* 2006;6(7):979–86.

131. Trampuz A, Piper KE, Jacobson MJ, Hanssen AD, Unni KK, Osmon DR et al. Sonication of removed hip and knee prostheses for diagnosis of infection. *N Engl. J Med.* 2007;357(7):654–63.

132. Corvec S, Portillo ME, Pasticci BM, Borens O, Trampuz A. Epidemiology and new developments in the diagnosis of prosthetic joint infection. *Int J Artif Organs.* 2012;35(10):923–34.

133. Coskun H, Bozkurt S. A case of asymptomatic fungal and bacterial colonization of an intragastric balloon. *World J Gastroenterol: WJG.* 2009;15(45):5751.

134. Sciubba DM, Stuart RM, McGirt MJ, Woodworth GF, Samdani A, Carson B et al. Effect of antibiotic-impregnated shunt catheters in decreasing the incidence of shunt infection in the treatment of hydrocephalus. *J Neurosurg: Pediatrics.* 2005;103(2):131–6.

135. Enger P, Svendsen F, Wester K. CSF shunt infections in children: Experiences from a population-based study. *Acta Neurochirurg.* 2003;145(4):243–8.

136. Elving GJ, van der Mei HC, van Weissenbruch R, Busscher HJ, Albers FW. Comparison of the microbial composition of voice prosthesis biofilms from patients requiring frequent versus infrequent replacement. *Ann Otol Rhinol Laryngol.* 2002;111(3):200–3.

137. Buijssen KJ, Harmsen HJ, van der Mei HC, Busscher HJ, van der Laan BF. Lactobacilli: Important in biofilm formation on voice prostheses. *Otolaryngology – Head Neck Surg.* 2007;137(3):505–7.

138. Klotz SA, Chasin BS, Powell B, Gaur NK, Lipke PN. Polymicrobial bloodstream infections involving *Candida* species: Analysis of patients and review of the literature. *Diagn Microbiol Infect Dis.* 2007;59(4):401–6.

139. Trampuz A, Widmer AF. Infections associated with orthopedic implants. *Curr Opin Infect Dis.* 2006;19(4):349–56.
140. Kojic EM, Darouiche RO. *Candida* infections of medical devices. *Clin Microbiol Rev.* 2004;17(2):255–67.
141. Wenzel RP. Nosocomial candidemia: Risk factors and attributable mortality. *Clin Infect Dis.* 1995;20(6):1531–4.
142. Tchekmedyian NS, Newman K, Moody MR, Costerton JW, Aisner J, Schimpff SC et al. Special studies of the Hickman catheter of a patient with recurrent bacteremia and candidemia. *Am J Med Sci.* 1986;291(6):419–24.
143. Tumbarello M, Fiori B, Trecarichi EM, Posteraro P, Losito AR, De Luca A et al. Risk factors and outcomes of candidemia caused by biofilm-forming isolates in a tertiary care hospital. *PloS ONE.* 2012;7(3):e33705.
144. Rajendran R, Sherry L, Nile CJ, Sherriff A, Johnson EM, Hanson MF et al. Biofilm formation is a risk factor for mortality in patients with *Candida albicans* bloodstream infection-Scotland, 2012–2013. *Clin Microbiol Infect.* 2016;22(1):87–93.
145. Ramage G, Williams C. The clinical importance of fungal biofilms. *Adv Appl Microbiol.* 2013;84:27–83.
146. Adam B, Baillie GS, Douglas LJ. Mixed species biofilms of *Candida albicans* and *Staphylococcus epidermidis.* *J Med Microbiol.* 2002;51(4):344–9.
147. Baena-Monroy T, Moreno-Maldonado V, Franco-Martinez F, Aldape-Barrios B, Quindos G, Sanchez-Vargas LO. *Candida albicans, Staphylococcus aureus* and *Streptococcus mutans* colonization in patients wearing dental prosthesis. *Med Oral Patol Oral Cirug Bucal.* 2005;10(Suppl 1):E27–39.
148. Tawara Y, Honma K, Naito Y. Methicillin-resistant *Staphylococcus aureus* and *Candida albicans* on denture surfaces. *Bull Tokyo Dent Coll.* 1996;37(3):119–28.
149. Perlroth J, Choi B, Spellberg B. Nosocomial fungal infections: Epidemiology, diagnosis, and treatment. *Med Mycol.* 2007;45(4):321–46.
150. Peters BM, Jabra-Rizk MA, O'May GA, Costerton JW, Shirtliff ME. Polymicrobial interactions: Impact on pathogenesis and human disease. *Clin Microbiol Rev.* 2012;25(1):193–213.
151. Peters BM, Ovchinnikova ES, Krom BP, Schlecht LM, Zhou H, Hoyer LL et al. *Staphylococcus aureus* adherence to *Candida albicans* hyphae is mediated by the hyphal adhesin Als3p. *Microbiology.* 2012;158(Pt 12):2975–86.
152. Peters BM, Noverr MC. *Candida albicans-Staphylococcus aureus* polymicrobial peritonitis modulates host innate immunity. *Infect Immun.* 2013;81(6):2178–89.
153. Schlecht LM, Peters BM, Krom BP, Freiberg JA, Hansch GM, Filler SG et al. Systemic *Staphylococcus aureus* infection mediated by *Candida albicans* hyphal invasion of mucosal tissue. *Microbiology.* 2015;161(Pt 1):168–81.
154. Nair N, Biswas R, Gotz F, Biswas L. Impact of *Staphylococcus aureus* on pathogenesis in polymicrobial infections. *Infect Immun.* 2014;82(6):2162–9.
155. Peters BM, Jabra-Rizk MA, Scheper MA, Leid JG, Costerton JW, Shirtliff ME. Microbial interactions and differential protein expression in *Staphylococcus aureus-Candida albicans* dual-species biofilms. *FEMS Immunol Medical Microbiol.* 2010;59(3):493–503.
156. Yi Jey Lin LA, Vogel F, Koppar S, Nevarez L, Auguste F, Seymour J, Syed A, Christoph K, Loomis JS. Interactions between *Candida albicans* and *Staphylococcus aureus* within mixed species biofilms. *BioOne.* 2013;84(1):30–9.
157. Harriott MM, Noverr MC. *Candida albicans* and *Staphylococcus aureus* form polymicrobial biofilms: Effects on antimicrobial resistance. *Antimicrob Agents Chemother.* 2009;53(9):3914–22.
158. Beaussart A, Herman P, El-Kirat-Chatel S, Lipke PN, Kucharikova S, Van Dijck P et al. Single-cell force spectroscopy of the medically important *Staphylococcus epidermidis-Candida albicans* interaction. *Nanoscale.* 2013;5(22):10894–900.

159. Harriott MM, Noverr MC. Ability of *Candida albicans* mutants to induce *Staphylococcus aureus* vancomycin resistance during polymicrobial biofilm formation. *Antimicrob Agents Chemother.* 2010;54(9):3746–55.

160. Carlson E. Effect of strain of *Staphylococcus aureus* on synergism with *Candida albicans* resulting in mouse mortality and morbidity. *Infect Immun.* 1983;42(1):285–92.

161. Carlson E, Johnson G. Protection by *Candida albicans* of *Staphylococcus aureus* in the establishment of dual infection in mice. *Infect Immun.* 1985;50(3):655–9.

162. Nash EE, Peters BM, Palmer GE, Fidel PL, Noverr MC. Morphogenesis is not required for *Candida albicans-Staphylococcus aureus* intra-abdominal infection-mediated dissemination and lethal sepsis. *Infect Immun.* 2014;82(8):3426–35.

163. Akiyama H, Oono T, Huh WK, Yamasaki O, Ogawa S, Katsuyama M et al. Actions of farnesol and xylitol against *Staphylococcus aureus. Chemotherapy.* 2002;48(3):122–8.

164. Jabra-Rizk MA, Meiller TF, James CE, Shirtliff ME. Effect of farnesol on *Staphylococcus aureus* biofilm formation and antimicrobial susceptibility. *Antimicrob Agents Chemother.* 2006;50(4):1463–9.

165. Unnanuntana A, Bonsignore L, Shirtliff ME, Greenfield EM. The effects of farnesol on *Staphylococcus aureus* biofilms and osteoblasts. An in vitro study. *J Bone Joint Surg* (US). 2009;91(11):2683–92.

166. Kuroda M, Nagasaki S, Ito R, Ohta T. Sesquiterpene farnesol as a competitive inhibitor of lipase activity of *Staphylococcus aureus. FEMS Microbiology Lett.* 2007;273(1):28–34.

167. Lin YJ, Alsad L, Vogel F, Koppar S, Nevarez L, Auguste F et al. Interactions between *Candida albicans* and *Staphylococcus aureus* within mixed species biofilms. *BIOS.* 2013;84(1):30–9.

168. Fehrmann C, Jurk K, Bertling A, Seidel G, Fegeler W, Kehrel BE et al. Role for the fibrinogen-binding proteins coagulase and Efb in the *Staphylococcus aureus-Candida* interaction. *Int J Med Microbiol:* IJMM. 2013;303(5):230–8.

169. Peters BM, Ward RM, Rane HS, Lee SA, Noverr MC. Efficacy of ethanol against *Candida albicans* and *Staphylococcus aureus* polymicrobial biofilms. *Antimicrob Agents Chemother.* 2013;57(1):74–82.

170. Sud IJ, Feingold DS. Action of antifungal imidazoles on *Staphylococcus aureus. Antimicrob Agents Chemother.* 1982;22(3):470–4.

171. Pammi M, Liang R, Hicks J, Mistretta TA, Versalovic J. Biofilm extracellular DNA enhances mixed species biofilms of *Staphylococcus epidermidis* and *Candida albicans. BMC Microbiol.* 2013;13:257.

172. Rajendran R, Sherry L, Lappin DF, Nile CJ, Smith K, Williams C et al. Extracellular DNA release confers heterogeneity in *Candida albicans* biofilm formation. *BMC Microbiol.* 2014;14(1):303.

173. Sapaar B, Nur A, Hirota K, Yumoto H, Murakami K, Amoh T et al. Effects of extracellular DNA from *Candida albicans* and pneumonia-related pathogens on *Candida* biofilm formation and hyphal transformation. *J Appl Microbiol.* 2014;116(6):1531–42.

174. Pammi M, Liang R, Hicks J, Mistretta T-A, Versalovic J. Biofilm extracellular DNA enhances mixed species biofilms of *Staphylococcus epidermidis* and *Candida albicans. BMC Microbiol.* 2013;13(1):257.

175. Vos T, Flaxman AD, Naghavi M, Lozano R, Michaud C, Ezzati M et al. Years lived with disability (YLDs) for 1160 sequelae of 289 diseases and injuries 1990–2010: A systematic analysis for the Global Burden of Disease Study 2010. *Lancet.* 2012;380(9859):2163–96.

176. Loesche WJ. Role of *Streptococcus mutans* in human dental decay. *Microbiol Rev.* 1986;50(4):353–80.

177. Badet C, Thebaud NB. Ecology of lactobacilli in the oral cavity: A review of literature. *Open Microbiol J.* 2008;2:38–48.

178. Belda-Ferre P, Alcaraz LD, Cabrera-Rubio R, Romero H, Simon-Soro A, Pignatelli M et al. The oral metagenome in health and disease. *ISME J.* 2012;6(1):46–56.

179. Simon-Soro A, Guillen-Navarro M, Mira A. Metatranscriptomics reveals overall active bacterial composition in caries lesions. *J Oral Microbiol.* 2014;6:25443.

180. Krasse B. The relationship between lactobacilli, *Candida* and streptococci and dental caries; examination of saliva and plaque material collected on the same occasion. *Odontologisk Revy.* 1954;5(4):241–61.

181. Koo H, Bowen WH. *Candida albicans* and *Streptococcus mutans*: A potential synergistic alliance to cause virulent tooth decay in children. *Fut Microbiol.* 2014;9(12):1295–7.

182. Metwalli KH, Khan SA, Krom BP, Jabra-Rizk MA. *Streptococcus mutans*, Candida albicans, and the human mouth: A sticky situation. *PLoS Pathog.* 2013;9(10):e1003616.

183. Moore WEC, Holdeman LV, Smibert RM, Good IJ, Burmeister JA, Palcanis KG et al. Bacteriology of experimental gingivitis in young-adult humans. *Infect Immun.* 1982; 38(2):651–67.

184. Syed SA, Loesche WJ. Bacteriology of human experimental gingivitis: Effect of plaque age. *Infect Immun.* 1978;21(3):821–9.

185. Kawamura Y, Hou XG, Sultana F, Miura H, Ezaki T. Determination of 16S rRNA sequences of *Streptococcus mitis* and *Streptococcus gordonii* and phylogenetic relationships among members of the genus *Streptococcus*. *Int J Syst Bacteriol.* 1995;45(2):406–8.

186. Diaz PI, Dupuy AK, Abusleme L, Reese B, Obergfell C, Choquette L et al. Using high throughput sequencing to explore the biodiversity in oral bacterial communities. *Mol Oral Microbiol.* 2012;27(3):182–201.

187. Dutton LC, Nobbs AH, Jepson K, Jepson MA, Vickerman MM, Aqeel Alawfi S et al. *O*-mannosylation in *Candida albicans* enables development of interkingdom biofilm communities. *mBio.* 2014;5(2):e00911.

188. Holmes AR, van der Wielen P, Cannon RD, Ruske D, Dawes P. *Candida albicans* binds to saliva proteins selectively adsorbed to silicone. *Oral Surg Oral Med Oral Pathol Oral Radiol Endodont.* 2006;102(4):488–94.

189. Takahashi N, Nyvad B. The role of bacteria in the caries process: Ecological perspectives. *J Dent Res.* 2011;90(3):294–303.

190. Jenkinson HF, Lala HC, Shepherd MG. Coaggregation of *Streptococcus sanguis* and other streptococci with *Candida albicans*. *Infect Immun.* 1990;58(5):1429–36.

191. Nasution O, Srinivasa K, Kim M, Kim YJ, Kim W, Jeong W et al. Hydrogen peroxide induces hyphal differentiation in *Candida albicans*. *Eukaryot Cell.* 2008;7(11):2008–11.

192. Jenkinson HF, Douglas LJ. Interactions between *Candida* species and bacteria in mixed infections. In Brogden K, Guthmiller J (eds), *Polymicrobial diseases* (pp. 357–74). Washington, DC: ASM Press; 2002.

193. Xu H, Sobue T, Thompson A, Xie Z, Poon K, Ricker A et al. Streptococcal co-infection augments *Candida* pathogenicity by amplifying the mucosal inflammatory response. *Cell Microbiol.* 2014;16(2):214–31.

194. Kolenbrander PE, Andersen RN, Blehert DS, Egland PG, Foster JS, Palmer RJ, Jr. Communication among oral bacteria. *Microbiol Mol Biol Rev: MMBR.* 2002;66(3):486–505.

195. Holmes AR, McNab R, Jenkinson HF. *Candida albicans* binding to the oral bacterium *Streptococcus gordonii* involves multiple adhesin-receptor interactions. *Infect Immun.* 1996;64(11):4680–5.

196. Bamford CV, d'Mello A, Nobbs AH, Dutton LC, Vickerman MM, Jenkinson HF. *Streptococcus gordonii* modulates *Candida albicans* biofilm formation through intergeneric communication. *Infect Immun.* 2009;77(9):3696–704.

197. Bamford CV, Nobbs AH, Barbour ME, Lamont RJ, Jenkinson HF. Functional regions of *Candida albicans* hyphal cell wall protein Als3 that determine interaction with the oral bacterium *Streptococcus gordonii*. *Microbiology.* 2015;161(Pt 1):18–29.

198. Gregoire S, Xiao J, Silva BB, Gonzalez I, Agidi PS, Klein MI et al. Role of glucos-yltransferase B in interactions of *Candida albicans* with *Streptococcus mutans* and with an experimental pellicle on hydroxyapatite surfaces. *Appl Environ Microbiol.* 2011;77(18):6357–67.

199. Al-Fattani MA, Douglas LJ. Biofilm matrix of *Candida albicans* and *Candida tropicalis*: Chemical composition and role in drug resistance. *J Med Microbiol.* 2006;55(Pt 8): 999–1008.

200. Taff HT, Nett JE, Zarnowski R, Ross KM, Sanchez H, Cain MT et al. A *Candida* biofilm-induced pathway for matrix glucan delivery: Implications for drug resistance. *PLoS Pathog.* 2012;8(8):e1002848.

201. Falsetta ML, Klein MI, Colonne PM, Scott-Anne K, Gregoire S, Pai CH et al. Symbiotic relationship between *Streptococcus mutans* and *Candida albicans* synergizes virulence of plaque biofilms in vivo. *Infect Immun.* 2014;82(5):1968–81.

202. Ramage G, Saville SP, Wickes BL, Lopez-Ribot JL. Inhibition of *Candida albicans* biofilm formation by farnesol, a quorum-sensing molecule. *Appl Environ Microbiol.* 2002;68(11):5459–63.

203. Koo H, Hayacibara MF, Schobel BD, Cury JA, Rosalen PL, Park YK et al. Inhibition of *Streptococcus mutans* biofilm accumulation and polysaccharide production by api-genin and tt-farnesol. *J Antimicrob Chemother.* 2003;52(5):782–9.

204. Jeon JG, Pandit S, Xiao J, Gregoire S, Falsetta ML, Klein MI et al. Influences of trans-trans farnesol, a membrane-targeting sesquiterpenoid, on *Streptococcus mutans* physiology and survival within mixed-species oral biofilms. *Int J Oral Sci.* 2011;3(2):98–106.

205. Vendeville A, Winzer K, Heurlier K, Tang CM, Hardie KR. Making 'sense' of metabolism: Autoinducer-2, LuxS and pathogenic bacteria. *Nat Rev Microbiol.* 2005; 3(5):383–96.

206. McNab R, Ford SK, El-Sabaeny A, Barbieri B, Cook GS, Lamont RJ. LuxS-based sig-naling in *Streptococcus gordonii*: Autoinducer 2 controls carbohydrate metabolism and biofilm formation with *Porphyromonas gingivalis. J Bacteriol.* 2003;185(1):274–84.

207. Jarosz LM, Deng DM, van der Mei HC, Crielaard W, Krom BP. *Streptococcus mutans* competence-stimulating peptide inhibits *Candida albicans* hypha formation. *Eukaryot cell.* 2009;8(11):1658–64.

208. Jack AA, Daniels DE, Jepson MA, Vickerman MM, Lamont RJ, Jenkinson HF et al. *Streptococcus gordonii* comCDE (competence) operon modulates biofilm formation with *Candida albicans. Microbiology.* 2015;161(Pt 2):411–21.

209. Ximenez-Fyvie LA, Haffajee AD, Socransky SS. Comparison of the microbiota of supra- and subgingival plaque in health and periodontitis. *J Clin Periodontol.* 2000; 27(9):648–57.

210. Shi B, Chang M, Martin J, Mitreva M, Lux R, Klokkevold P et al. Dynamic changes in the subgingival microbiome and their potential for diagnosis and prognosis of peri-odontitis. *mBio.* 2015;6(1):e01926–14.

211. Canabarro A, Valle C, Farias MR, Santos FB, Lazera M, Wanke B. Association of subgingival colonization of *Candida albicans* and other yeasts with severity of chronic periodontitis. *J Periodont Res.* 2013;48(4):428–32.

212. Sardi JC, Duque C, Mariano FS, Marques MR, Hofling JF, Goncalves RB. Adhesion and invasion of *Candida albicans* from periodontal pockets of patients with chronic periodontitis and diabetes to gingival human fibroblasts. *Med Mycol.* 2012;50(1):43–9.

213. Hammad MM, Darwazeh AM, Idrees MM. The effect of glycemic control on *Candida* colonization of the tongue and the subgingival plaque in patients with type II diabetes and periodontitis. *Oral Surg Oral Med Oral Pathol Oral Radiol.* 2013;116(3):321–6.

214. Zakout YM, Salih MM, Ahmed HG. Frequency of *Candida* species in Papanicolaou smears taken from Sudanese oral hormonal contraceptives users. *Biotech Histochem* 2012;87(2):95–7.

215. Spinillo A, Capuzzo E, Nicola S, Baltaro F, Ferrari A, Monaco A. The impact of oral contraception on vulvovaginal candidiasis. *Contraception.* 1995;51(5):293–7.
216. Kazi YF, Saleem S, Kazi N. Investigation of vaginal microbiota in sexually active women using hormonal contraceptives in Pakistan. *BMC Urol.* 2012;12:22.
217. Brusca MI, Rosa A, Albaina O, Moragues MD, Verdugo F, Ponton J. The impact of oral contraceptives on women's periodontal health and the subgingival occurrence of aggressive periodontopathogens and *Candida* species. *J Periodontol.* 2010;81(7):1010–8.
218. Thein ZM, Samaranayake YH, Samaranayake LP. Effect of oral bacteria on growth and survival of *Candida albicans* biofilms. *Arch Oral Biol.* 2006;51(8):672–80.
219. Nair RG, Anil S, Samaranayake LP. The effect of oral bacteria on *Candida albicans* germ-tube formation. *APMIS: Acta Pathol Microbiol Immunol Scand.* 2001;109(2):147–54.
220. Nair RG, Samaranayake LP. The effect of oral commensal bacteria on candidal adhesion to human buccal epithelial cells in vitro. *J Med Microbiol.* 1996; 45(3):179–85.
221. Tamai R, Sugamata M, Kiyoura Y. *Candida albicans* enhances invasion of human gingival epithelial cells and gingival fibroblasts by *Porphyromonas gingivalis. Microbial Pathog.* 2011;51(4):250–4.
222. Grimaudo NJ, Nesbitt WE. Coaggregation of *Candida albicans* with oral *Fusobacterium* species. *Oral Microbiol Immunol.* 1997;12(3):168–73.
223. Jabra-Rizk MA, Falkler WA, Jr., Merz WG, Kelley JI, Baqui AA, Meiller TF. Coaggregation of *Candida dubliniensis* with *Fusobacterium nucleatum. J Clin Microbiol.* 1999;37(5):1464–8.
224. Hogan DA, Kolter R. *Pseudomonas-Candida* interactions: An ecological role for virulence factors. *Science.* 2002;296(5576):2229–32.
225. Gibson J, Sood A, Hogan DA. *Pseudomonas aeruginosa-Candida albicans* interactions: Localization and fungal toxicity of a phenazine derivative. *Appl Environ Microbiol.* 2009;75(2):504–13.
226. Morales DK, Jacobs NJ, Rajamani S, Krishnamurthy M, Cubillos-Ruiz JR, Hogan DA. Antifungal mechanisms by which a novel *Pseudomonas aeruginosa* phenazine toxin kills *Candida albicans* in biofilms. *Mol Microbiol.* 2010;78(6):1379–92.
227. Hogan DA, Vik A, Kolter R. A *Pseudomonas aeruginosa* quorum-sensing molecule influences *Candida albicans* morphology. *Mol Microbiol.* 2004;54(5):1212–23.
228. Mowat E, Rajendran R, Williams C, McCulloch E, Jones B, Lang S et al. *Pseudomonas aeruginosa* and their small diffusible extracellular molecules inhibit *Aspergillus fumigatus* biofilm formation. *FEMS Microbiol Lett.* 2010;313(2):96–102.
229. Ader F, Jawhara S, Nseir S, Kipnis E, Faure K, Vuotto F et al. Short term *Candida albicans* colonization reduces *Pseudomonas aeruginosa*-related lung injury and bacterial burden in a murine model. *Crit Care* (London). 2011;15(3):R150.
230. Mear JB, Gosset P, Kipnis E, Faure E, Dessein R, Jawhara S et al. *Candida albicans* airway exposure primes the lung innate immune response against *Pseudomonas aeruginosa* infection through innate lymphoid cell recruitment and interleukin-22–associated mucosal response. *Infect Immun.* 2014;82(1):306–15.
231. Cugini C, Calfee MW, Farrow JM, III, Morales DK, Pesci EC, Hogan DA. Farnesol, a common sesquiterpene, inhibits PQS production in *Pseudomonas aeruginosa. Mol Microbiol.* 2007;65(4):896–906.
232. Sibley CD, Duan K, Fischer C, Parkins MD, Storey DG, Rabin HR et al. Discerning the complexity of community interactions using a *Drosophila* model of polymicrobial infections. *PLoS Pathog.* 2008;4(10):e1000184.
233. Sibley CD, Parkins MD, Rabin HR, Duan K, Norgaard JC, Surette MG. A polymicrobial perspective of pulmonary infections exposes an enigmatic pathogen in cystic fibrosis patients. *Proceedings of the Natl Acad Sci U S A.* 2008;105(39):15070–5.

234. Moree WJ, Phelan VV, Wu CH, Bandeira N, Cornett DS, Duggan BM et al. Interkingdom metabolic transformations captured by microbial imaging mass spectrometry. *Proc Natl Acad Sci U S A*. 2012;109(34):13811–6.
235. Bandara HM, Lam OL, Watt RM, Jin LJ, Samaranayake LP. Bacterial lipopolysaccharides variably modulate in vitro biofilm formation of *Candida* species. *J Med Microbiol*. 2010;59(Pt 10):1225–34.
236. Bandara HM, Cheung BP, Watt RM, Jin LJ, Samaranayake LP. Secretory products of *Escherichia coli* biofilm modulate *Candida* biofilm formation and hyphal development. *J Invest Clin Dent*. 2013;4(3):186–99.
237. Trautner BW, Hull RA, Darouiche RO. *Escherichia coli* 83972 inhibits catheter adherence by a broad spectrum of uropathogens. *Urology*. 2003;61(5):1059–62.
238. Samaranayake YH, Bandara HM, Cheung BP, Yau JY, Yeung SK, Samaranayake LP. Enteric gram-negative bacilli suppress *Candida* biofilms on Foley urinary catheters. *APMIS: Acta Pathol Microbiol Immunol Scand*. 2014;122(1):47–58.
239. Burd RS, Raymond CS, Dunn DL. Endotoxin promotes synergistic lethality during concurrent *Escherichia coli* and *Candida albicans* infection. *J Surg Res*. 1992;52(6):537–42.
240. Klaerner HG, Uknis ME, Acton RD, Dahlberg PS, Carlone-Jambor C, Dunn DL. *Candida albicans* and *Escherichia coli* are synergistic pathogens during experimental microbial peritonitis. *J Surg Res*. 1997;70(2):161–5.
241. Levison ME, Pitsakis PG. Susceptibility to experimental *Candida albicans* urinary tract infection in the rat. *J Infect Dis*. 1987;155(5):841–6.
242. De Brucker K, Tan Y, Vints K, De Cremer K, Braem A, Verstraeten N et al. Fungal beta-1,3-glucan increases ofloxacin tolerance of *Escherichia coli* in a polymicrobial *E. coli/Candida albicans* biofilm. *Antimicrob Agents Chemother*. 2015;59(6):3052–8.
243. Mason KL, Erb Downward JR, Mason KD, Falkowski NR, Eaton KA, Kao JY et al. *Candida albicans* and bacterial microbiota interactions in the cecum during recolonization following broad-spectrum antibiotic therapy. *Infect Immun*. 2012;80(10):3371–80.
244. Siqueira JF, Jr, Rocas IN. Diversity of endodontic microbiota revisited. *J Dent Res*. 2009;88(11):969–81.
245. Siqueira JF, Jr., Sen BH. Fungi in endodontic infections. *Oral Surg Oral Med Oral Pathol Oral Radiol Endodont*. 2004;97(5):632–41.
246. Sen BH, Safavi KE, Spangberg LS. Growth patterns of *Candida albicans* in relation to radicular dentin. *Oral Surg Oral Med Oral Pathol Oral Radiol Endodont*. 1997;84(1):68–73.
247. Baumgartner JC, Watts CM, Xia T. Occurrence of *Candida albicans* in infections of endodontic origin. *J Endodont*. 2000;26(12):695–8.
248. Peciuliene V, Reynaud AH, Balciuniene I, Haapasalo M. Isolation of yeasts and enteric bacteria in root-filled teeth with chronic apical periodontitis. *Int Endodont J*. 2001;34(6):429–34.
249. Hermann C, Hermann J, Munzel U, Ruchel R. Bacterial flora accompanying *Candida* yeasts in clinical specimens. *Mycoses*. 1999;42(11–12):619–27.
250. Fox EP, Cowley ES, Nobile CJ, Hartooni N, Newman DK, Johnson AD. Anaerobic bacteria grow within *Candida albicans* biofilms and induce biofilm formation in suspension cultures. *Curr Biol: CB*. 2014;24(20):2411–6.
251. Cruz MR, Graham CE, Gagliano BC, Lorenz MC, Garsin DA. *Enterococcus faecalis* inhibits hyphal morphogenesis and virulence of *Candida albicans*. *Infect Immun*. 2013;81(1):189–200.
252. Garsin DA, Lorenz MC. *Candida albicans* and *Enterococcus faecalis* in the gut: Synergy in commensalism? *Gut Microbes*. 2013;4(5):409–15.
253. Swidergall M, Ernst AM, Ernst JF. *Candida albicans* mucin Msb2 is a broad-range protectant against antimicrobial peptides. *Antimicrob Agents Chemother*. 2013;57(8):3917–22.

254. Young G, Krasner RI, Yudkofsky PL. Interactions of oral strains of *Candida albicans* and lactobacilli. *J Bacteriol*. 1956;72(4):525–9.
255. Kumar S, Singhi S, Chakrabarti A, Bansal A, Jayashree M. Probiotic use and prevalence of candidemia and candiduria in a PICU. *Pediatr Crit Care Med*. 2013;14(9):e409–15.
256. Mendonca FH, Santos SS, Faria Ida S, Goncalves e Silva CR, Jorge AO, Leao MV. Effects of probiotic bacteria on *Candida* presence and IgA anti-*Candida* in the oral cavity of elderly. *Brazil Dent J*. 2012;23(5):534–8.
257. Strus M, Kucharska A, Kukla G, Brzychczy-Wloch M, Maresz K, Heczko PB. The in vitro activity of vaginal *Lactobacillus* with probiotic properties against *Candida*. *Infect Dis Obstet Gynecol*. 2005;13(2):69–75.
258. Martinez RC, Seney SL, Summers KL, Nomizo A, De Martinis EC, Reid G. Effect of *Lactobacillus rhamnosus* GR-1 and *Lactobacillus reuteri* RC-14 on the ability of *Candida albicans* to infect cells and induce inflammation. *Microbiol Immunol*. 2009;53(9):487–95.
259. Orsi CF, Sabia C, Ardizzoni A, Colombari B, Neglia RG, Peppoloni S et al. Inhibitory effects of different lactobacilli on *Candida albicans* hyphal formation and biofilm development. *J Biol Regul Homeostat Agents*. 2014;28(4):743–52.
260. Bilhan H, Sulun T, Erkose G, Kurt H, Erturan Z, Kutay O et al. The role of *Candida albicans* hyphae and *Lactobacillus* in denture-related stomatitis. *Clin Oral Invest*. 2009;13(4):363–8.
261. Jiang Q, Stamatova I, Kari K, Meurman JH. Inhibitory activity in vitro of probiotic lactobacilli against oral *Candida* under different fermentation conditions. *Benef Microbes*. 2015;6(3):361–8.
262. Jeganathan S, Lin CC. Denture stomatitis: A review of the aetiology, diagnosis and management. *Austral Dent J*. 1992;37(2):107–14.
263. Gendreau L, Loewy ZG. Epidemiology and etiology of denture stomatitis. *J Prosthodont*. 2011;20(4):251–60.
264. Nikawa H, Hamada T, Yamamoto T. Denture plaque – Past and recent concerns. *J Dent*. 1998;26(4):299–304.
265. Ramage G, Tomsett K, Wickes BL, Lopez-Ribot JL, Redding SW. Denture stomatitis: A role for *Candida* biofilms. *Oral Surg Oral Med O*. 2004;98(1):53–9.
266. Bagg J, Sweeney MP, Lewis MA, Jackson MS, Coleman D, Al MA et al. High prevalence of non-*albicans* yeasts and detection of anti-fungal resistance in the oral flora of patients with advanced cancer. *Palliat Med*. 2003;17(6):477–81.
267. Coleman D, Sullivan D, Harrington B, Haynes K, Henman M, Shanley D et al. Molecular and phenotypic analysis of *Candida dubliniensis*: A recently identified species linked with oral candidosis in HIV-infected and AIDS patients. *Oral Dis*. 1997;3(Suppl 1):S96–101.
268. Li L, Redding S, Dongari-Bagtzoglou A. *Candida glabrata*: An emerging oral opportunistic pathogen. *J Dent Res*. 2007;86(3):204–15.
269. Redding SW, Marr KA, Kirkpatrick WR, Coco BJ, Patterson TF. *Candida glabrata* sepsis secondary to oral colonization in bone marrow transplantation. *Med Mycol*. 2004;42(5):479–81.
270. Coco BJ, Bagg J, Cross LJ, Jose A, Cross J, Ramage G. Mixed *Candida albicans* and *Candida glabrata* populations associated with the pathogenesis of denture stomatitis. *Oral Microbiol Immunol*. 2008;23(5):377–83.
271. McCulloch E, Lucas C, Ramage G, Williams C. Improved early diagnosis of *Pseudomonas aeruginosa* by real-time PCR to prevent chronic colonisation in a paediatric cystic fibrosis population. *J Cyst Fibros*. 2011;10(1):21–4.
272. Dagistan S, Aktas AE, Caglayan F, Ayyildiz A, Bilge M. Differential diagnosis of denture-induced stomatitis, *Candida*, and their variations in patients using complete denture: A clinical and mycological study. *Mycoses*. 2009;52(3):266–71.

273. Ramage G, VandeWalle K, Lopez-Ribot JL, Wickes BL. The filamentation pathway controlled by the Efg1 regulator protein is required for normal biofilm formation and development in *Candida albicans*. *FEMS Microbiol Lett*. 2002;214(1):95–100.

274. Verran J, Jackson S, Coulthwaite L, Scallan A, Loewy Z, Whitehead K. The effect of dentifrice abrasion on denture topography and the subsequent retention of microorganisms on abraded surfaces. *J Prosth Dent*. 2014;112(6):1513–22.

275. O'Donnell LE, Robertson D, Nile CJ, Cross LJ, Riggio M, Sherriff A et al. The oral microbiome of denture wearers is influenced by levels of natural dentition. *PloS ONE*. 2015;10(9):e0137717.

276. Ribeiro DG, Pavarina AC, Dovigo LN, Machado AL, Giampaolo ET, Vergani CE. Prevalence of *Candida* spp. associated with bacteria species on complete dentures. *Gerodontology*. 2012;29(3):203–8.

277. Marcos-Arias C, Eraso E, Madariaga L, Aguirre JM, Quindos G. Phospholipase and proteinase activities of *Candida* isolates from denture wearers. *Mycoses*. 2011; 54(4):e10–6.

278. Ramage G, Zalewska A, Cameron DA, Sherry L, Murray C, Finnegan MB et al. A comparative in vitro study of two denture cleaning techniques as an effective strategy for inhibiting *Candida albicans* biofilms on denture surfaces and reducing inflammation. *J Prosthodont*. 2012;21(7):516–22.

279. Silva S, Henriques M, Hayes A, Oliveira R, Azeredo J, Williams DW. *Candida glabrata* and *Candida albicans* co-infection of an in vitro oral epithelium. *J Oral Pathol Med*. 2011;40(5):421–7.

280. Alves CT, Wei XQ, Silva S, Azeredo J, Henriques M, Williams DW. *Candida albicans* promotes invasion and colonisation of *Candida glabrata* in a reconstituted human vaginal epithelium. *J Infect*. 2014;69(4):396–407.

281. Nett JE, Marchillo K, Spiegel CA, Andes DR. Development and validation of an in vivo *Candida albicans* biofilm denture model. *Infect Immun*. 2010;78(9):3650–9.

282. McLean RJ. Normal bacterial flora may inhibit *Candida albicans* biofilm formation by Autoinducer-2. *Front Cell Infect Microbiol*. 2014;4:117.

3 Oral Biofilms and Their Implication in Oral Diseases

Georgios N. Belibasakis and Nagihan Bostanci

CONTENTS

INTRODUCTION

Microorganisms and the host live together in a symbiotic and inseparable relationship, when colonising the human host. Endogenous oral microorganisms tend to form complex biofilm communities on the surface of teeth and the oral mucosa, which are their natural habitats. Normally, this intimate interaction is commensurate with health. However, should microecological changes occur in these specific niches of the oral cavity, some of the microorganisms in the biofilm will become more prolific and may act as opportunistic pathogens, therefore inflicting disease. In fact the most common oral diseases, including dental caries, endodontic infections, periodontal diseases and peri-implant diseases, are almost exclusively of microbial biofilm etiology. Hence, it is the aim of this chapter to review the current knowledge on the ecological considerations and microbial composition of various oral biofilm communities, and to elaborate their implication in the associated oral diseases.

ORAL MICROBIAL ECOLOGY AND THE ORAL MICROBIOTA

The oral cavity is the beginning of the digestive system and forms an intersection with the respiratory system. It is inhabited by a plethora of microorganisms that are collectively referred to as the 'oral microbiota' or the 'oral microbiome'. Most bacteria are transiting through the oral cavity rather than successfully residing in it. Physiological factors, such as salivary flow and shearing forces, or microecological factors, such as redox potential, partial oxygen pressure, pH and nutrient availability, define whether a microorganism is suitable for surviving in the environment of the oral cavity. Host-related factors, such as the local immune response, hormonal changes, aging, smoking and drug consumption may also influence the composition of the oral microbiota. The capacity of a microorganism to adhere onto, for instance, a tooth surface is an important initial step, but its ability to grow onto that surface is instrumental for its survival and adaptation into the oral cavity. Hence, despite their large diversity, oral microbes in fact exhibit a high tropism for their particular ecological niche.

The various microanatomical niches of the oral cavity are defined by its structural tissues: the soft oral mucosal surfaces (including gingiva, cheeks, lips, palate, tongue and tonsils) and the teeth. Saliva is the fluidic milieu of the oral cavity that lubricates the mucosa and teeth, provides buffering capacity and food clearance, and contains various mineral elements, serum components, antimicrobials and nutrients. The salivary pellicle that coats the tooth surfaces is mediating the attachment of oral bacteria onto these surfaces. In addition, oral bacteria can metabolise nutrients contained in saliva, for the benefit of their growth.

Despite the unbarred interaction of the oral cavity with the aerobic environment, several of the microorganisms that reside in it are strictly anaerobic or aerotolerant. More than 1,000 different taxa have been identified by metagenomic sequencing at various anatomical niches of the oral cavity (approximately only half of them cultivable) [1,2]. This microbial affluence and combinatory possibilities result in a very complex microbial flora that can vary between individuals, or even between different oral niches of the same individual.

BIOFILMS AND ORAL PHYSIOLOGY

Microorganisms in nature tend to grow on surfaces, and only transiently exist in planktonic single cell form. Hence, they form 'biofilms', which are microorganism communities embedded into a polymeric matrix consisting of their own released metabolic products and components of the environment in which they grow. In principle, the phenotypic properties of microbes in a biofilm are fundamentally different from their planktonic counterparts. Their growth slows down but they coaggregate, benefitting from each other's metabolic products and exchanging communication (molecular) signals. This enables them to sense their microcommunity more efficiently. In fact, 'microgradients' are established within the mass of a biofilm, selectively favouring the growth and survival of the most well-adapted species. These microgradients can be physicochemical (e.g. temperature, redox potential, oxygen partial pressure and pH), or molecular (e.g. penetration of nutrients, diffusion of secreted communication molecules, etc.). In terms of medical importance, a striking behavioural difference of biofilms compared to planktonic microbial cells is that the former are extremely tolerant to antimicrobial agents (even at a magnitude of 1,000-fold), and to components of the immune system.

The dental plaque forming on the tooth surfaces is most often used synonymously with the terms 'dental biofilm' or 'oral biofilm'. In fact, dental plaque possesses all the required traits to be considered a polymicrobial biofilm [3]. Indeed, it can form on biological or artificial surfaces, such as natural teeth, or dental prosthetic and implant restorations, respectively. Hundreds of different microbial species can contribute to the formation of an oral biofilm. When considering the localisation on tooth surfaces, oral biofilms that grow above the gingival margin are defined as 'supragingival', whereas ones that form below the gingival margin are termed subgingival.

It is beyond question that the oral microbiota is imperative for a healthy oral cavity. Despite their great diversity, they are marked by a very high stability among the constituent species and their interaction with the host [4], establishing a homeostatic relationship. A functional and metabolic redundancy also exists between the microorganisms of a biofilm. This ensures the coverage of the same metabolic role by several microorganisms within that unique community. Hence, when one of the constituent microbes undergoes elimination in a biofilm, its role is likely to be covered by other members of that same community. In principle, the greater the species' diversity in a microbial biofilm, the higher its functional stability, owing to their overlapping metabolic capacities. This stability may be an important factor to ensure a healthy state status of the host.

One may say that controlled colonisation of the mucosal and tooth surfaces by commensal microbiota is commensurate to health. They act to (a) prime, without overstimulating the immune system, (b) out-compete the colonisation and invasion of the oral tissues by exogenous pathogens and (c) ensure health-compatible microenvironmental conditions that prevent endogenous opportunistic pathogens from outgrowing and prevailing. Characteristic microorganisms of supragingival biofilms associated with oral health rather than disease are streptococci, particularly of the mitis group, and *Leptotrichia buccalis* (Figure 3.1), as well as various *Actinomyces* spp., *Veillonella* spp. and *Neisseria* spp.

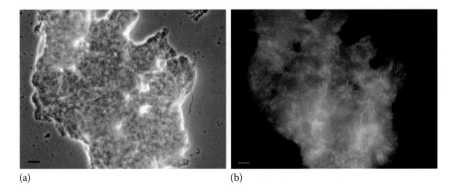

(a)   (b)

FIGURE 3.1 Image of a supragingival biofilm sample obtained from a disease-free tooth site, as viewed under direct light microscopy (a). The sample was processed by fluorescence *in situ* hybridisation (FISH), using 16S rRNA-targeting oligonucleotide probes for the genus *Streptococcus* (green) and the species *Leptotrichia buccalis* (red), and was viewed by epifluorescence microscopy (b). Notice the presence of the small streptococci (green) within the biofilm mass and the long filamentous *Leptotrichia buccallis* (red). Scale bars = 10 μm.

BIOFILMS AND ORAL PATHOLOGY

The most contemporary hypothesis proposed on the relationship between oral bio-films and oral diseases is the 'ecological plaque hypothesis', according to which there is a tight equilibrium between the local oral microbiota and the host response. Microbes typically associated with the disease may still be present at a healthy site, albeit at too low numbers and proportions to be deleterious. Changes in the local microenvironmental conditions may cause breakage in this homeostatic equilibrium and result in a shift of the biofilm's microbial composition. Under the newly established conditions, quiescent opportunistic pathogens can now become prolific and more virulent, leading to oral disease. Oral diseases of biofilm etiology include dental caries, endodontic infections, periodontal diseases and peri-implant infections. These are the most exclusive and common oral diseases, and recent epidemiological surveys indicate that their treatment has a severe global economic impact, amounting to almost half a trillion US dollars annually [5].

DENTAL CARIES

Dental caries is a very common oral disease of biofilm etiology. It is characterised by the localised destruction of the mineral tissue of the teeth, starting as white lesions and progressing as excessive cavitations. The different anatomical sites of the tooth (e.g. fissures, cervical region and proximal surfaces) have different susceptibilities in cariogenic biofilm formation. The fissures of the occlusal surfaces of posterior teeth are the sites most prone to foster cariogenic biofilms and hence more likely to develop dental caries.

   The demineralisation of the enamel and dentin occurring in dental caries is a consequence of a local drop in pH, caused by bacteria of the biofilm. Evidently, supragingival biofilms are directly exposed to the openness of the oral cavity and the affluent sugar availability in our nutrition. Given the appropriate fermentable carbohydrates, overgrowth and maturation of a supragingival biofilm will result in the domination of aerobic, or aerotolarant, and saccharolytic lactic acid–producing bacteria. As such, acidogenic and aciduric members of the mutans streptococci and lactobacilli are most well adapted to grow under these conditions, and their presence correlates well with caries. These bacteria adhere by means of cell surface adhesins to the receptors which are present on the saliva-coated tooth [6]. They degrade the carbohydrates derived from foods and form organic acids such as lactic, formic, acetic and/or succinic acid. Subsequently, the supragingival plaque pH falls to around 4 in several minutes. In particular, *Streptococcus mutans* is the dominating cariogenic species, followed by *Streptococcus sobrinus* and various members of the *Lactobacillus* spp. [7]. On the other hand, an inverse relationship between dental caries and other members of the *Streptococcus* spp. has also been reported, in particular *Streptococcus sanguinis*. *S. sanguinis* is capable of oxidising thiocyanate (SCN-) in saliva to hypothiocyanite (OSCN-), thereby repressing the glycolytic activity of mutans [8]. A number of *Actinomyces* spp. have been associated with the root cementum caries. This is a form of the disease that occurs in periodontitis-affected teeth, in which the root surface is exposed due to gingival recession. It is also proposed that the hard-tissue specificity (e.g. enamel, dentin or cementum) may influence the establishment of a caries-specific biofilm microflora [9,10].

By the use of high-throughput metagenomic sequencing methods, additional microbial genera have been identified in biofilms obtained from dental carious lesions, including *Bifidobacterium*, *Propionibacterium*, *Scardovia*, *Atopobium*, *Prevotella* and *Veillonella* [10,11]. Such studies not only show large variations in the microbial genera detected in biofilms from carious lesions, but also denote that an overlapping degree of metabolic activities must exist between them, despite their phylogenetic distance.

ENDODONTIC INFECTIONS

Progression of dental caries results in microbial invasion into the pulp chamber and root canal space. Eventually, the contained pulp tissue becomes infected, and within that confined space it is not immunologically efficient to tackle the evolving infection. If the infection is not handled clinically by removal of the affected pulp tissue, the subsequent necrosis will lead to infection of the entire root canal space, forcing the host defence front to establish at the periapical tissue region (i.e. surrounding apex of the root of the tooth). This is frequently accompanied by the formation of a periapical bone lesion, which is visible radiographically and is defined clinically as apical periodontitis.

Endodontic infections are clearly of polymicrobial nature, and the magnitude of the microbial load may be proportional to the extent of the periapical host response. Although not completely established, there is circumstantial, yet convincing, evidence that the microbial challenge that causes the immunological response in the periapical region is organised in the form of biofilms [12,13].

The microbial composition of endodontic infections is largely characterised by Gram-negative anaerobic species belonging to the *Bacteroidetes* phylum [14,15], or Gram-positive facultative anaerobic enterococci, particularly *Enterococcus faecalis*. *E. faecalis* has been implicated in about 24–77% of endodontic lesions. *E. faecalis* possesses various survival and virulence factors such as its ability to compete with other microorganisms, invade dentinal tubules and resist nutritional deprivation [16]. However, high-throughput molecular studies have revealed an even greater diversity of the microbiota in the infected root canals. This mosaic includes uncultivable members of the phyla *Spirochaetes*, *Deferribacteres*, *Synergistetes*, *Firmicutes*, *Bacteroidetes*, *Actinobacteria* and *Proteobacteria* [17–20]. There are interindividual variations in the microbial spectrum of infected root canals, that is, the microbial communities in infected root canals of different individuals are not exactly the same [17,19,21–24], and may also differ according to the location of the affected tooth [25,26]. Even within a single infected root canal, the microbial composition in the apical and coronal regions differs: the former typically has a higher level of microbial diversity than the latter, and the dominant microbes are different (the apical area mainly contains obligate anaerobes) [17,27]. Shifts in the microbial composition occur at different phases of endodontic infections (i.e. chronic versus acute), which also indicates underlying differences in the immunological responses at the affected regions [28].

PERIODONTAL DISEASES

Periodontal diseases, along with dental caries, are the most common oral diseases in humans. Gingivitis is the initial inflammatory reaction of the gingiva to a developing supragingival biofilm on the tooth surface. Periodontitis is a progressed stage of periodontal disease, and the primary cause of tooth loss in adults. The pathogenesis of periodontitis entails the process of inflammatory destruction of the tooth-supporting (periodontal) tissues, in response to a subgingival biofilm developing on the juxtaposed tooth surface. The development of a subgingival biofilm within a periodontal pocket is an unwanted clinical/histopathological outcome, and a sign of progressing periodontal disease. The environment of a periodontal pocket is an oxygen-restricted one, which is continuously enriched by the protein-rich exudate of the inflamed gingival tissue, the gingival crevicular fluid (GCF). The proteineous nutrional source and the low oxygen microenvironmental conditions favour the proliferation of anaerobic and proteolytic microorganisms such as *Porphyromonas, Tannerella, Treponema, Prevotella, Fusobacterium, Campylobacter* and *Eubacterium* spp. in the subgingival biofilms. Indeed, it has long been known that conversion from health to periodontitis is associated with Gram-negative, anaerobic and motile microbial flora [29–32]. Representative images demonstrating the morphological diversity of the microorganisms present within a periodontitis-associated subgingival biofilm are shown in Figure 3.2. The most well-established and characterised periodontal pathogens, according to their prevalence and association with disease severity, are the 'red complex' species, namely *Porphyromonas gingivalis, Tannerella forsythia* and *Treponema denticola* [30], all of which are strict anaerobes and proteolytic. Other biofilm species closely associated with periodontitis are *Prevotella intermedia, Eikenella corrodens, Campylobacter rectus, Fusobacterium nucleatum* and *Aggregatibacter actinomycetemcomitans*, the latter one particularly in aggressive

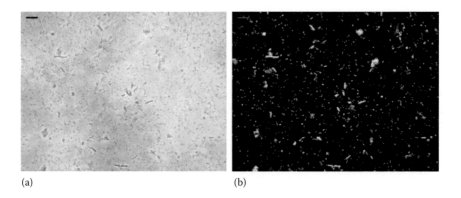

(a)   (b)

FIGURE 3.2   Image of a subgingival biofilm sample obtained from a periodontal pocket, as viewed under direct light microscopy (a). The sample was processed by fluorescence *in situ* hybridisation (FISH), using a 16S rRNA-targeting oligonucleotide probe for all eubacteria (red), and was then viewed by epifluorescence microscopy (b). Notice the great morphological diversity among the biofilm species, including cocci, rods of various sizes, fusiforms and spirochetes (all red). Scale bars = 10 μm.

forms of the disease [11,30]. Biofilm species associated with periodontal health rather than disease are *S. sanguinis, S. mitis* and various *Actinomyces* spp. [33,34].

Contemporary culture-independent metagenomic approaches based on 16S rRNA cloning and sequencing have revealed a further complex mosaic of the biofilm microbiota associated with periodontitis. Newly identified periodontitis-associated bacteria include the species *Peptostreptococcus stomatis, Filifactor alocis* and members of the genera *Desulfolobulus, Dialister, Megasphaera* or the phyla *Synergistetes, Deferribacteres* and TM7 [35–38]. A recent systematic review of the available metagenomics literature has identified that at least 17 novel individual species or phylotypes, beyond the well-characterised ones, may be associated with periodontitis [39]. As changes in the clinical periodontal status are associated with shifts in the microbial composition of the subgingival biofilm community, it is postulated that more species are 'lost' or 'gained' in subjects whose clinical status has changed over time. Therefore, there is an evolving concept that measuring 'microbial stability', rather than screening for individual species, may be useful in the clinical diagnosis of periodontitis and prognosis of its treatment [38].

PERI-IMPLANT DISEASES

Peri-implant diseases are a new form of oral infections that have arisen with the emergence of dental implants as a routine treatment option in restorative dentistry. Failure of functional dental implants is primarily associated with chronic infection of their peri-implant tissues, as a result of biofilm colonisation. The associated biofilm forms on the implant surface, within a peri-implant pocket (a pathological structure analogous to the periodontal pocket). These biofilms are best defined as 'submucosal'.

The periodontal and the peri-implant pocket potentially share similar microenvironmental conditions (e.g. anaerobic). The initial form of peri-implant infection is peri-implant mucositis, characterised by inflammation of the soft peri-implant mucosa, but with no evidence of destruction of the supporting bone. Progression of inflammation deeper into the implant-supporting bone manifests as peri-implantitis. Peri-implant mucositis and peri-implantitis are considered as the peri-implant variants of gingivitis and periodontitis. Yet, the clinical features of peri-implantitis are much more aggressive, rapidly progressing and difficult to treat, compared to periodontitis. In this sense, the patho-mechanisms of peri-implantitis may be distinct to those of periodontitis, even though they display qualitative similarities [40]. A good description of the relationship between peri-implantitis and periodontitis is that they are 'fraternal' infections [41].

The biofilm microbiota of healthy peri-implant sites resemble that of healthy periodontal sites. The switch to peri-implant mucositis is associated with increased presence of cocci, motile bacilli and spirochetes, comparable to that in gingivitis, whereas progression to peri-implantitis is associated with a switch to Gram-negative, motile and anaerobic species highly resembling periodontitis [42,43]. In essence, the qualitative microbial composition of peri-implantitis-associated biofilms resembles that of periodontitis. Nevertheless, some microorganisms identified in submucosal biofilms are not common in subgingival ones, including staphylococci, aerobic Gram-negative bacilli (e.g. Enterobacteriaceae, *Pseudomonas* spp., etc.), *Helicobacter pylori*, as well as *Candida* spp. fungi [44–48]. Current molecular methods, such as broad-range polymerase chain reaction (PCR) and pyrosequencing, have helped us increase our knowledge on the composition of submucosal biofilms [49–52]. We now start to understand that the peri-implant and periodontal biofilm microbiomes may have similarities, but also distinctive differences [53].

CONCLUDING REMARKS

Oral biofilms form naturally on tooth and mucosal surfaces. The interaction between their component organisms and the host is a crucial homeostatic mechanism for the maintenance of health. Yet, changes in the microenvironmental conditions may cause shifts in the endogenous microbial flora of the biofilm into an opportunistic one, thereby causing disease. The most common oral diseases, including dental caries, endodontic, periodontal and peri-implant infections, are of biofilm aetiology. Importantly, these are polymicrobial infections and therefore no one biofilm microorganism alone can be singled out as their principal causative factor. A summary of the major microbial taxa found to be associated with these infections is provided in Table 3.1. Rather, the disease process is perceived as the deregulated crosstalk between a more virulent biofilm community and an insufficient host immune response. Therefore, future preventive and therapeutic strategies for oral diseases

TABLE 3.1
Summary of Major Microbial Taxa Involved in Biofilm-Associated Oral Infections

Dental Caries	Endodontic Infections	Periodontal Infections	Peri-Implant Infections
Streptococcus mutans	*Enterococcus faecalis*	*Porphyromonas gingivalis*	Various periodontal pathogens
Streptococcus sobrinus	*Actinomyces* spp.	*Tannerella forsythia*	*Staphylococcus* spp.
Actinomyces spp.	*Fusobacterium* spp.	*Treponema* spp.	*Enterobacter* spp.
Lactobacillus spp.	*Treponema* spp	*Prevotella* spp.	*Escherichia* spp.
Bifidobacterium spp.	*Synergistetes* phylum	*Fusobacterium* spp.	*Klebsiella* spp.
Propionibacterium spp.	*Deferribacteres* phylum	*Campylobacter* spp.	*Pseudomonas* spp.
Scardovia spp.	*Firmicutes* phylum	*Eubacterium* spp.	*Helicobacter* spp.
Atopobium spp.	*Bacteroidetes* phylum	*Aggregatibacter actinomycetemcomitans*	*Candida* spp.
Prevotella spp.		*Desulfolobulus* spp.	
Veillonella spp.		*Dialister* spp.	
		Synergistetes spp.	
		Megasphaera spp.	
		Deferribacteres phylum	
		TM7 phylum	

should aim at controlling the ecological parameters that drive biofilm formation, rather than eliminating completely the associated oral microbial flora.

ACKNOWLEDGEMENTS

The authors would like to thank Mrs. Helga Lüthi-Schaller (University of Zürich) for her technical assistance in obtaining the FISH images.

CORRESPONDING AUTHOR

Georgios N. Belibasakis
Department of Dental Medicine
Karolinska Institute
Stockholm, Sweden
George.Belibasakis@zzm.uzh.ch

REFERENCES

1. Dewhirst FE, Chen T, Izard J, Paster BJ, Tanner AC, Yu WH et al. The human oral microbiome. *J Bacteriol.* 2010;192(19):5002–17.
2. Keijser BJ, Zaura E, Huse SM, van der Vossen JM, Schuren FH, Montijn RC et al. Pyrosequencing analysis of the oral microflora of healthy adults. *J Dent Res.* 2008;87(11):1016–20.
3. Schaudinn C, Gorur A, Keller D, Sedghizadeh PP, Costerton JW. Periodontitis: An archetypical biofilm disease. *J Am Dent Assoc.* 2009;140(8):978–86.
4. Peterson SN, Snesrud E, Liu J, Ong AC, Kilian M, Schork NJ et al. The dental plaque microbiome in health and disease. *PLoS ONE.* 2013;8(3):e58487.
5. Listl S, Galloway J, Mossey PA, Marcenes W. Global economic impact of dental diseases. *J Dent Res.* 2015;94(10):1355–61.
6. Kolenbrander PE, London J. Adhere today, here tomorrow: Oral bacterial adherence. *J. Bacteriol.* 1993;175(11):3247–52. Epub 1993/06/01.
7. Caufield PW, Schon CN, Saraithong P, Li Y, Argimon S. Oral lactobacilli and dental caries: A model for niche adaptation in humans. *J Dent Res.* 2015;94(9 Suppl):110S–8S.
8. Carlsson J, Iwami Y, Yamada T. Hydrogen peroxide excretion by oral streptococci and effect of lactoperoxidase-thiocyanate-hydrogen peroxide. *Infect Immun.* 1983;40(1):70–80.
9. Belda-Ferre P, Williamson J, Simon-Soro A, Artacho A, Jensen ON, Mira A. The human oral metaproteome reveals potential biomarkers for caries disease. *Proteomics.* 2015;15(20):3497–507.
10. Simon-Soro A, Mira A. Solving the etiology of dental caries. *Trends Microbiol.* 2015;23(2):76–82.
11. Wade WG. The oral microbiome in health and disease. *Pharmacol Res.* 2013;69(1): 137–43.
12. Schaudinn C, Carr G, Gorur A, Jaramillo D, Costerton JW, Webster P. Imaging of endodontic biofilms by combined microscopy (FISH/cLSM - SEM). *J Microsc.* 2009;235(2):124–7.
13. Nair PN. Apical periodontitis: A dynamic encounter between root canal infection and host response. *Periodontol 2000.* 1997;13:121–48.

14. Sundqvist G. Associations between microbial species in dental root canal infections. *Oral Microbiol Immunol.* 1992;7(5):257–62.
15. Sundqvist G. Ecology of the root canal flora. *J Endod.* 1992;18(9):427–30.
16. Stuart CH, Schwartz SA, Beeson TJ, Owatz CB. *Enterococcus faecalis*: Its role in root canal treatment failure and current concepts in retreatment. *J Endod.* 2006;32(2):93–8.
17. Siqueira JF Jr, Rocas IN, Cunha CD, Rosado AS. Novel bacterial phylotypes in endodontic infections. *J Dent Res.* 2005;84(6):565–9.
18. Siqueira JF, Jr., Rocas IN, Paiva SS, Magalhaes KM, Guimaraes-Pinto T. Cultivable bacteria in infected root canals as identified by 16S rRNA gene sequencing. *Oral Microbiol Immunol.* 2007;22(4):266–71.
19. Siqueira JF Jr, Rocas IN. Diversity of endodontic microbiota revisited. *J Dent Res.* 2009;88(11):969–81.
20. Fernandes Cdo C, Rechenberg DK, Zehnder M, Belibasakis GN. Identification of Synergistetes in endodontic infections. *Microb Pathog.* 2014;73:1–6.
21. Machado de Oliveira JC, Gama TG, Siqueira JF, Jr., Rocas IN, Peixoto RS, Rosado AS. On the use of denaturing gradient gel electrophoresis approach for bacterial identification in endodontic infections. *Clin Oral Invest.* 2007;11(2):127–32.
22. Santos AL, Siqueira JF, Jr., Rocas IN, Jesus EC, Rosado AS, Tiedje JM. Comparing the bacterial diversity of acute and chronic dental root canal infections. *PLoS ONE.* 2011;6(11):e28088.
23. Siqueira JF, Jr., Alves FR, Rocas IN. Pyrosequencing analysis of the apical root canal microbiota. *J Endod.* 2011;37(11):1499–503.
24. Siqueira JF Jr, Rocas IN, Debelian GJ, Carmo FL, Paiva SS, Alves FR et al. Profiling of root canal bacterial communities associated with chronic apical periodontitis from Brazilian and Norwegian subjects. *J Endod.* 2008;34(12):1457–61.
25. Rocas IN, Alves FR, Santos AL, Rosado AS, Siqueira JF Jr. Apical root canal microbiota as determined by reverse-capture checkerboard analysis of cryogenically ground root samples from teeth with apical periodontitis. *J Endod.* 2010;36(10):1617–21.
26. Siqueira JF Jr, Rocas IN, Alves FR, Silva MG. Bacteria in the apical root canal of teeth with primary apical periodontitis. *Oral Surg Oral Med Oral Pathol Oral Radiol Endod.* 2009;107(5):721–6.
27. Ozok AR, Persoon IF, Huse SM, Keijser BJ, Wesselink PR, Crielaard W et al. Ecology of the microbiome of the infected root canal system: A comparison between apical and coronal root segments. *Int Endod J.* 2012;45(6):530–41.
28. Zehnder M, Belibasakis GN. On the dynamics of root canal infections – What we understand and what we don't. *Virulence.* 2015;6(3):216–22.
29. Moore WE, Moore LV. The bacteria of periodontal diseases. *Periodontol 2000.* 1994;5: 66–77.
30. Socransky SS, Haffajee AD. Periodontal microbial ecology. *Periodontol 2000.* 2005;38: 135–87.
31. Listgarten MA, Levin S. Positive correlation between the proportions of subgingival spirochetes and motile bacteria and susceptibility of human subjects to periodontal deterioration. *J Clin Periodontol.* 1981;8(2):122–38.
32. Listgarten MA, Levin S, Schifter CC, Sullivan P, Evian CI, Rosenberg ES. Comparative differential dark-field microscopy of subgingival bacteria from tooth surfaces with recent evidence of recurring periodontitis and from nonaffected surfaces. *J Periodontol.* 1984;55(7):398–401.
33. Roberts FA, Darveau RP. Beneficial bacteria of the periodontium. *Periodontol 2000.* 2002;30:40–50.
34. Roberts FA, Darveau RP. Microbial protection and virulence in periodontal tissue as a function of polymicrobial communities: Symbiosis and dysbiosis. *Periodontol 2000.* 2015;69(1):18–27.

35. Brinig MM, Lepp PW, Ouverney CC, Armitage GC, Relman DA. Prevalence of bacteria of division TM7 in human subgingival plaque and their association with disease. *Appl Environ Microbiol.* 2003;69(3):1687–94.
36. Kumar PS, Griffen AL, Barton JA, Paster BJ, Moeschberger ML, Leys EJ. New bacterial species associated with chronic periodontitis. *J Dent Res.* 2003;82(5):338–44.
37. Kumar PS, Griffen AL, Moeschberger ML, Leys EJ. Identification of candidate periodontal pathogens and beneficial species by quantitative 16S clonal analysis. *J Clin Microbiol.* 2005;43(8):3944–55.
38. Kumar PS, Leys EJ, Bryk JM, Martinez FJ, Moeschberger ML, Griffen AL. Changes in periodontal health status are associated with bacterial community shifts as assessed by quantitative 16S cloning and sequencing. *J Clin Microbiol.* 2006;44(10):3665–73.
39. Perez-Chaparro PJ, Goncalves C, Figueiredo LC, Faveri M, Lobao E, Tamashiro N, et al. Newly identified pathogens associated with periodontitis: A systematic review. *J Dent Res.* 2014;93(9):846–58.
40. Belibasakis GN. Microbiological and immuno-pathological aspects of peri-implant diseases. *Arch Oral Biol.* 2014;59(1):66–72.
41. Robitaille N, Reed DN, Walters JD, Kumar PS. Periodontal and peri-implant diseases: Identical or fraternal infections? *Mol Oral Microbiol.* 2016;31(4):285–301.
42. Mombelli A, Decaillet F. The characteristics of biofilms in peri-implant disease. *J Clin Periodontol.* 2011;38(Suppl 11):203–13.
43. Mombelli A, van Oosten MA, Schurch E, Jr., Land NP. The microbiota associated with successful or failing osseointegrated titanium implants. *Oral Microbiol Immunol.* 1987;2(4):145–51.
44. Rams TE, Link CC Jr. Microbiology of failing dental implants in humans: Electron microscopic observations. *J Oral Implantol.* 1983;11(1):93–100.
45. Leonhardt A, Dahlen G, Renvert S. Five-year clinical, microbiological, and radiological outcome following treatment of peri-implantitis in man. *J Periodontol.* 2003;74(10): 1415–22.
46. Renvert S, Roos-Jansaker AM, Lindahl C, Renvert H, Rutger Persson G. Infection at titanium implants with or without a clinical diagnosis of inflammation. *Clin Oral Implants Res.* 2007;18(4):509–16.
47. Charalampakis G, Leonhardt A, Rabe P, Dahlen G. Clinical and microbiological characteristics of peri-implantitis cases: A retrospective multicentre study. *Clin Oral Implants Res.* 2012;23(9):1045–54.
48. Belibasakis GN, Charalampakis G, Bostanci N, Stadlinger B. Peri-implant infections of oral biofilm etiology. *Adv Exp Med Biol.* 2015;830:69–84.
49. Charalampakis G, Belibasakis GN. Microbiome of peri-implant infections: Lessons from conventional, molecular and metagenomic analyses. *Virulence.* 2015;6(3):183–7.
50. Kumar PS, Mason MR, Brooker MR, O'Brien K. Pyrosequencing reveals unique microbial signatures associated with healthy and failing dental implants. *J Clin Periodontol.* 2012;39(5):425–33.
51. Tsigarida AA, Dabdoub SM, Nagaraja HN, Kumar PS. The influence of smoking on the peri-implant microbiome. *J Dent Res.* 2015;94(9):1202–17.
52. Heuer W, Kettenring A, Stumpp SN, Eberhard J, Gellermann E, Winkel A et al. Metagenomic analysis of the peri-implant and periodontal microflora in patients with clinical signs of gingivitis or mucositis. *Clin Oral Invest.* 2012;16(3):843–50.
53. Dabdoub SM, Tsigarida AA, Kumar PS. Patient-specific analysis of periodontal and peri-implant microbiomes. *J Dent Res.* 2013;92(12 Suppl):168S–75S.

4 Composition and Diversity of Human Oral Microbiome

Preethi Balan, Chaminda Jayampath Seneviratne and Wim Crielaard

CONTENTS

INTRODUCTION

Our understanding of the human microbiota has evolved over a period of nearly five centuries, since the observation of microorganisms in human dental plaque by Antonie van Leeuwenhoek [1]. Today, it is known that the human body surfaces and cavities are inhabited by a complex and dynamic consortium of microorganisms which reside harmoniously with the host in health. Yet they are capable of eliciting disease under certain circumstances [2]. These microbial communities were thought to be approximately 10 times more abundant than human cells, together making us a 'superorganism' [3]. However, recently some have suggested the ratio of microbial to human cells is less than what was previously thought [4].

The term *microbiome* was proposed by Nobel laureate Joshua Lederberg to signify the ecological community of commensal, symbiotic and pathogenic microorganisms that literally share our body space [5]. Hence, the microbiome is the totality of microbes, their genetic elements (genomes) and environmental interactions in a particular environment [5]. However, the term microbiome may be confused or even used interchangeably with the term *microbiota*, which is the microbial taxa associated with humans [6]. The microbiome has evolved through thousands of years of coinhabiting in a microbial–human symbiosis with mutual benefits [7]. The overall human microbiome is contributed by the various microhabitats throughout the body. Each microhabitat forms a unique ecosystem with its distinct atmospheric and nutritional compositions [8,9]. The oral cavity harbours one such extremely diverse and complex microbial community, with more than 700 bacterial species [10,11]. The oral microbiota mostly lies within the protective consortium of biofilm which can be formed on the hard surfaces of teeth as well as the soft tissue of the oral mucosa. However, oral microbiota can also exist in the 'free-floating' or the 'planktonic' mode in the oral fluidic environment such as saliva and gingival crevicular fluid. In health, the microbial composition and activity in the oral microbiome remain stable and maintain oral homeostasis. However, a dysbiosis, or disruption to the microbial homeostasis, can turn the once harmonious microbiota into a potential source of infection in the oral cavity [12]. Moreover, biofilm cells may also disperse and gain access to the circulation, causing systemic effects at distant body sites.

In the past, research on microbial pathogenesis was largely focussed on single pathogenic organisms. However, with the advent of high-throughput omics biology techniques, it has become feasible to study the whole microbial community, that is, microbiota or microbiome in health and disease [13]. For example, oral microbiota have been shown to be associated with a number of systemic diseases, including cardiovascular disease, respiratory tract infections, gastrointestinal diseases and adverse gestational outcomes [14]. In this context, it becomes a prerequisite to enhance our current knowledge on the oral microbiome in health and disease states. In this chapter, we attempt to briefly discuss the composition and diversity of human oral microbiome. The novel gene sequencing tools which have been used for the microbial profiling are also elaborated. Knowledge of the oral microbiome will also help readers to understand the framework and diversity of the microbiome of other body sites such as gut and vagina.

HUMAN ORAL MICROBIOME

As the oral cavity is at the junction of entrance into the enteric and respiratory systems, the acquisition of oral microbiome is unique. The oral cavity is in constant contact with the environmental microbes via food intake or mouth breathing, which contribute to the diverse oral microbial community. The oral microbiome is one of the most diverse and complex microbiomes in the human body [15,16] (Figure 4.1). The oral microbial community is formed mainly by a diverse range of bacteria and much less characterised members which include fungi, viruses and archaea. The microbiome can survive in a planktonic state as in saliva or remain adhered to hard and soft tissues forming biofilms. The two types of microbiome that exist across body habitats are variable microbiome and core microbiome [17]. The variable microbiome is subject specific, and is acquired in response to lifestyle, genotypic and phenotypic factors. The core microbiome is the predominant overlapping microbiome profile shared among different healthy individuals [10,18]. The identification of key members of variable and core microbiome will allow us to understand the metabolic network existing among host and microbial interactions [19]. Although individuals share microbiota at similar sites of the body, there are varying differences at the species and strain levels of the microbiome. This can be as inimitable to the individual as is the fingerprint [20]. The core microbiome of the oral cavity is summarised in Figure 4.2.

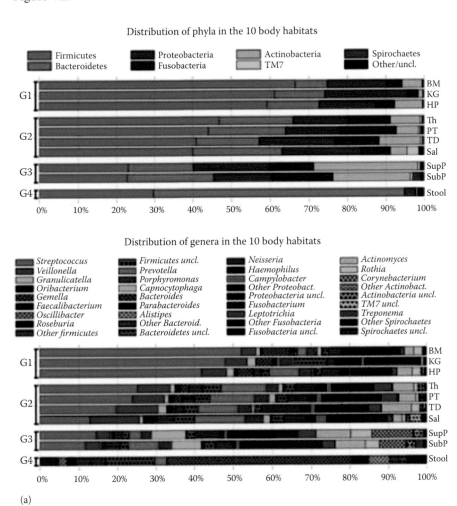

(a)

FIGURE 4.1 Taxonomic composition of the microbiota from 10 digestive tract body habitats. (a) Microbiota from the 10 habitats are grouped based on the ratio of Firmicutes to Bacteroidetes as follows: Group 1 (G1), buccal mucosa (BM), keratinized gingiva (KG) and hard palate (HP); Group 2 (G2), throat (Th), palatine tonsils (PT), tongue dorsum (TD) and saliva (Sal); Group 3 (G3), supragingival (SupP) and subgingival plaques (SubP); and Group 4 (G4), stool (Stool).   *(Continued)*

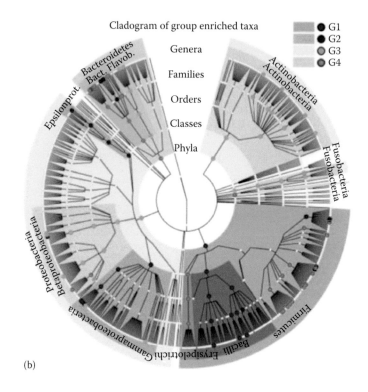

(b)

FIGURE 4.1 (CONTINUED) Taxonomic composition of the microbiota from 10 digestive tract body habitats. (b) Circular cladogram reporting taxa consistently differential among the body habitats in at least one group detected using Linear discriminant analysis Effect Size (LEfSe). (From Segata, N. et al., Composition of the adult digestive tract bacterial microbiome based on seven mouth surfaces, tonsils, throat and stool samples. *Genome Biol.* 2012;13(6):R42.)

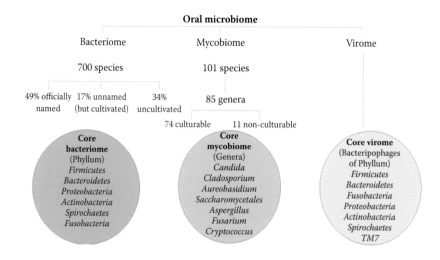

FIGURE 4.2 Summary of oral microbiome.

Oral Bacteriome

Of the different members constituting the oral microbiome, the oral bacteriome is the most extensively studied group of the microbial community. Rapid advances in molecular identification techniques in the past few decades have given us an insight into the phylogenetic evolution of the oral bacteriome, their diversity at different niches and their role in health and disease states.

Traditional culture-dependent techniques have identified approximately 280 oral bacterial species [21]. However, culture-dependent techniques limit the isolation and characterisation of cultivable bacteria, which are less than half of the species present in the oral cavity [22]. The fastidious growth, morphological variations and unusual biochemical reactions may account for limited capacity of the culture-dependent identification methods. Subsequent development of microbial DNA-based identification technologies such as checkerboard assays and microarrays have aided the identification of more oral bacterial species, which were not possible with culture-dependent methods.

Using whole genomic DNA probes and checkerboard DNA–DNA hybridisation, Socransky et al. characterised the periodontal microbial communities into color-coded complexes. Accordingly, the group of 'red complex' bacteria (*Porphyromonas gingivalis*, *Treponema denticola* and *Tannerella forsythia*) were found to be strongly associated with periodontitis [23]. However, microbial identification based on the aforementioned DNA techniques requires prior knowledge of the organism to construct species-specific primers and probes [24].

The development of 16S ribosomal RNA (16S rRNA) gene sequencing techniques has completely revolutionised our capacity to understand the composition and diversity of oral microbiome. The 16S rRNA is a component of 30S ribosomal subunit of prokaryotes. The nucleotide sequence (gene) that encodes 16S rRNA is called 16S rDNA. 16S rDNA is highly conserved within the same genus and species of bacteria and archaea because of the slow rate of evolution [25]. On the contrary, 16S rDNA has hypervariable regions that vary among different species. Therefore, 16S rRNA gene sequencing has been a useful strategy to construct bacterial phylogenies [26]. Based on rRNA sequence characterisation, Woese and collegaues proposed a classification of the three domains of life – Bacteria, Archaea, and Eukarya – as opposed to the traditional classification of prokaryotes and eukaryotes [27]. The relatively shorter length of 16S rRNA gene (1.5 kb) has made sequencing faster and less costly as compared to many other unique bacterial genes. Most of the sequencing work based on 16S rDNA has been carried out in bacteria. In addition to determining the phylogenetic relationships, 16S rDNA sequencing has also helped discovery and classification of novel uncultivable bacteria. Moreover, it has aided the reclassification and renaming of numerous known bacterial genera and species.

The first DNA sequencing method was developed by Gilbert in 1973 and Sanger in 1975 [28,29]. Aas and colleagues used the Sanger sequencing method to identify more than 700 16S rDNA sequences of oral bacteria in health and disease [10]. These sequences were later deposited in GenBank, a comprehensive database that contains publicly available nucleotide sequences. Only fewer than half of this number are from species that have been cultivated and characterised [30]. Several new methods for DNA sequencing were developed in 1990s and were implemented in commercial DNA sequencers (Table 4.1).

Next-generation sequencing (NGS) is the latest advancement in sequencing technologies, allowing massive sequencing with much higher throughput than Sanger sequencing. Pyrosequencing is the first alternative to the conventional Sanger method for *de novo* DNA sequencing. The pyrosequencing technique eliminates the need for cloning and sequencing by amplifying a single DNA molecule [31,32]. Roche 454 pyrosequencing generates up to one million copies in a run with a read lengths of 500–600 bases [24]. This results in very large sampling depth and allows detection of even the rare bacterial taxa present in low abundance [33]. Several studies have employed pyrosequencing platforms to analyse the diversity of the oral microbiome [34,35]. A study utilising the pyrosequencing technique revealed an estimated number of approximately 19,000 phylotypes, which is considerably higher than what was previously reported [34]. The most outstanding advantage of Roche 454 is its speed but the high cost of reagents remains a challenge [36]. Recently, the first gene catalogue of the dental plaque microbiota was assembled via shotgun metagenomics using a combination of 454 and Illumina sequencing platforms [37]. Illumina GAIIx and HiSeq 2000 instrument have also helped unveil more than 175 bacterial species at >90% accuracy in human saliva, which included bacteria *Haemophilus influenzae*, *Neisseria meningitidis*, *Streptococcus pneumoniae*, and *Gammaproteobacteria* [38]. The SOLiD system, which is based on sequencing by ligation of dye-labeled oligonucleotides, can generate 4 Gb of sequence but the reads are only 35 nucleotides [31]. In contrast, the Pacific Biosystem system allows very long reads (>1,000 nucleotides) but it has the highest error rate (approx. 17%) of all NGS systems [39]. However, 16S rDNA sequencing only provides the taxonomic details of the sample under investigation, but does not provide functional characterisation [40].

TABLE 4.1
Generations of Gene Sequencing Technologies

Generation	Sequencer	Sequencing Principle
I Generation	AB70	Sanger method: chain termination
II Generation/next-generation sequencing (NGS)	454 GS	Pyrosequencing: chemiluminescent enzymatic reactions
	Illumina	Polymerase-based sequence by synthesis
	Sequencing by oligonucleotide ligation and detection (SOLiD)	Sequencing by ligation
	Ion torrent	Ion semiconductor sequencing
III Generation sequencing	PacBio RS	Single molecule real-time sequencing (SMRT) sequencing
	MinION	DNA nanopore sequencing

HUMAN ORAL MICROBIOME PROJECT

The National Institutes of Health (NIH)-funded Human Microbiome Project (HMP) employed pyrosequencing technique and shotgun sequencing using the Illumina GAIIx platform to characterise the human microbiome at different body sites. The HMP included a population of 242 healthy subjects who were sampled at 15–18 body sites [41]. Of these, nine samples were collected from the oral cavity which included saliva, keratinised gingiva, tongue, buccal mucosa, palate, throat, tonsils and supragingival and subgingival dental plaque [42]. About 5,177 microbial taxonomic profiles and more than 3.5 Tb of metagenomic sequences have been generated from these resources. In parallel, approximately 800 reference strains isolated from the human body have been sequenced [41]. Moreover, HMP elucidated that each body habitat harbours unique microbiome. Interestingly, each body habitat shows significant diversity among individuals.

The efforts of HMP together with other metagenomics studies collectively made available thousands of oral 16S rDNA sequences which were deposited into GenBank without any taxonomic anchor [43]. Thus, a need to establish a provisional taxonomic scheme for the unnamed human oral bacterial isolates and phylotypes which could be made publicly available to the scientific community was recognised and the Human Oral Microbiome Database (HOMD) (www.homd.org) was developed. Dewhirst and colleagues established the HOMD based on the analysis of 16S rRNA gene sequences [11]. When a 16S rDNA sequence did not match the named species, a novel 16S rDNA gene-based phylotype was created. A phylotype was defined as a cluster of full-length 16S rDNA sequences having greater than 98.5% similarity to one another and less than 98.5% similarity to neighbouring species or phylotypes [11]. Each species and phylotype was assigned a human oral taxon (HOT) number, starting at 001. In the first version of HOMD, there were 619 taxa which belong to 293 (47.3%) named species, 113 (18.3%) unnamed cultivable taxa and 213 (34.4%) unnamed uncultivable taxa. Currently, HOMD contains comprehensive information on approximately 700 bacterial species that reside in human oral cavity. To date, from this curated database, approximately 49% are officially named, 17% are unnamed but cultivated and 34% are known only as uncultivated phylotypes (as accessed www.homd.org on 1 August 2016). An increasing number of genome sequences for oral bacteria are being resolved progressively, primarily through the efforts of HMP and other sequencing projects. They are being deposited to HOMD, thereby competently moulding the data set.

COMPOSITION AND DIVERSITY OF THE ORAL BACTERIOME

The compilation of HOMD has revealed that the human oral microbiome comprises approximately 700 bacterial species, including officially named and unnamed as well as culturable and non-culturable phylotypes. The oral microbiome is composed mainly of bacteria which belong to well-known phyla – Firmicutes, Proteobacteria, Bacteroidetes, Actinobacteria, Spirochaetes, Fusobacteria, Tenericutes and Chylamydiae – as well as the lesser-known phyla or candidate divisions, including Synergistetes, TM7, Chlorobi, Chloroflexi, GN02, SR1 and WPS-2 [44]. The majority of oral representatives (about 96%) permeated into the phyla Firmicutes, Proteobacteria, Actinobacteria, Bacteroidetes, Spirochaetes and Fusobacteria (as accessed www.homd.org on 15 June 2016) (Figure 4.3).

Comprehensive reports from several sequencing studies have shown that each body habitat has a unique microbial community because every human body surface has a unique environment that shapes niche-specific microbiota. According to Whittaker, the total species diversity in an environment (gamma diversity) is reliant on two factors, namely, the mean species diversity in a particular site or habitat, known as alpha diversity, and the species differentiation between those habitats or sites, known as beta diversity. As compared to all other human microbial habitats, the oral cavity is unique owing to the presence of two types of microbial colonisation sites: shedding surfaces (mucosa) and non-shedding surfaces (teeth or dentures) [18,45]. The oral microbiota preferentially colonises the different habitats in the oral cavity depending on the optimal conditions each niche offers to the populating microbes [46].

In one of the earliest studies on the human oral microbiome, Aas and colleagues analysed nine oral sites from five clinically healthy subjects to determine the site and subject specificity of bacterial colonisation using ABI 3100 DNA sequencer [10]. The species that were found to be common to all oral sites belonged to the genera *Streptococcus*, *Veillonella*, *Gemella*, and *Granulicatella*. However, some species were site specific. The predominant species on the tooth surface were *Streptococcus* sp. clone EK048, *S. sanguinis*, and *S. gordonii*, and *Rothia dentocariosa*, *G. hemolysans*, *G. adiacens*, *Actinomyces* sp. clone BL008 and *Abiotrophia defectiva*. In subgingival plaque, several species of *Streptococcus* and *Gemella* were often detected. *S. mitis* biovar 2 was present at the lateral side of the tongue while being absent on the tongue dorsum. On the hard palate, the predominant bacterial species included *S. mitis*, *S. mitis* biovar 2, *Streptococcus* sp. clone FN051, *Streptococcus infantis*, *Granulicatella elegans*, *G. hemolysans*, and *Neisseria subflava*. On the soft palate, *S. mitis*, other cultivable and not-yet-cultivable species of *Streptococcus*, *G. adiacens* and *G. hemolysans* were predominant. Following this study, Egija Zaura and colleagues examined the diversity and uniqueness of individual oral microbiomes using pyrosequencing for the first time [18]. In this study it was observed that the cheek samples were the least diverse while the dental samples showed the highest diversity. Principal component analysis discriminated the profiles of the samples originating from shedding mucosal surfaces from the samples that were obtained from the non-shedding surfaces [18].

The oral microbiota continuously slough into the saliva, rendering salivary microbiome as a blueprint of the oral microbiome [45]. Saliva has the highest median alpha diversities of operational taxonomic units (OTUs) but one of the lowest beta diversities. In other words, each individual's saliva is observed to be ecologically rich, but members of the population share similar salivary organisms [42]. Saliva and other oral samples, for instance dental plaque, clustered distinctly in the principal coordinates analysis based on OTU abundance, indicating that the bacterial community of subgingival plaque is distinct from those present in saliva [47]. (Figure 4.4 depicts unpublished data from Dr. Seneviratne's laboratory.) The microbiomes associated with health and diseased states are shown to be very distinctive. For example, the species involved in dental caries or periodontal disease are not detected in

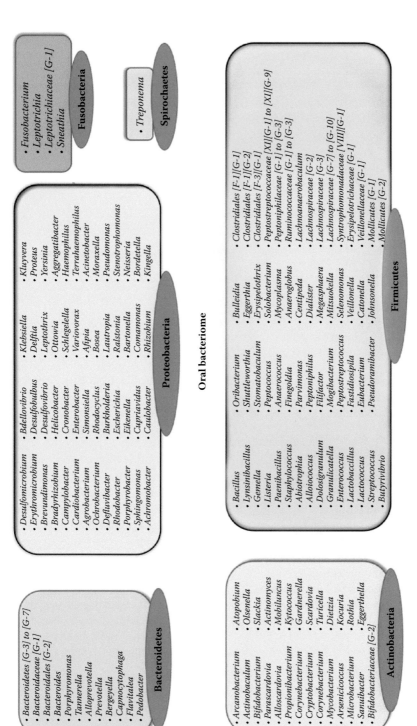

FIGURE 4.3 Composition of the oral bacteriome (as accessed www.homd.org on 16 June 2016).

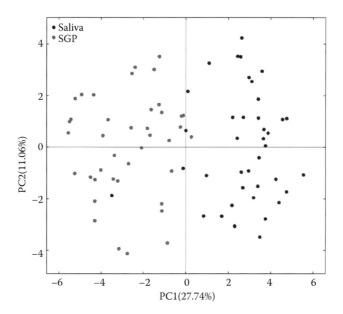

FIGURE 4.4   Principal coordinates analysis based on OTU abundance shows distinct clustering of saliva and subgingival plaque (SGP) samples.

supragingival and subgingival plaques from clinically healthy teeth [10]. Therefore, it is vital to have an insight into the oral microbiome at a resolution of NGS to obtain a deeper understanding of the microbial role in health and disease.

ORAL MYCOBIOME

The term *mycobiome* represents the fungal component of the microbiome community [48]. Being as low as 0.1% of the total microbiome, the mycobiome is often ignored as a constituent of the microbial community [49]. The term microbiome is often used synonymously to represent exclusively the bacterial component of the community. The pioneering HMP and related research consortium have also entirely focussed on the bacteriome in their publications on human microbiome [50]. However, with the commencement of increased recent studies on the human mycobiome, the recovery of information on fungal species populating the microbiome has become increasing available. High-throughput sequencing technologies have begun to untangle the diversity and dynamics of fungal community and are elucidating their role as commensals and pathogens, similar to their bacterial counterparts. The mycobiome is now regarded to play a vital role in maintaining the structure, metabolism and interactions of the microbiome [51].

COMPOSITION AND DIVERSITY OF THE ORAL MYCOBIOME

Sample collection is the first step in the identification and characterisation of fungal isolates.

However, during mycobiome analysis, sample collection poses several challenges. First, fungi are in lesser abundance as compared to bacteria in human niches. Second, there are chances of contamination of samples by human or animal cells. Moreover, the isolation of quality genetic material from fungi could be more challenging than isolating it from the bacterial or animal cells [51]. The sampling of the oral mycobiome is usually carried out using oral rinses, as this enables the collection of organisms from the entire oral mucosal environment [52,53]. Whole saliva collection and swabbing of gingival or buccal tissue are other techniques that may be used for the collection of oral fungal samples [54,55]. Each method has its own merits and disadvantages, and the choice of sampling technique depends primarily on the type of analysis and accessibility of the lesion.

Fungi can be identified based on the traditional culture techniques using the growth media. However, slower growth characteristics of fungi may result in slower recovery of the organisms, especially from the clinical specimens [56]. The development of chromogenic media along with rapid screening tests has enabled the identification of the multiple fungal species in mixed-species infections [57]. However, these techniques may not be sufficient to identify emerging fungal pathogens [58]. These commercial products are organised micro-well format and are based on the principle of substrate utilisation. Substrate utilisation is discerned by increased turbidity and generation of coloured or fluorescent products. Some kits are read manually while others are read automatically. The test results are provided in the form of numerical codes which can be compared against the database to identify the test organism [58,59]. Analysing genetic variability using methods such as restriction fragment length polymorphism (RFLP), denaturing gradient gel electrophoresis (DGGE) and oligonucleotide fingerprinting of rRNA genes (OFRG) has revealed greater complexity in fungal community compared to the results obtained from culture-dependent methods. However, these techniques underachieve when it comes to identifying specific fungal species [60].

The latest tools in mycobiome research are the molecular identification techniques based on high-throughput sequencing of rRNA gene. Polymerase chain reaction (PCR) amplification and sequencing of target genes have provided more accurate and rapid identification of sizeable number of culturable and unculturable fungal species. The fungal ribosome is composed of a small subunit (SSU: 16S/18S) and a large subunit (LSU: 23S/25S/28S) [61]. The genes encoding for these subunits are separated by the internal transcribed spacer regions (ITS), namely ITS1 and ITS2 [62,63]. Of these, 18S rRNA FFgene and ITS regions are the most frequently used for fungal sequencing studies.

The highly conserved rDNA is present in multiple copies in fungal genomes. This enhances the sensitivity of PCR assays as compared to the single-copy targets to amplify the wide range of taxa [64]. rDNAs are also the most frequent fungal DNA sequences available in the public databases, making it easier for sequence homology searches [58]. To obtain information at the phylogenetic level, the internal transcribed spacer (ITS) region has been particularly attractive because it does not code for ribosome components, making it highly variable; with a few exceptions [29]. The evaluation of ITS polymorphism has shown to be reliable in the identification of 40 species of clinically significant yeasts [65]. The sequencing data acquired from these platforms can be compared with the numerous public databases for identifying sequence homology. The most prevailing database is GenBank (http://www.ncbi .nlm.nih.gov/entrez/), which extensively covers a large number of sequences including fungal rDNA sequences. However, the sequences available in GenBank represent only a fraction of the fungal speices, which may be as little as 1% considering the enmormous diversity of fungal species [60].

The fungal species of the oral cavity were previously considered to be relatively less in terms of number and biodiversity. The oral fungal population was reported to be composed primarily of *Candida*, *Saccharomyces*, *Penicillium*, *Aspergillus*, *Scopulariopsis*, *Hormodendrum Geotrichum* and *Hemispora* [66–68]. However, this representation is an underestimated number of fungal inhabitants of the oral cavity, as these studies relied on culture-dependent or genus/species-focused culture-independent methods to confirm the identity of the species.

The first insight into the basal mycobiome of the oral cavity in health came from study by Ghannoum et al. in 2010 [52]. In this study, the oral mycobiome was characterised in 20 healthy individuals using pan-fungal ITS primers and multitag pyrosequencing (Roche 454) methodologies. The identification of 85 fungal genera, including 74 culturable and 11 non-culturable genera, unveiled the diversity of mycobiome in the oral cavity. Of the 74 culturable genera identified, 61 represented one species each, while 13 genera comprised between 2 and 6 different species. The total number of culturable species identified were 101 and each individual harboured species in the range of 9–23. The seven genera which shaped the core mycobiome of oral cavity included *Candida* species (isolated from 75% of participants), followed by *Cladosporium* (65%), *Aureobasidium*, *Saccharomycetales* (50% for both), *Aspergillus* (35%), *Fusarium* (30%) and *Cryptococcus* (20%). Although *Candida* is a known commensal organism in human oral cavities, the actual percentage is much higher than previously reported from culture-based studies. *Candida albicans* was in abundance in 40% of the subjects, followed by *C. parapsilosis* (15%), *C. tropicalis* (15%), *C. khmerensis* (5%) and *C. metapsilosis* (5%). Another important finding was the discovery that nearly one third of the detected fungi were not culturable (Figure 4.5). More recently, Dupuy et al. (2014) reconfirmed presence of the seven consensus members of the core mycobiome despite the differences in the methodologies employed [69]. The shared genera from the studies by Ghannoum et al. and Dupuy et al. included *Candida*, *Pichia Cladosporium*, *Davidiella*, *Alternaria*, *Lewia*, *Aspergilllus*, *Emericella*, *Eurotium*, *Fusarium*, *Gibberella*, *Cryptococcus*, *Filobasidiella* and *Aureobasidium*. However, some components of the core mycobiome (*Saccharomycetales*, *Dothioraceae*, *Glomus* and *Teratosphaeria*) identified by Ghannoum et al. were absent in the study by Dupuy et al. The most noticeable feature of the latter study was the discovery of the skin commensal and pathogen *Malassezia* spp. as a prominent commensal in saliva.

Similar to the bacterial microbiota, the fungal mycobiota also varies among different body sites and diversifies over time and with disease state. The oral cavity holds a significantly larger and more diverse fungal population when compared to the mycobiome of skin or other mucosal sites [60]. These two pioneering studies [52,69] have exemplified the diversity of the oral mycobiome with the discovery of

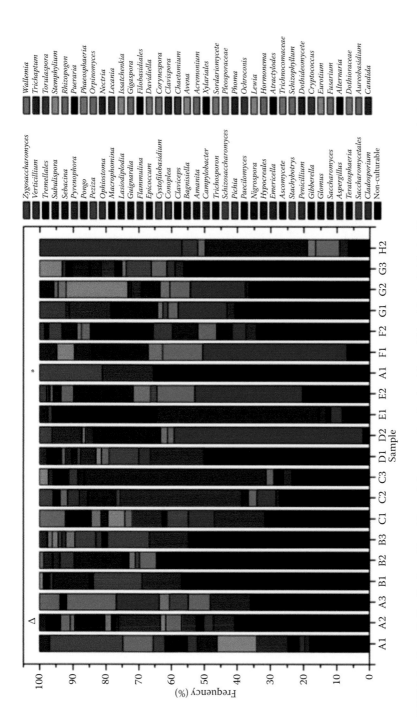

FIGURE 4.5 Overall distribution of fungi in oral rinse samples obtained from 20 healthy individuals. The symbols Δ and * indicate samples containing 16 and 3 fungal genera, respectively. (From Ghannoum MA, Jurevic RJ, Mukherjee PK, Cui F, Sikaroodi M, Naqvi A et al. Characterization of the oral fungal microbiome (mycobiome) in healthy individuals. *PLoS Pathog.* 2010;6:e1000713.)

101 fungal species across various micro niches in the oral cavity. As these studies were based on the oral rinse samples, they represented the washed out microbes from the oral mucosal environment. The ecological niches of periodontal pockets were forfeited in these oral rinse samples. The fact that fungi may form biofilms with bacteria within the anaerobic environment of gingival sulci and periodontal pocket suggests that the diversity of oral mycobiome still remains underestimated [70].

The distribution of fungal community has been shown to vary greatly among different individuals. Monteiro-da-Silva et al. demonstrated a high interindividual variability of the oral fungal population [71]. However, the frequency and quantification of each fungal taxon over the 30-week observation period was observed to be stable, suggesting that the fungal mycobiome maintains an intraindividual stability over time.

Some of the earlier studies have suggested the possibility of global differences in oral yeast colonisation. For instance, the Chinese population demonstrated a greater number and diversity of yeast species in the oral cavity as compared to the population from eastern North America [72]. In addition, *Candida albicans*, which is the predominant commensal and etiologic species of candidiasis in Europe and the Western Hemisphere, was relatively rare in China. Moreover, oral fungal diversity can vary among different races and ethnic populations as well as between genders [52]. Hence, the fungal microbiome was found to differ significantly between Caucasian and Asian men, whereas women showed a tendency to co-cluster irrespective of race or ethnicity. However, this trend needs to be confirmed with a larger population size to draw definite conclusions.

ORAL VIROME

Viruses are integral members of the human oral microbiome [73]. They are dependent biologic entities that can replicate only within a living host cell. The viruses that replicate inside bacteria, known as bacteriophages, attack the bacteria in order to integrate into their genetic material for reproduction. In the oral microbiome, bacteriophages constitute a significant population as compared to the eukaryotic viruses which are also members of the microbiome [74,75]. The predominance of bacteriophages could possibly be secondary to the abundant bacterial cells, which is known to exist in 35 times higher numbers than viruses [76,77]. Relatively very little is known about the role of these viral communities. But the intimate association of bacteriophage and bacteria suggests their active role in shaping and determining the structure of oral microbiome. The bacterial–viral interaction impacts the microbial ecosystem by implementing selection pressures [78], 'kill-the-winner' dynamics [79], stimulating evolutionary change in bacterial hosts [80] and thus maintaining and accelerating bacterial diversity.

COMPOSITION AND DIVERSITY OF THE ORAL VIROME

The classical method of isolating viruses is by culturing. Similar to work with bacteria and fungi, appropriate culture conditions for the virus and the host is a requisite for obtaining a successful cultivation [81]. Electron microscopy has been used in some of the earlier studies to detect the presence of bacteriophage in the dental plaque, based on the detection of virus-like particles (VLPs) [82]. However, these methods were not able to characterise the phage taxonomically.

PCR and culture-based approaches require prior knowledge about the virus to be investigated, thereby narrowing the scope of analysis and effective information obtained [83]. Viral nucleic acids can be enriched using techniques such as micro-array and subsequently sequenced to obtain information about the viral genomes. However, enrichment techniques can be biased against certain viruses [84]. Low-abundance viruses may be lost during the enrichment process also. High-throughput, deep sequencing technology is revolutionary, because it provides an unbiased approach that can detect even rare components of a microbial community.

The discovery of clustered regularly interspaced short palindromic repeats (CRISPR) has provided an alternative approach to detect unidentified viruses in a given environment. Broadly, CRISPR are DNA segments containing short repetitions of base sequences with each repetition followed by short segments of spacer DNA [85]. When a bacterium is invaded by a bacteriophage for the first time, the bacterium acquires short sequences of exogenous DNA from the invading virus and integrates the segment into its CRISPR loci as a novel spacer. These sequences are used to resist subsequent exposures to those viruses through nucleic acid interference. To be more precise, CRISPR sequences constitute a 'genetic memory' of previous infections and exposure to bacteriophage [86]. Metagenomic analysis based on CRISPR has been suggested to be a valuable approach to detect phage–bacteria interaction in complex communities [87]. Taking advantage of this phenomenon, various studies have tracked viral exposure in the oral cavity to understand the evolution of microbiota [88,89]. One approach to estimate the biodiversity of the virome from the contig spectrum of shotgun sequence data is by means of an online computational tool known as PHACCS (PHAge Communities from Contig Spectrum). PHACCS can mathematically analyse the viral shotgun libraries and gain insights about viral ecology and population dynamics [90]. PHACCS analysis has shown the critical role that assemblers play in estimating phage community diversity, by demonstrating that certain assemblers may provide significantly different estimations of community diversity. Despite the limitations imposed in the assembly process, estimates of phage diversity in human saliva suggest that there are hundreds to thousands of different phage genotypes that are relatively evenly distributed in the oral environment [74].

As mentioned earlier, the viral population of the oral microbiome is made up predominantly of bacteriophages of the oral bacteria. In general, bacteriophages may have a lytic or a lysogenic life cycle [91]. In the lytic phage, the bacteriophase replicates and lyse the bacterial cell while in the lysogenic phage, the viral genome integrates with bacterial DNA. As many of the oral bacteriophages have been identified to have lysogenic lifestyles, they have the capability to alter the oral bacteriome substantially. In addition, oral viruses tend to live in a dynamic equilibrium with the bacterial host because the virions of lysogenic viruses are stable components of the oral ecosystem [92,93]. Thus, bacteriophage may have roles both as 'commensals' [94] and as 'pathogens' [95]. Although the gut bacteriome is considered to be more populous than the mouth, the oral microbiome has a higher degree of mobile genetic elements (including viruses, plasmids and transposons) as compared to that of stool [96]. Healthy humans harbour a persistent community of double-stranded DNA viruses in their saliva, with the exclusive identification of bacteriophage as the most abundant virus types [74]. Studies based on epifluorescence microscopy have visualised VLPs to an approximate concentration of 10^8 VLPs/mL of fluid from oropharyngeal swabs [81], 10^8 VLPs/mL of saliva [74] and 10^7 VLPs/mg of dental plaque [97].

Using the patterns of homologous sequences, a study attempted to envisage the putative hosts of bacteriophages [74]. It revealed members of Firmicutes (includes *Streptococcus, Granulicatella* and *Veillonella*), Bacteroidetes (includes *Prevotella*), Fusobacteria (includes *Leptotrichia*), Proteobacteria (includes *Neisseria*), Actinobacteria, Spirochaetes and members of the TM7 phylum as putative hosts [74,77]. The genetic makeup of the bacteriophages suggests their existence as prophages within their respective hosts. This further corroborates the presence of lysogenic viruses in the oral microbial community [74]. Although in relative minority, metagenomics studies have also identified some eukaryotic viruses which includes torque teno viruses, circoviruses, herpesviruses (HSV) and Epstein–Barr virus (EBV) among a few others in the oral cavity [74,76,89,97].

Human oral viruses have also been found to be highly specific to an individual, and to co-evolve with the bacterial host. They also tend to form a persistent community of the oral microbiome [76]. The existence of the same virus in an individual over time could be due to the shared characteristics, for instance virulence factors, among the different viruses. On the contrary, the disparity in the profile among the individuals suggests the role of environmental factors in determining the viral community [74,76]. Unrelated subjects belonging to the same household share a similar living environment and have been shown to have significantly higher proportions of shared viromes than those subjects belonging to different households. The sharing of viruses could be either by via direct personal contact or through environmental reservoirs for viruses [89]. Other factors which may contribute in shaping the oral virome include oral health and/or medical conditions, diet and age [76]. In addition to the personalised and persistent behaviour of oral virome, they also tend to be strongly associated with the sex of the individual. Abeles et al. put forth the first evidence of sex-specific differences in the oral virome community [76]. The hormone driven factors influencing the bacterial microbiota are also known to govern the gender specificities in the viral communities [92].

INTERACTION OF THE HUMAN ORAL MICROBIOME AND HOST IN HEALTH AND DISEASE

The human microbiome, in general, exhibits a phenomenon known as commensalism in which microbes coexist based on a mutually beneficial relationship. The commensal organisms reside at various anatomical locations in the body according to the conditions which favour their growth and proliferation. Although there are ample opportunities for the exchange of bacteria, each site maintains its own microbial profile. Despite their ubiquitous presence in the body, they remain confined to their inherent location because of the presence of physical and immunomodulatory barriers, thereby maintaining the sterility of underlying tissues and human health [98]. Thus a state of equilibrium exists among microorganisms by means of mutualism, commensalism and parasitism for their coexistence. These interactions maintain the balance and stability of the microbial community. However, perturbations in this balance results in microbial shifts leading to disease states.

Microbiome profiles generated by 'omics' approaches are being used extensively to explore the co-occurrence and co-exclusion patterns in oral communities. A study on fungal–bacterial ecological interactions has revealed that the diversity of salivary microbiome decreases with increasing load of *Candida*. The composition of saliva changes towards dominance by Bacilli (streptococci and lactobacilli) and disappearance of genera within class Fusobacteria and Bacteroidia [99]. Similarly, several researchers have studied the viral bacterial interaction in context of oral diseases. The viral activity in periodontal tissues may impact the local immune response in a way that benefits opportunistic bacteria and thus leads to aggravated symptoms [100]. Bacteriophages also play a role in driving bacterial diversity in dental plaque biofilms. A study by Ly et al. demonstrated that subgingival crevices of periodontitis patients have significantly more myoviruses than healthy individuals [101]. They proposed the myoviruses may have an impact on the bacterial diversity in the subgingival pocket in the disease state.

The associations inferred from these analyses sheds light on the synergistic or antagonistic interactions among the different branches of the microbial tree inhabiting the oral cavity. The clinical implications of these polymicrobial biofilm interactions primarily relate to recalcitrance to antimicrobial treatment strategies. Elucidation of these interactions among microbial communities at a molecular level will explain the influence of the constituent microbiome on the health and disease state which eventually impacts the clinical outcome. This would in turn determine how we can translate this knowledge to improve patient management.

CORRESPONDING AUTHOR

Chaminda Jayampath Seneviratne
Discipline of Oral Sciences
Faculty of Dentistry
National University of Singapore
Singapore
jaya@nus.edu.sg

REFERENCES

1. Jorth P, Turner KH, Gumus P, Nizam N, Buduneli N, Whiteley M. Metatranscriptomics of the human oral microbiome during health and disease. *mBio*. 2014;5(2):e01012–4.
2. Goodman AL, Gordon JI. Our unindicted co-conspirators: Human metabolism from a microbial perspective. *Cell Metab*. 2010;12(2):111–6.
3. Gill SR, Pop M, DeBoy RT, Eckburg PB, Turnbaugh PJ, Samuel BS et al. Metagenomic analysis of the human distal gut microbiome. *Science* (New York). 2006;312(5778):1355–9.

4. Abbott, A. Scientists bust myth that our bodies have more bacteria than human cells in Nature News. Nature Publishing Group. 08 January 2016. doi:10.1038/nature .2016.19136.

5. Lederberg J, McCray AT. 'Ome sweet 'omics – A genealogical treasury of words. *Scientist.* 2001;15(8):10.

6. Ursell LK, Metcalf JL, Parfrey LW, Knight R. Defining the human microbiome. *Nutr Rev.* 2012;70(Suppl 1):S38–S44.

7. Hooper LV, Gordon JI. Commensal host-bacterial relationships in the gut. *Science* (New York). 2001;292(5519):1115–8.

8. Zarco MF, Vess TJ, Ginsburg GS. The oral microbiome in health and disease and the potential impact on personalized dental medicine. *Oral Dis.* 2012;18(2):109–20.

9. Badger J, Ng P, Venter JC. The human genome, microbiomes, and disease. In: Nelson KE (ed), *Metagenomics of the human body* (pp. 1–14). New York: Springer Science+Business Media; 2011.

10. Aas JA, Paster BJ, Stokes LN, Olsen I, Dewhirst FE. Defining the normal bacterial flora of the oral cavity. *J Clin Microbiol.* 2005;43(11):5721–32.

11. Dewhirst FE, Chen T, Izard J, Paster BJ, Tanner AC, Yu WH et al. The human oral microbiome. *J Bacteriol.* 2010;192(19):5002–17.

12. Flemmig TF, Beikler T. Control of oral biofilms. *Periodontol 2000.* 2011;55(1):9–15.

13. Ahn J, Chen CY, Hayes RB. Oral microbiome and oral and gastrointestinal cancer risk. *Cancer Causes Contr: CCC.* 2012;23(3):399–404.

14. Han YW, Wang X. Mobile microbiome: Oral bacteria in extra-oral infections and inflammation. *J Dent Res.* 2013;92(6):485–91.

15. D'Argenio V, Salvatore F. The role of the gut microbiome in the healthy adult status. *Clin Chim Acta.* 2015;451, Part A:97–102.

16. Segata N et al. Composition of the adult digestive tract bacterial microbiome based on seven mouth surfaces, tonsils, throat and stool samples. *Genome Biol.* 2012;13(6):R42.

17. Turnbaugh PJ, Ley RE, Hamady M, Fraser-Liggett CM, Knight R, Gordon JI. The human microbiome project. *Nature.* 2007;449(7164):804–10.

18. Zaura E, Keijser BJ, Huse SM, Crielaard W. Defining the healthy "core microbiome" of oral microbial communities. *BMC Microbiol.* 2009;9:259.

19. Shafquat A, Joice R, Simmons SL, Huttenhower C. Functional and phylogenetic assembly of microbial communities in the human microbiome. *Trends Microbiol.* 2014;22(5):261–6.

20. Dethlefsen L, McFall-Ngai M, Relman DA. An ecological and evolutionary perspective on human-microbe mutualism and disease. *Nature.* 2007;449(7164):811–8.

21. Paster BJ, Olsen I, Aas JA, Dewhirst FE. The breadth of bacterial diversity in the human periodontal pocket and other oral sites. *Periodontol 2000.* 2006;42:80–7.

22. Daskalaki A. *Informatics in oral medicine: Advanced techniques in clinical and diagnostic technologies.* Hershey, PA: IGI Global; 2010.

23. Kornman KS, Loesche WJ. The subgingival microbial flora during pregnancy. *J Periodont Res.* 1980;15(2):111–22.

24. Lamont RJ, Hajishengallis G, Jenkinson HF. *Oral microbiology and immunology*, 2nd ed. 2013. Washington, DC: ASM Press.

25. Woo PC, Lau SK, Teng JL, Tse H, Yuen KY. Then and now: Use of 16S rDNA gene sequencing for bacterial identification and discovery of novel bacteria in clinical microbiology laboratories. *Clin Microbiol Infect.* 2008;14(10):908–34.

26. Woese CR, Fox GE. Phylogenetic structure of the prokaryotic domain: The primary kingdoms. *Proc Natl Acad Sci U S A.* 1977;74(11):5088–90.

27. Woese CR, Kandler O, Wheelis ML. Towards a natural system of organisms: Proposal for the domains Archaea, Bacteria, and Eucarya. *Proc Natl Acad Sci USA.* 1990;87(12):4576–9.

28. Yeo A, Smith MA, Lin D, Riche EL, Moore A, Elter J et al. *Campylobacter rectus* mediates growth restriction in pregnant mice. *J Periodontol.* 2005;76(4):551–7.
29. Fardini Y, Chung P, Dumm R, Joshi N, Han YW. Transmission of diverse oral bacteria to murine placenta: Evidence for the oral microbiome as a potential source of intrauterine infection. *Infect. Immun.* 2010;78(4):1789–96.
30. Kumar PS, Griffen AL, Moeschberger ML, Leys EJ. Identification of candidate periodontal pathogens and beneficial species by quantitative 16S clonal analysis. *J Clin Microbiol.* 2005;43(8):3944–55.
31. Blencowe H, Cousens S, Chou D, Oestergaard M, Say L, Moller AB et al. Born too soon: The global epidemiology of 15 million preterm births. *Reprod Health.* 2013;10 (Suppl 1):S2.
32. von Bubnoff A. Next-generation sequencing: The race is on. *Cell.* 2008;132(5):721–3.
33. Siqueira JF, Jr., Fouad AF, Rocas IN. Pyrosequencing as a tool for better understanding of human microbiomes. *J Oral Microbiol.* 2012;4. doi:10.3402/jom.v4:0.10743.
34. Keijser BJ, Zaura E, Huse SM, van der Vossen JM, Schuren FH, Montijn RC et al. Pyrosequencing analysis of the oral microflora of healthy adults. *J Dent Res.* 2008;87(11):1016–20.
35. Belda-Ferre P, Alcaraz LD, Cabrera-Rubio R, Romero H, Simon-Soro A, Pignatelli M et al. The oral metagenome in health and disease. *ISME J.* 2012;6(1):46–56.
36. Ling ZJ, Lian WB, Ho SK, Yeo CL. Parental knowledge of prematurity and related issues. *Singapore Med J.* 2009;50(3):270–7.
37. Xie G, Chain PS, Lo CC, Liu KL, Gans J, Merritt J et al. Community and gene composition of a human dental plaque microbiota obtained by metagenomic sequencing. *Mol Oral Microbiol.* 2010;25(6):391–405.
38. Han YW, Redline RW, Li M, Yin L, Hill GB, McCormick TS. *Fusobacterium nucleatum* induces premature and term stillbirths in pregnant mice: Implication of oral bacteria in preterm birth. *Infect Immun.* 2004;72(4):2272–9.
39. Challis JR, Lockwood CJ, Myatt L, Norman JE, Strauss JF, 3rd, Petraglia F. Inflammation and pregnancy. *Reprod Sci.* 2009;16(2):206–15.
40. Gomez R, Romero R, Edwin SS, David C. Pathogenesis of preterm labor and preterm premature rupture of membranes associated with intraamniotic infection. *Infect Dis Clin North Am.* 1997;11(1):135–76.
41. Human Microbiome Project C. A framework for human microbiome research. *Nature.* 2012;486(7402):215–21.
42. Human Microbiome Project C. Structure, function and diversity of the healthy human microbiome. *Nature.* 2012;486(7402):207–14.
43. Chen T, Yu W-H, Izard J, Baranova OV, Lakshmanan A, Dewhirst FE. The Human Oral Microbiome Database: A web accessible resource for investigating oral microbe taxonomic and genomic information. *Database: J Biol Databases Curat.* 2010; doi: 10.1093database/baq013.
44. Camanocha A, Dewhirst FE. Host-associated bacterial taxa from Chlorobi, Chloroflexi, GN02, Synergistetes, SR1, TM7, and WPS-2 Phyla/candidate divisions. *J Oral Microbiol.* 2014;6. doi:10.3402/jom.v6.25468.
45. He J, Li Y, Cao Y, Xue J, Zhou X. The oral microbiome diversity and its relation to human diseases. *Folia Microbiol.* 2015;60(1):69–80.
46. Avila M, Ojcius DM, Yilmaz O. The oral microbiota: Living with a permanent guest. *DNA Cell Biol.* 2009;28(8):405–11.
47. Li Y, Feng X, Xu L, Zhang L, Lu R, Shi D et al. Oral microbiome in chinese patients with aggressive periodontitis and their family members. *J Clin Periodontol.* 2015;42(11):1015–23.
48. Ghannoum M, Mukherjee P. The human mycobiome and its impact on health and disease. *Curr Fungal Infect Rep.* 2013;7(4):345–50.

49. Qin J, Li R, Raes J, Arumugam M, Burgdorf KS, Manichanh C et al. A human gut microbial gene catalogue established by metagenomic sequencing. *Nature.* 2010;464(7285):59–65.

50. TC. W. Is the human microbiome too bacteriocentric? *Microbe.* 2009;4(12):536.

51. Seed PC. The human mycobiome. *Cold Spring Harbor Perspect Med.* 2015;5(5):a019810.

52. Ghannoum MA, Jurevic RJ, Mukherjee PK, Cui F, Sikaroodi M, Naqvi A et al. Characterization of the oral fungal microbiome (mycobiome) in healthy individuals. *PLoS Pathog.* 2010;6:e1000713.

53. Mukherjee PK, Chandra J, Retuerto M, Sikaroodi M, Brown RE, Jurevic R et al. Oral mycobiome analysis of HIV-infected patients: Identification of *Pichia* as an antagonist of opportunistic fungi. *PLoS Pathog.* 2014;10(3):e1003996.

54. Marsh PD MM. Oral fungal infections. In: *Oral microbiology* (p. 179). Edinburgh, UK: Churchill Livingstone; 2009.

55. Oliver DE, Shillitoe EJ. Effects of smoking on the prevalence and intraoral distribution of *Candida albicans. J Oral Pathol.* 1984;13(3):265–70.

56. Alexander BD, Pfaller MA. Contemporary tools for the diagnosis and management of invasive mycoses. *Clin Infect Dis.* 2006;43(Suppl 1):S15–27.

57. Freydiere AM, Buchaille L, Gille Y. Comparison of three commercial media for direct identification and discrimination of *Candida* species in clinical specimens. *Eur J Clin Microbiol Infect Dis.* 1997;16(6):464–7.

58. Pincus DH, Orenga S, Chatellier S. Yeast identification – Past, present, and future methods. *Med Mycol.* 2007;45(2):97–121.

59. Ellepola AN, Morrison CJ. Laboratory diagnosis of invasive candidiasis. *J Microbiol.* 2005;43 Spec No: 65–84.

60. Underhill DM, Iliev ID. The mycobiota: Interactions between commensal fungi and the host immune system. *Nat Rev Immunol.* 2014;14(6):405–16.

61. Baskaradoss JK, Geevarghese A, Al Dosari AA. Causes of adverse pregnancy outcomes and the role of maternal periodontal status: A review of the literature. *Open Dent J.* 2012;6:79–84.

62. Dollive S, Peterfreund GL, Sherrill-Mix S, Bittinger K, Sinha R, Hoffmann C et al. A tool kit for quantifying eukaryotic rRNA gene sequences from human microbiome samples. *Genome Biol.* 2012;13(7):R60.

63. White JR, Maddox C, White O, Angiuoli SV, Fricke WF. CloVR-ITS: Automated internal transcribed spacer amplicon sequence analysis pipeline for the characterization of fungal microbiota. *Microbiome.* 2013;1(1):6.

64. McGaw T. Periodontal disease and preterm delivery of low-birth-weight infants. *J Can Dent Assoc.* 2002;68(3):165–9.

65. Chen Y-C, Eisner JD, Kattar MM, Rassoulian-Barrett SL, Lafe K, Bui U et al. Polymorphic internal transcribed spacer region 1 DNA sequences identify medically important yeasts. *J Clin Microbiol.* 2001;39(11):4042–51.

66. Schuster GS. Oral flora and pathogenic organisms. *Infect Dis Clin North Am.* 1999;13(4):757–74.

67. Salonen JH, Richardson MD, Gallacher K, Issakainen J, Helenius H, Lehtonen OP et al. Fungal colonization of haematological patients receiving cytotoxic chemotherapy: Emergence of azole-resistant *Saccharomyces cerevisiae. J Hosp Infect.* 2000;45(4):293–301.

68. Jabra-Rizk MA, Ferreira SM, Sabet M, Falkler WA, Merz WG, Meiller TF. Recovery of *Candida dubliniensis* and other yeasts from human immunodeficiency virus-associated periodontal lesions. *J Clin Microbiol.* 2001;39(12):4520–2.

69. Dupuy AK, David MS, Li L, Heider TN, Peterson JD, Montano EA et al. Redefining the human oral mycobiome with improved practices in amplicon-based taxonomy: Discovery of *Malassezia* as a prominent commensal. *PLoS ONE.* 2014;9(3):e90899.

70. Xu H, Dongari-Bagtzoglou A. Shaping the oral mycobiota: Interactions of opportunistic fungi with oral bacteria and the host. *Curr Opin Microbiol.* 2015;26:65–70.
71. Monteiro-da-Silva F, Araujo R, Sampaio-Maia B. Interindividual variability and intraindividual stability of oral fungal microbiota over time. *Med Mycol.* 2014;52(5):498–505.
72. Xu J, Mitchell TG. Geographical differences in human oral yeast flora. *Clin Infect Dis.* 2003;36(2):221–4.
73. Liu L, Johnson HL, Cousens S, Perin J, Scott S, Lawn JE et al. Global, regional, and national causes of child mortality: An updated systematic analysis for 2010 with time trends since 2000. *Lancet.* 2012;379(9832):2151–61.
74. Pride DT, Salzman J, Haynes M, Rohwer F, Davis-Long C, White RA 3rd et al. Evidence of a robust resident bacteriophage population revealed through analysis of the human salivary virome. *ISME J.* 2012;6(5):915–26.
75. De Vlaminck I, Khush KK, Strehl C, Kohli B, Luikart H, Neff NF et al. Temporal response of the human virome to immunosuppression and antiviral therapy. *Cell.* 2013;155(5):1178–87.
76. Abeles SR, Robles-Sikisaka R, Ly M, Lum AG, Salzman J, Boehm TK et al. Human oral viruses are personal, persistent and gender-consistent. *ISME J.* 2014;8(9):1753–67.
77. Edlund A, Santiago-Rodriguez TM, Boehm TK, Pride DT. Bacteriophage and their potential roles in the human oral cavity. *J Oral Microbiol.* 2015;7:27423.
78. Donlan RM. Preventing biofilms of clinically relevant organisms using bacteriophage. *Trends Microbiol.* 2009;17(2):66–72.
79. Rodriguez-Valera F, Martin-Cuadrado AB, Rodriguez-Brito B, Pasic L, Thingstad TF, Rohwer F et al. Explaining microbial population genomics through phage predation. *Nat Rev Microbiol.* 2009;7(11):828–36.
80. Pal C, Macia MD, Oliver A, Schachar I, Buckling A. Coevolution with viruses drives the evolution of bacterial mutation rates. *Nature.* 2007;450(7172):1079–81.
81. Haynes M, Rohwer FL. The human virome. In: Nelson KE (ed), *Metagenomics of the human body.* New York: Springer Science+Business Media; 2011.
82. Brady JM, Gray WA, Caldwell MA. The electron microscopy of bacteriophage-like particles in dental plaque. *J Dent Res.* 1977;56(8):991–3.
83. Carta G, Persia G, Falciglia K, Iovenitti P. Periodontal disease and poor obstetrical outcome. *Clin Experimental Obstetrics & Gynecology.* 2004;31(1):47–9.
84. Howson CP, Kinney MV, McDougall L, Lawn JE. Born too soon: Preterm birth matters. *Reproductive health.* 2013;10(Suppl 1):S1.
85. Gursoy M, Kononen E, Gursoy UK, Tervahartiala T, Pajukanta R, Sorsa T. Periodontal status and neutrophilic enzyme levels in gingival crevicular fluid during pregnancy and postpartum. *J Periodontol.* 2010;81(12):1790–6.
86. Marraffini LA, Sontheimer EJ. CRISPR interference: RNA-directed adaptive immunity in bacteria and archaea. *Nat Rev Genet.* 2010;11(3):181–90.
87. Collins JG, Windley HW, 3rd, Arnold RR, Offenbacher S. Effects of a *Porphyromonas gingivalis* infection on inflammatory mediator response and pregnancy outcome in hamsters. *Infect Immun.* 1994;62(10):4356–61.
88. Pride DT, Salzman J, Relman DA. Comparisons of CRISPRs and viromes in human saliva reveal bacterial adaptations to salivary viruses. *Environ Microbiol.* 2012;14(9):2564–76.
89. Robles-Sikisaka R, Ly M, Boehm T, Naidu M, Salzman J, Pride DT. Association between living environment and human oral viral ecology. *ISME J.* 2013;7(9):1710–24.
90. Angly F, Rodriguez-Brito B, Bangor D, McNairnie P, Breitbart M, Salamon P et al. PHACCS, an online tool for estimating the structure and diversity of uncultured viral communities using metagenomic information. *BMC Bioinformat.* 2005;6(1):1–9.
91. Canchaya C, Fournous G, Chibani-Chennoufi S, Dillmann ML, Brussow H. Phage as agents of lateral gene transfer. *Curr Opin Microbiol.* 2003;6(4):417–24.

92. Abeles SR, Pride DT. Molecular bases and role of viruses in the human microbiome. *J Mol Biol.* 2014;426(23):3892–906.

93. Kunin V, He S, Warnecke F, Peterson SB, Garcia Martin H, Haynes M et al. A bacterial metapopulation adapts locally to phage predation despite global dispersal. *Genome Res.* 2008;18(2):293–7.

94. Bachrach G, Leizerovici-Zigmond M, Zlotkin A, Naor R, Steinberg D. Bacteriophage isolation from human saliva. *Lett Appl Microbiol.* 2003;36(1):50–3.

95. Stevens RH, Preus HR, Dokko B, Russell DT, Furgang D, Schreiner HC et al. Prevalence and distribution of bacteriophage phi Aa DNA in strains of *Actinobacillus actinomycetemcomitans. FEMS Microbiol Lett.* 1994;119(3):329–37.

96. Zhang Q, Rho M, Tang H, Doak TG, Ye Y. CRISPR-Cas systems target a diverse collection of invasive mobile genetic elements in human microbiomes. *Genome Biol.* 2013;14(4):R40.

97. Naidu M, Robles-Sikisaka R, Abeles SR, Boehm TK, Pride DT. Characterization of bacteriophage communities and CRISPR profiles from dental plaque. *BMC Microbiol.* 2014;14:175.

98. Li X, Kolltveit KM, Tronstad L, Olsen I. Systemic diseases caused by oral infection. *Clin Microbiol Rev.* 2000;13(4):547–58.

99. Kraneveld EA, Buijs MJ, Bonder MJ, Visser M, Keijser BJF, Crielaard W et al. The relation between oral *Candida* load and bacterial microbiome profiles in Dutch older adults. *PLoS ONE.* 2012;7(8):e42770.

100. Lin D, Smith MA, Elter J, Champagne C, Downey CL, Beck J et al. *Porphyromonas gingivalis* infection in pregnant mice is associated with placental dissemination, an increase in the placental Th1/Th2 cytokine ratio, and fetal growth restriction. *Infect Immun.* 2003;71(9):5163–8.

101. Ly M, Abeles SR, Boehm TK, Robles-Sikisaka R, Naidu M, Santiago-Rodriguez T et al. Altered oral viral ecology in association with periodontal disease. *mBio.* 2014;5(3):e01133–14.

Candida Biofilms
*Properties, Antifungal
Resistance and Novel
Therapeutic Options*

Chaminda Jayampath Seneviratne,
Thuyen Truong and Yue Wang

CONTENTS

INTRODUCTION

Candida is a group of commensal fungi that inhabit various niches of the human body, including the oral cavity, gastrointestinal tract, vagina, and skin of healthy individuals [1,2]. *Candida* is a eukaryotic organism which has been included in the kingdom Fungi. *Candida* is classified in the order Saccharromycetaeceae and the class Hemiascomycetes. Although more than 200 *Candida* spp. have been identified, only a few of them are associated with human or animal infections [3,4]. These include *C. albicans, C. glabrata, C. tropicalis, C. krusei, C. parapsilosis,* among others. Under certain circumstances, transition of innocuous commensal *Candida* to the disease-causing 'parasitic' form causes infection, or candidiasis, which can range from superficial mucous membrane infection to life-threatening systemic disease [1].

C. albicans is a major cause of nosocomial infections, causing severe mucosal infections such as oral candidiasis, onychomycoses and vulvovaginal candidiasis, as well as systemic mycoses with high mortality rates (Figure 5.1) [5–7]. Candidiasis is reported to be the third or fourth leading cause of nosocomial infection in the United States, which ranks higher than some common bacterial infections [8,9]. Certain compromised population groups such as patients with HIV/ AIDS, transplant recipients, and patients receiving chemotherapy are especially vulnerable to *Candida* infections [10]. Candidiasis is, in fact, the most common fungal infection in both child and adult HIV/AIDS patients [11]. *Candida* is a major pathogen in solid organ transplant recipients with a mortality that can be as high as 50% [12,13]. Moreover, *Candida* infections are associated with the highest crude mortality rate among vascular catheter-related infections [14]. Therefore, understanding of the pathogenic mechanisms of *Candida* infections is a priority in the healthcare field.

Most epidemiological studies have reported *C. albicans* as the most commonly identified pathogenic *Candida* spp. [3,15,16]. *C. albicans* is also the most prevalent fungal pathogen in lethal bloodstream infections in humans [17]. *C. albicans* is also the most frequently isolated species in various host populations, including adults and children [18,19]. However, recent studies have also shown the escalation of the incidence of non-*albicans Candida* species such as *C. glabrata*, *C. parapsilosis* and *C. tropicalis* [20–23]. Of these, *C. glabrata* accounts for 5–20% of all *Candida* infections and often ranks as the second most prevalent *Candida* pathogen [24–28]. *C. glabrata* has a lower susceptibility to azole antifungals and may also be resistant to antifungals including echinocandins [29,30]. Moreover, some studies have reported more than a single *Candida* species coinfecting the host [31].

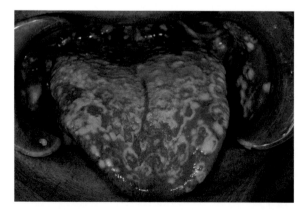

FIGURE 5.1 Clinical appearance of oral candidiasis. (Courtesy of Dr. Intekhab Islam, Faculty of Dentistry, National University of Singapore.)

CANDIDA BIOFILMS

One of the major factors contributing to the virulence of *Candida* is its versatility in adapting to a variety of different habitats for growth and formation of surface-attached microbial communities known as 'biofilms' [32]. Biofilms are defined as surface-attached microbial communities encased in a matrix of extracellular polymeric substances (EPS) and display phenotypic features that differ from those of their planktonic or free-floating counterparts [33]. *Candida* forms biofilms on abiotic surfaces such as implanted medical devices as well as biotic surfaces such as mucosa and skin [34]. *Candida* biofilms are known to be highly resistant to existing antifungal agents. Therefore, indwelling medical devices infected with *Candida* biofilms often have to be removed [35]. Therefore, greater understanding of *Candida* biofilm formation is necessary to develop novel therapeutic options.

Candida Biofilm Structure

Our understanding of *Candida* biofilm structure is based mainly on the observations made using various techniques such as scanning electron microcopy, fluorescence microscopy and confocal scanning laser microscopy as well as growth kinetics assays. In general, biofilm formation of *Candida* spp. is similar to the sequence of events taking place in bacterial biofilms [32]. In brief, planktonic yeast forms of *Candida* come into contact with the surface and adhere. This is followed by micro-colony formation. *C. albicans* biofilm has a unique feature as it contains different morphological forms such as yeast and pseudohyphal and hyphal cells [32] (Figure 5.2). Next, biofilm cells

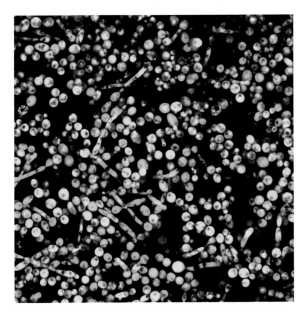

FIGURE 5.2 Biofilm of *Candida albicans* which contains different morphological forms such as yeast, pseudohyphae and hyphae.

secrete EPS which encase the cells. Finally, maturation of biofilm results in three-dimensional, spatially arranged biofilm structure. Some biofilm cells may disperse from the mature biofilms as described in the introduction chapter.

Candida biofilms grown in in vitro models usually consist of several layers. Candida biofilms can be either thicker or thinner than bacterial biofilms depending on the species and the environmental conditions. Hence, biofilm thickness may range from a few to several hundred micrometers. A summary of the events taking place during the formation of a typical Candida biofilm is given in the text that follows. In laboratory protocols, Candida in the planktonic mode is capable of adhering to a surface by one to two hours [36,37]. As described in Chapter 1, the adhesion process is initiated between cells and the surface by non-specific interactions through hydrophobic and electrostatic forces. Thereafter, in the next stage, expression of the specific adhesion molecules facilitates stronger adhesion to the surface. The cell wall of Candida is composed mainly of carbohydrates such as glucan, chitin and mannose [38]. Adhesins are glycosylated cell-wall proteins (CWP) located at the exterior side of the cell wall. Most of the adhesion proteins have the glycosyl-phosphatidyl-inositol (GPI) anchor [39,40]. In C. albicans, the three gene families encoding for adhesion properties are ALS, HWP and IFF/HYR. The agglutinin-like sequence (ALS) gene family is the most studied in C. albicans adhesion [41]. C. glabrata has adhesins encoded by the EPA (epithelial adhesion) gene family, and Epa proteins are structurally similar to Als proteins of C. albicans [42]. Hwp1 and Epa1 are two adhesins present in C. albicans that promote colonisation. Epa1, an adhesin unique to C. albicans, facilitates adhesion to abiotic surfaces and biofilm formation [43]. On the other hand, Ywp1, a yeast-specific protein of C. albicans, is known to negatively regulate the adhesion [44]. Ywp1 is not present in the hyphal or chlamydospores forms, and yeast cells lacking Ywp1 are more adhesive and form thicker biofilms, implying an anti-adhesive activity for Ywp1.

Chandra et al. described the classical biofilm formation process of C. albicans biofilm formation on polymethylmethacrylate strips. On the observations made, biofilm formation was divided into three overlapping phases: early (0–11 h), intermediate (12–30 h) and maturation (38–72 h) phases [45]. The early stage is characterised by adherence and development of blastospores into distinct microcolonies. By 18–24 h, the Candida biofilm community appears as a bilayered structure comprising a mixture of yeasts, germ tubes and young hyphae. In parallel, production of EPS was also observed, which became thick with the maturation of the biofilms. EPS encased a dense network in which yeasts, pseudohyphae and hyphae are embedded. Some studies have suggested the presence of water channels among biofilm cells which may aid the diffusion of nutrients from outside environment to the inner cell layers while taking the microbial waste products out of the biofilm community. Candida in vivo biofilms may follow a similar sequence of events [46]. In vivo Candida biofilms mature faster and exhibit thicker biomass and EPS compared to in vitro biofilms. For instance, the thickness of in vitro Candida biofilms may range from 25 to 450 μm [45,47,48], whereas in vivo models have shown biofilm thickness of greater than 100 μm [46].

Dispersal is the least understood and perhaps the most complicated process involved in both fungal and bacterial biofilms. As a part of their life cycle, members of the *Candida* biofilm community singly or as a group may detach from the biofilm and disseminate through a fluid phase to seed new sites. Genome-wide studies have shown that Set3, an NAD-dependent histone deacetylation complex, modulates the expression of *NRG1* [49], which encodes a transcriptional regulator of biofilm dispersal [50]. Nrg1 is a well-known transcriptional repressor of filamentation [51], and Set3 complex mutants are hyperfilamentous [52]. The typical dispersal of *C. albicans* cells from biofilms is found to be in the yeast form, possibly due to the effect of Nrg1 and Set3 complex [50]. Thus, manipulations that increase filamentous cells and decrease yeast-form cells may reduce biofilm dispersal [53]. Studies by Murad et al. revealed that the dispersal stage of the fungal biofilm has an association with disease progression. In *C. albicans*, deletion of the *NRG1* gene completely attenuated virulence in a murine model of systemic candidiasis [54]. However, as deleting *NRG1* causes a constitutive filamentous growth of *C. albicans* cells, it is not certain that the effect is due solely to biofilm dispersal. If targeted well, blocking the biofilm dispersal stage may provide an alternative strategy for developing novel therapeutic options in the future for controlling *Candida* biofilm–associated infections.

BIOFILM FORMATION OF DIFFERENT *CANDIDA* SPECIES

Biofilm formation ability may differ among *Candida* species. Some studies reported that *C. albicans*, *C. parapsilosis and C. tropicalis* have more biofilm formation ability than other species [23,55,56]. However, the conclusions from these studies should be interpreted with caution for several reasons. First, there is a considerable variation in the biofilm formation ability among strains even in the same *Candida* species [32,57,58]. It has been shown that strains with 'strong' and 'weak' biofilm-forming ability exist within each *Candida* species [58,59]. Second, studies may have interpreted the biofilm formation ability on the basis of their methodology, which varies among different studies. For instance, some studies have reported biofilm formation ability in terms of the commonly used XTT reduction assay whereas others may have used counting colony-forming units (CFUs). In addition, biofilm formation of clinical *Candida* isolates may be significantly different from that in laboratory isolates. Therefore, researchers working on *Candida* biofilm should consider including laboratory as well as clinical strains in their studies to obtain clinically relevant information.

   Candida spp. reside as mixed-species biofilms on mucosal habitats such as the oral cavity and the vagina. *Candida* spp. have been shown to form mixed-species biofilms with one another as well as with bacterial species [60,61]. Multiple *Candida* species such as *C. albicans*, *C. tropicalis*, *C. glabrata* and *C. krusei* have all been recovered either in combination or with other bacterial species such as *Enterobacter* species, *Pseudomonas aeruginosa* and *Klebsiella pneumoniae*. A recent study on oral candidiasis patients reported that the proportion of mixed colonisation with more than one *Candida* species was 18% of total cases [23].

PROTOCOL FOR *CANDIDA* BIOFILM FORMATION

The protocols that have been used for *Candida* biofilm studies vary among different research groups. The common factors that may differ between studies include the strain used, culture conditions and biofilm harvesting time. Herein, we describe a simple, straightforward methodology which will enable researchers to form *Candida* biofilms on polystyrene surfaces [62–64]. In brief, *Candida* strains should be subcultured on Sabouraud dextrose agar (SDA; Gibco, Paisley, UK) and maintained at 4°C prior to the biofilm formation experiments. Before usage, the purity of the culture should be verified by Gram-stain visualisation and the germ tube test. Single colonies are picked from the SDA plate to prepare a broth culture in liquid yeast nitrogen base (YNB; Difco) medium supplemented with 50 mM glucose. After overnight culture in a rotary shaker at 75 rpm, the yeasts are harvested in the late exponential growth phase and washed twice with 20 mL of 0.1 M phosphate-buffered saline (PBS; pH 7.2) prior to use in the biofilm studies. *Candida* cells are then resuspended in YNB supplemented with 100 mM glucose to prepare a standard inoculum of 1×10^7 cells/mL for a biofilm experiment using optical density (OD). The inoculum is then used immediately to develop biofilms on presterilised 96-well polystyrene plates (IWAKI, Tokyo, Japan). One hundred microliters of the *Candida* cell suspension is pipetted into each well of a microtitre plate. Each microtitre plate should control a few negative controls to which no *Candida* suspension is added. This protocol includes a 1.5-h 'adhesion phase' in which yeast cells are allowed to adhere to the surface of the material. For this purpose, the set-up is incubated for 1.5 h at 37°C in a shaker at 75 rpm. Following the adhesion phase, medium containing *Candida* cells is aspirated. Loosely adhering *Candida* cells are removed by gently washing the wells of the microtitre plate with 100 µL of PBS. Then, wells are replenished with 200 µL of medium, and the set-up is further incubated until harvesting biofilms. According to this protocol, biofilm maturation occurs by 24–48 h, depending on the strain used for the study. These biofilms can be used for downstream analysis such as quantification, imaging and molecular work.

QUANTIFICATION OF *CANDIDA* BIOFILMS

Candida biofilm formation is divided into several phases by the observations taken from growth kinetics assays and microscopic evaluations over a period of time. Growth kinetics of *Candida* biofilms have been recorded using various techniques such as CFU counting, dry weight measurement, colourimetric assays and radio-labelling. Of these, colourimetric assays remain the mainstay of biofilm quantification. Enumeration of CFUs has been the 'gold standard' method for planktonic culture-based microbiology studies. *C. albicans* biofilms may contain different morphological forms such as yeast, pseudohyphae and hyphal cells. Therefore, CFU counting of *C. albicans* biofilms may produce variable results. Dry weight measurement of the total biomass is another simple and straightforward method employed by several workers to quantify *Candida* biofilms [47,57,65]. For dry weight measurement, *Candida* biofilm is scraped off the substrate and transferred to preweighed cellulose nitrate filters. Thereafter, the biofilms are dried in an oven and the dry weight is taken. The dry weight of the biomass contains both biofilm cells and EPS and hence does not represent the active cellular component of the biofilm [47,57,65].

Chemical compounds which produce colourimetric changes on 'metabolic activity' have been used extensively for quantification of *Candida* biofilms [57,58,66–68].

These include XTT, MTT 3-(4,5-dimethylthiazol-2-yl)-2,5-diphenyltetrazolium bromide reduction assays, ATP bioluminescence assay, crystal violet (CV) assay and fluorescence-based assays. CV assay is another early colourimetric method used in biofilm experiments. Here, 1% crystal violet is used to measure the OD of the biofilms. Previous studies have found a good correlation between this assay and other colourimetric assays for the quantification of *C. albicans* biofilms [58,67,69]. However, crystal violet also stains both cellular and matrix components of the biofilms. Therefore, it should not be used as the sole method to quantify *Candida* biofilms.

The main colourimetric technique which has been used for the quantification of *Candida* biofilms is XTT [2, 3-bis (2-methoxy-4-nitro-5-sulphophenyl)-5-[(phenylamino) carbonyl]-2H-tetrazoliumhydroxide], a tetrazolium salt [70]. XTT reflects the metabolic activity of the biofilm cells. Hence, *Candida* cells in the biofilm community convert XTT to coloured formazan by the mitochondrial succino-oxidase and cytochrome P450 systems and flavoprotein oxidases [71]. Formazon is water soluble and accumulates in the supernatants. Subsequently the colour change of the wells containing biofilms can be compared with the negative controls using either a microtitre plate reader or a spectrophotometer at 490–492 nm [72].

Some studies have used the ATP bioluminescence assay to quantify *Candida* biofilms [73–75]. Others have used techniques such as the fluorescein diacetate (FDA) assay, resazurin assay, 1.9-dimethyl methylene blue (DMMB), and SYTO-9 assay. Colourimetric assays are relatively easy to perform and considerably accurate in reflecting the active status of the *Candida* biofilms. Therefore, the XTT reduction assay has become the standard technique to quantify *Candida* biofilms. It is particularly used to evaluate the antifungal activity against *Candida* biofilms [70]. However, some limitations of the XTT reduction assay should be kept in mind when arriving at conclusions [71]. For instance, there are interspecific and interstrain variations among *Candida* in the ability to metabolise XTT which should be noted when comparing growth kinetics of different species based on XTT readings [47,65,71]. Furthermore, at high cell densities, kinetics curves of XTT are known to be distinctly non-linear.

Although growth kinetics assays provide basic information on the *Candida* biofilms, a visual inspection of the features is mandatory to arrive at conclusions. In the past, various microscopic techniques have been used to study the architectural features of *Candida* biofilms. The commonly used microscopic techniques include scanning electron microscopy (SEM) and confocal scanning laser microscopy (CSLM) [45,59]. Here, we describe a protocol to obtain SEM images for *Candida* biofilms [63]. In brief, biofilm specimens formed on various surfaces such as polystyrene and acrylic should first be gently rinsed with PBS and placed in 1% osmium tetraoxide for one hour. Samples are subsequently washed in distilled water, dehydrated in a series of ethanol washes (70% for 10 min, 95% for 10 min and 100% for 20 min) and air-dried in a desiccator prior to sputter coating with gold. Thereafter, biofilm samples are mounted on aluminium stubs with copper tape and coated with gold in a low-pressure atmosphere with an ion sputter coater (JEOL JFC1 100: JEOL, Tokyo, Japan). The topographic features of the *Candida* biofilm can be visualised with appropriate SEM.

We also present a simple protocol to obtain CSLM images of *Candida* biofilms. Briefly, *Candida* biofilms are gently washed twice with PBS as described earlier. Thereafter, biofilms can be stained using the Molecular Probes' Live/Dead BacLight Viability kit comprising SYTO-9 and propidium iodide (PI) (Molecular Probes, Eugene, OR). SYTO-9 is a green fluorescent nucleic acid stain, generally labelling both live and dead cells. PI, in contrast, is a red fluorescent nucleic acid stain and penetrates only the cells with damaged membranes, thus visualising only the dead microbes. Biofilms are incubated with SYTO-9 and PI for 20 min in the dark at 30°C before the CSLM examination. Subsequently, images of stained biofilms can be captured using a CSLM system. A series of images can be obtained for each position at 1-µm intervals in the z section for a three-dimensional view of the biofilm (from the substratum to the top of the biofilm). At least five randomly selected positions from each corner and the middle of the coupons should be examined for each sample.

SEM enables researchers to inspect the topographic features of *Candida* biofilms. However, the major drawback of SEM imaging is the qualitative nature of the information. Software capable of quantifying SEM images has not been adequately developed. On the other hand, several types of software such as COMSTAT and Fuji which make use of mathematical modelling to analyse the CSLM images have been developed [76–78]. Confocal image analyses have many advantages over SEM, such as the ability to obtain real-time data without disruption to the structure of the biofilm and the ability to produce quantitative results. COMSTAT and Fuji analyses have been used successfully in *Candida* biofilm studies [63,79]. However, a major drawback of COMSTAT analysis is its inability to generate data on live/dead cell ratio, or, in other words, the cellular viability of the biofilm. There are newer software tools that can overcome this drawback. For instance, bioImage_L, an image analysis software, is able to calculate biofilm structural parameters stained with dual-channel fluorescent markers [80]. It has been shown that this software identifies tonality intensity *in situ*, independently processes the colour subpopulations and characterises the viability and metabolic activity of biofilms. This software has been used to analyse *C. albicans* biofilms [79].

DIFFUSION OF MOLECULES ACROSS *CANDIDA* BIOFILMS

Diffusion of molecules such as nutrients and antifungals across multilayered biofilm is an important process for the biofilm community [81]. A few studies have examined the diffusion of nutrients such as sugars across *Candida* biofilms [82]. It has been assumed that biofilms developing under the sugar 'excess' conditions exhibit different properties than sugar-starved biofilms. Diffusion of antifungal across the *Candida* biofilms has also been explored occasionally [83,84]. Diffusion efficiency of the antifungal seems to be dependent on the nature of the biofilm as well as physiochemical properties of antifungal agents. One study found amphotericin B penetrates through *Candida* biofilms poorly compared to flucytosine and fluconazole [84]. Conversely, another study claimed all the tested antifungals including amphotericin B diffuse rapidly in monospecific *Candida* biofilms compared to mixed-species biofilms [83]. There is an inherent technical difficulty in measuring diffusion through *Candida* biofilms. A few methods have been described in the literature, which merit further development in future studies [82,85]. We have used a model of artificial *Candida* biofilms to determine the diffusion coefficient (De) of simple sugars using the horizontal attenuated total reflectance–Fourier transform infrared (HATR-FTIR) technique. Under the given conditions, galactose has a higher De than glucose and sucrose in both the cell-free agarose films and artificial *Candida* biofilms, implying that galactose diffuses more efficiently across the biofilms. In addition, the higher percentage obstruction of galactose compared to glucose and sucrose suggests that galactose molecules are more effectively retained within the biomass. This implies that the nutrient (galactose) is likely to be available throughout the thickness of the biofilm from the top to the bottom layers. Taken together, these observations are in agreement with those of Hawser and Douglas [57], who claimed that galactose favours *Candida* biofilm formation over glucose. However, artificial biofilm models do not fully mimic the natural mechanisms operating in the natural *Candida* biofilms. Therefore, further research is warranted to develop proper models to study molecular diffusion across *Candida* biofilms.

Ex Vivo Model of Oral *Candida* Biofilms

Reconstituted human oral epithelium (RHOE) has been developed as a viable *ex vivo* model to study oral candidiasis. The RHOE model has been used to investigate the host interaction with *ex vivo Candida* biofilms [79]. Commercially available RHOE (Skinethic Laboratory Nice, France) is reconstituted by incubation for 24 h in serum-free, MCDB 153 defined medium in tissue culture plates. Thereafter, tissues can be infected with standard *Candida* inoculum and incubated at 37°C in 5% CO_2 for the desired time point. Samples are harvested by washing gently to remove non-adherent *Candida* cells and are fixed in 4% paraformaldehyde (Sigma) in PBS for 1 h at room temperature. The fixed tissues can then be taken and processed for periodic acid–Schiff (PAS) staining to visualise the *Candida* biofilm formation and tissue invasion (Figure 5.3).

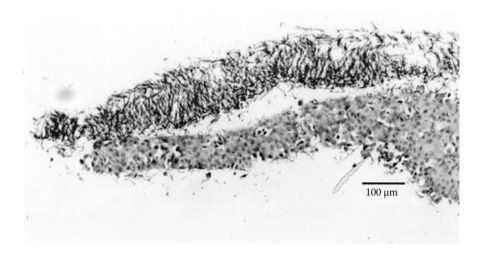

100 μm

FIGURE 5.3 Reconstituted human oral epithelium (RHOE) model for *ex vivo Candida* biofilms.

In Vivo Model of Oral Candida Biofilms

In vivo mouse model of oral candidiasis is a very useful tool to examine *Candida* biofilms under real-time conditions. In brief, selected strains of specific pathogen-free mice at ages 6–8 weeks can be used to develop oral candidiasis on tongue surfaces. Immunosuppression of mice is induced by subcutaneous injections of prednisolone prior to the *Candida* infection. On the day of infection, mice are inoculated with a standard inoculum of *Candida* by rubbing a cotton swab inside of the mouth to establish oral candidiasis. Mice are monitored twice a day for temperature, body weight, changes in oral mucosa and presence of candidiasis for a preselected time point (Figure 5.4).

Novel C. albicans 'Haploid Biofilm Model' and Its Implications

Historically, *C. albicans* has been thought to be an obligate diploid. Almost all the biofilm studies on this species have been carried out using diploid *C. albicans* strains. However, a recent ground-breaking discovery of 'haploid' *C. albicans* cells provides new opportunities to study the biofilms. In this chapter, we provide a brief account of the discovery of haploid *C. albicans* strains, the development of novel haploid biofilm models and their implications in future drug discovery.

In eukaryotes, the term 'ploidy' refers to the number of sets of chromosomes in a biological cell [86]. Cells containing two sets of chromosomes in their genome are called diploid cells whereas those with only one set of chromosomes are called haploid cells. In the eukaryotic model organism, the budding yeast *Saccharomyces cerevisiae*, haploid and diploid cells are the two forms that can survive and proliferate [87]. The haploid form is the sexual form of *S. cerevisiae*, and haploid cells undergo a simple life cycle of mitosis and proliferation. Haploid cells of the opposite mating types can mate and generate diploid cells. *S. cerevisiae* haploids have a lower tolerance to unfavourable environments and tend to die under stress conditions. In contrast, the diploid cells are the asexual form of *S. cerevisiae*. Under certain stress

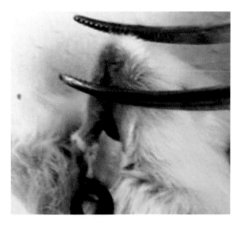

FIGURE 5.4 *In vivo* mouse model to examine *Candida* biofilms on tongue surfaces.

conditions, diploid cells undergo sporulation, producing four haploid spores via meiosis [86].

In *C. albicans*, however, diploid was believed to be the only mode of life [88,89]. Studies supporting the diploid nature of the microorganism include a genome size similar to that of the diploid *S. cerevisiae*, the requirement to delete two copies of the gene to create a null mutant [90,91] and a genome sequence of *C. albicans* which demonstrated heterozygosity throughout the entire genome [92,93]. Together with the predominantly diploid clonal nature of *C. albicans* within an individual host [94], it was assumed that the organism spends most, if not all, of its life cycle in the diploid state. The diploid nature of all clinical isolates and laboratory strains of *C. albicans* greatly hindered forward genetics research, the most reliable and unbiased approach in novel gene identification [95]. To date, around 4,500 open reading frames in the organism remains uncharacterised. This is a considerable challenge to identify the genetic regulators related to *C. albicans* biofilms.

In a ground-breaking discovery, Hickman and colleagues isolated viable haploid cells of *C. albicans*, changing the 'obligate' diploid concept in *C. albicans* [96]. *C. albicans* haploid cells are estimated to occur at a rate of 1–3 in 100,000 cells of the reference laboratory strain SC5314. In addition, similar to their diploid parent, haploid strains exhibit several key characteristics which define the species such as yeast–hyphae transition, white-opaque switching and chlamydospore formation [96]. The availability of *C. albicans* haploids greatly facilitates experimental approaches such as the classical genetic screen for recessive alleles and single-round gene-knockout phenotyping, which have been difficult tasks in diploids. However, as the haploid strains were generated through loss of one set of chromosomes from a highly heterozygous diploid, recessive mutations might be unmasked resulting in a different genetic background from their parent strain. Indeed, the haploid strains exhibit reduced growth rate and diminished virulence as compared to their diploid parent. Autodiploisation is also a major concern, which may affect result consistency and interpretation [96]. However, despite these limitations, promising studies have been conducted which demonstrated the utility of *C. albicans* haploids in biofilm research.

Taking advantage of the aforementioned discovery, we recently established a novel haploid *C. albicans* biofilm model [79]. We demonstrated that *C. albicans* haploid strains GZY792 and GZY803 are relatively stable and maintained their ploidy for at least 96 h as free-floating planktonic cells as well as in their biofilm mode of growth. Also, despite a slower biofilm development rate at earlier stages, the haploid cells were capable of forming mature biofilms to the same level as the diploids by 72 h in both *in vitro* and *ex vivo* models. *In vitro* haploid and diploid biofilms were structurally similar, with comparable spatial arrangements of yeast and hyphal cells embedded in extracellular matrix giving the classical three-dimensional appearance of *C. albicans* biofilms (Figure 5.5). By 72 h, haploids were also able to construct biofilms with an average height of approximately 13 μm, which was comparable with that of diploid biofilms. Consistent with the observations on *in vitro* biofilm formation, the haploid strains were able to form comparable biofilms on *ex vivo* reconstituted human oral epithelia, albeit at a slower rate as compared to the diploid strains. The diploid strains formed a thick layer of mature biofilm on the oral

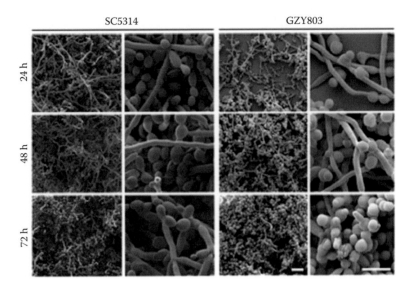

FIGURE 5.5 *Candida* biofilms of diploid SC5314 strain and 'new haploid' GZY803 strain.

epithelial surface by 48 h, whereas the haploid biofilm exhibited the same by 72 h. Fungal invasion into the tissues could be detected as early as in 24-h biofilm, which was more obvious in diploid strains. Tissue invasion by GZY803 cells became obvious by 48–72 h [79]. Taken together, these observations indicate that the haploid biofilm is a suitable model, as it displays key features of the mature biofilm formed by diploid *C. albicans.*

Understanding the genetic contribution to biofilm formation is a great challenge and a critical research gap in *C. albicans* research. Hence, next, we demonstrated the use of the novel haploid *C. albicans* biofilm model as a screening toolbox to uncover key biofilm regulators [79]. We generated a library of GTPase mutants from the *C. albicans* haploid and examined their role in biofilm formation. The screen identified *IRA2*, a negative regulator of the GTPase Ras1 [97], as a critical determinant of biofilm formation. Deletion of *IRA2* in the haploid strain resulted in diminished biofilm biomass with reduced structural complexity, and reinsertion of the *IRA2* gene largely restored the biofilm formation features. The phenotype was also confirmed in *IRA2* deletion mutants in the diploid strain. Hence, this finding not only opens up a new view to the role of GTPase in biofilm development but also justifies the reliability of the haploid model in *C. albicans* biofilm research [79].

The feasibility to carry out genetic screening to accelerate the discovery of new genes or pathways and to speed up identification of novel antifungal drug targets is an undeniable strength of *C. albicans* haploids. In addition, as haploids are capable of forming mature biofilms with key features similar to those of *C. albicans* diploids, employing the haploid as a model to uncover other features related to the organism's biofilms is a possible application. It is well known that *C. albicans* biofilms are resistant to many antifungal agents [98]; however, the molecular insights into antifungal tolerance and resistance of biofilms are still limited. Furthermore, the contribution to persister population generation is another interesting aspect of *C. albicans* biofilm which remains to be examined [99,100]. By exploiting the haploid toolbox, we recently identified *AHP1* as a critical gene that accounts for the persister population of *C. albicans* that resist amphotericin B treatment (unpublished data). Therefore, the novel haploid *C. albicans* biofilm model will certainly facilitate future studies in this field.

ANTIFUNGAL ACTIVITY AGAINST *CANDIDA* BIOFILMS

Only a few classes of antifungal drugs are available for the treatment of *Candida* infections. All current antifungal agents have various limitations, and none matches all the characteristics of an ideal agent. Currently there are few classes of antifungal agents that differ in their mechanism of action. In general, antifungal agents can be classified into four main groups: the azoles (ketoconazole, miconazole, clotrimazole, itraconazole, fluconazole, voriconazole, posaconazole), the polyenes (nystatin and amphotericin B), the echinocandins (caspofungin, micafungin and anidulafungin) and other miscellaneous classes of drugs such as the DNA analogue 5-fluorocytosine (5-FC).

Polyenes such as nystatin and amphotericin B interact with ergosterol of the fungal cell membrane and affect membrane-selective permeability. This results in leakage of intracellular potassium and magnesium and the loss of the proton gradient across the cell membrane [101]. In addition, amphotericin B may generate reactive oxygen species and cause oxidative damages to the fungal cell membrane [102]. Both nystatin and amphotericin B have been widely used in clinical practice. Nystatin is used mainly to treat superficial candidiasis and amphotericin B is used for systemic candidiasis. However, acute and chronic toxicities of amphotericin B limit its use; up to 80% of patients receiving the drug develop infusion-related toxicity or nephrotoxicity [103]. New versions of polyene antifungals such as the liposomal formulation of amphotericin B have enhanced tolerability, although infusion-related reactions and renal dysfunction are still commonplace [104,105].

Azoles are classified into two groups: imidazoles (ketoconazole, fenticonazole, miconazole, clotrimazole and econazole) and the triazoles (fluconazole, itraconazole, voriconazole and posaconazole). Azoles inhibit the fungal cytochrome P450 enzyme 14α-demethylase which converts 14α-demethylsterol to ergoaterol, which interrupt the cell membrane synthesis [106,107]. This results in compromised plasma membrane activity in the fungal cells. In addition, imidazoles interfere with fungal oxidative enzymes, leading to lethal accumulation of hydrogen peroxide [107].

The newest addition to the antifungal regime is the echinocandins, which inhibit β-1,3-glucan synthesis of the *Candida* cell wall [108]. Specifically, they bind to β-1,3-glucan synthase, an enzyme complex within the fungal cell wall [109]. β-1,3-D-glucan is a vital component in cell wall integrity, and inhibition of this process leads to osmotic lysis of the cell. Hence, echinocandins are fungicidal in nature. Several members of the echinocandins are currently available for clinical use [109]. These include caspofungin, micafungin and anidulafungin. In general, echinocandins are well tolerated and have fewer side effects than polyenes. Miscellaneous classes of antifungal agents include flucytosine, which is a DNA analogue. Flucytosine is a potent inhibitor of thymidylate synthase, an enzyme involved in DNA synthesis and nuclear division [106,107]. Because flucytosine has only a fungistatic effect, it is usually used in combination with other antifungals such as amphotericin B for systemic candidiasis. In addition, various other antifungal agents have also been reported or are under development [110].

It is generally regarded that 65–80% of all microbial infections are related to biofilms [111]. As mentioned previously, *Candida* forms biofilms on both abiotic and biofilm surfaces, in particular on medical devices [34]. The major clinical problem associated with *Candida* biofilms is the high resistance to antifungal agents. The first report of higher antifungal resistance of *Candida* in the biofilm growth mode came from the work of Hawser and Douglas in 1995. They observed *Candida* biofilms are 30–2,000 times as resistant as the planktonic cells to antifungals such as amphotericin B, fluconazole, itraconazole and ketoconazole [68]. Thereafter, many studies have corroborated these findings [62,70,112]. For instance, *Candida* biofilms can be resistant to fluconazole as much as 250–400 times that of planktonic cells *in vitro* [70,112]. These observations have been confirmed by *in vivo* studies [46]. Researchers have reported some success using relatively newer antifungal agents, such as echinocandins and liposomal formulations of amphotericin B, against *Candida* biofilms [65,113]. On the contrary, other studies have shown that some *Candida* strains form biofilms that are resistant to the aforementioned antifungal agents [62,114].

ANTIFUNGAL SUSCEPTIBILITY TESTING FOR *CANDIDA* BIOFILMS

Conventionally, antifungal susceptibility testing is performed on planktonic cultures of *Candida*. Expert communities such as the Clinical Laboratory Standard Institute (CLSI), USA and European Committee on Antimicrobial Susceptibility Testing (EUCAST) have provided certain protocols and cutoff values for antifungal susceptibility testing. However, the minimum inhibitory concentrations (MICs) from these assays are determined for the planktonic cultures, not for the biofilm cultures. Therefore, researchers have developed the commonly used XTT reduction assay as an option for the determination of MIC values for *Candida* biofilms [115,116]. However, researchers must be careful when comparing biofilm MIC values with CLSI-derived planktonic MIC values of *Candida*. CLSI microdilution assays employ a standard concentration of the planktonic mode of *Candida* (0.5×10^3 cells/mL) compared to the considerably higher cell numbers that exist in *Candida* biofilms. Therefore, both planktonic and biofilm cultures should be prepared to obtain approximately equal cell numbers in a comparative analysis as described previously [62].

FACTORS CONTRIBUTING TO THE ANTIFUNGAL RESISTANCE OF *CANDIDA* BIOFILMS

Several factors have been proposed to account for the higher antifungal resistance seen in *Candida* biofilms. These include altered growth, the presence of EPS, expression of resistance genes/proteins and 'persister' populations. Early studies on bacterial biofilms have suggested that the biofilm mode of growth has a reduced metabolic and growth rate, which accounts for their higher drug resistance [117]. However, subsequent studies found biofilm resistance of *Candida* biofilms may not be related to the growth rate [112,118]. Biofilms consist of a heterogeneous population of cells with different growth rates [119]. Therefore, a subpopulation of cells with a slower metabolic rate may be contributory to the antifungal resistance, which needs to be investigated for firm conclusions.

The formation of the EPS by biofilm cells and its role in drug resistance has been discussed in the preceding chapters of this book. Previous work has identified a prominent role for the *Candida* matrix in the development of the drug-resistant phenotype associated with the biofilm mode of growth [120,121]. For instance, one study showed that *C. albicans* biofilms formed under a constant flow of liquid with increased matrix synthesis significantly enhance resistance to amphotericin B [122]. Moreover, another study demonstrated the survival of cells in *Candida* biofilms against amphotericin B decreased by as much as 20% when the EPS was removed [123]. In contrast, *Candida* biofilm cells grown statically in the presence of minimal matrix exhibited the same level of drug resistance to the antifungals flucytosine, fluconazole, and amphotericin B as did cells grown in a shaker with a large amount of matrix [124]. Therefore, it can be assumed that the amount of EPS is not the sole reason for the higher drug resistance in *Candida* biofilms.

The EPS of *Candida* biofilms is composed of carbohydrates, proteins, lipids and DNA. A recent comprehensive study on *C. albicans* EPS, using state-of-the-art 'omic' tools including glycomics, proteomics and lipidomics, identified 55% protein, 25% carbohydrate, 15% lipid and 5% nucleic acid in the *C. albicans* biofilm matrix [120]. Surprisingly, this study found that the most abundant polysaccharides are α-1,2 branched α-1,6-mannans (87%) associated with unbranched β-1,6-glucans (13%) in an apparent mannan–glucan complex (MGCx), compared to the previously thought of β-1,3-glucan as the most abundant matrix carbohydrate. The study also revealed 458 functional proteins in the matrix. The matrix lipids consisted of neutral glycerolipids (89.1%), polar glycerolipids (10.4%) and sphingolipids (0.5%) [125]. Interestingly, they also discovered that the extracellular DNA (eDNA) in *C. albicans* biofilm is almost exclusively composed of random noncoding sequences.

The *C. albicans* zinc-response transcription factor Zap1 has been identified as a negative regulator of a major matrix component, soluble β-1,3 glucan, using *in vitro* as well as *in vivo* biofilm models [121]. Furthermore, the authors found Zap1 target genes through expression profiling and full genome chromatin immunoprecipitation. In addition, two glucoamylases, Gca1, Gca2, and Adh5 were found to have positive roles in matrix production whereas Csh1 and Ifd6 have negative roles. They proposed that alcohol dehydrogenases generate quorum-sensing aryl and acyl alcohols that in turn govern the regulatory circuit of *Candida* biofilm formation and matrix development. The presence of β-1,3 glucan in EPS has also been linked to the antifungal resistance, as it is capable of sequestering antifungals [126].

Some studies have suggested that a higher expression of classical drug resistance genes in the biofilm mode may play a role in the higher resistance in *Candida* biofilms. For instance, involvement of ATP-binding cassette (ABC) and major facilitator superfamily (MFS) drug efflux pumps have been suggested as a possible reason for azole resistance in *Candida* biofilms [127]. *MDR1*, *CDR1* and *CDR2* genes have been shown to be up-regulated in *Candida* biofilms. However, deletion of the aforementioned genes did not make *Candida* biofilms susceptible to azoles. A study using a microarray showed that *MDR* and *CDR* gene expression contributes to the azole resistance only in the early phase of *Candida* biofilm formation [128]. An *in vivo Candida* biofilm study demonstrated that *CDR1* and *CDR2* expression is significantly up-regulated in biofilms compared with planktonic cells, but *EFG11* and *MDR1* expression is similar in both biofilm and planktonic cells [46]. Therefore, it is unlikely that a single or few genes solely regulate the higher drug resistance in *Candida* biofilms.

One of the interesting concepts that has been proposed to explain the higher drug resistance in microbial biofilms is the presence of persister cells. Persister cells are a subpopulation of highly drug-resistant cells in the biofilm mode. These cells are not mutants, but rather phenotypic variants of wild-type cells [129]. Persisters are capable of surviving exceedingly high drug concentrations compared to the rest of the biofilm cells. *Candida* biofilms have been shown to contain persister cell populations [130,131]. A detailed discussion on biofilm persisters is provided in Chapter 8. This area of research in biofilm biology warrants further exploratory studies to unravel the complex molecular mechanisms that contribute to this intriguing phenomenon.

NOVEL ANTI-BIOFILM ANTIFUNGAL STRATEGIES AGAINST *CANDIDA* BIOFILMS

In general, drug discovery is a lengthy process and takes approximately 14 years for the launching of a new systemic antibiotic onto the market after its initial discovery via high-throughput screening [132]. Despite numerous efforts invested in drug discovery and development, only approximately 20% of all projects proceed to clinical trials, and 10% of these successfully pass through the subsequent hurdles [133]. These failures are mainly biological (poorly validated hits) and/or chemical (undesirable chemical properties that lead to toxicity) [133].

Therefore, various strategies have been used to develop anti-biofilm antifungal agents. However, most of the strategies have resulted in only limited success. Here, we succinctly describe some of them, including photodynamic therapy, nanotherapy, probiotics, plant extracts with active compounds, quorum sensing molecules and small-molecule-based drug discovery [134]. Small-molecule-based drug discovery is given more focus.

Researchers have attempted to use nanoparticles to generate new antifungals with better properties than the existing ones for *Candida* biofilms [135]. The silver nanomaterial is a good example of this technology. It inhibits fungal multiplication by interfering with DNA replication. Silver ions can also lead to protein denaturation and cell death because of their reaction with nucleophilic amino acid residues in proteins and their attachment to thiol, amino, imidazole, phosphate and carboxyl groups of membrane proteins or enzymes [136]. Silver nanoparticles have a well-tolerated tissue response with less cytotoxicity or genotoxicity and lower propensity to induce microbial resistance [137]. Recently, antifungal activity and an inhibitory effect on adhesion and biofilm formation by denture base resin containing nano-silver have been demonstrated [138,139]. The nano-silver's antifungal activity is higher against *C. glabrata* than *C. albicans*. Nano-silver particles are also more effective in inhibiting biofilm formation than controlling established biofilms [140]. *In vitro* studies have also demonstrated potent antifungal effects of nano-silver coating of denture base material, as shown by inhibition of *Candida* adherence to the surface and deformation of the normal morphology of *Candida*. Further attempts to apply silver nano-particle-coated denture base materials for clinical use are expected.

Probiotic microbes are defined as organisms that may be ingested in various formulations to improve either human or animal health. Lactic acid bacteria including bifidobacteria, lactobacilli and enterococci are the most typical probiotic bacteria. Animal studies carried out to assess the therapeutic potential of probiotic bacteria on candidiasis have shown promising results. We have devoted a separate chapter (Chapter 10) to discuss the effect of probiotics on oral biofilms, including that of *Candida*.

In antimicrobial drug discovery, small molecules are defined as non-peptide organic compounds that are synthetic or from natural product extracts with a low molecular weight (approx. 200–500 Daltons) according to Lipinski's rule [141]. These molecules bind to biopolymers such as proteins and nucleic acids and alter their normal functions [142–145]. Small molecules are also used in these disciplines to probe biological pathways and gain new insights into unclear mechanisms [145,146]. The data on small molecules obtained from probing assays, including chemical structure and predicted solubility, are now stored in open databases, such as ChemBank, PubChem (currently contains information of more than 700,000 compounds) [147,148] and ChemDB (contains more than 4 million small molecules) [149]. Both phenotype-based and target-based drug discovery approaches involve the screening of small-molecule libraries. Modern high-throughput screening (HTS) technologies enable rapid hit identification and accelerate early stage drug discovery. Subsequently, with careful hit-to-lead process and lead optimisation, eventually the ideal antifungal agent can be discovered [150,151]. HTS of small molecules has many advantages. (I) The utilisation of small molecules can bridge drug discovery with chemical biology to understand biological processes of the pathogens. (II) Synthetic organic chemistry and combinatorial chemistry have allowed the rapid and cost-effective generation of a large amount of compounds with diverse structures [152,153]. (III) Most importantly, high-throughput phenotype-based screening of small molecules with antifungal activity could allow the identification of hits that target multiple proteins [142].

HTS of a small-molecule library has been used for identifying anti-biofilm antifungal agents. LaFleur and colleagues identified 19 *C. albicans* biofilm inhibitors (effective alone or in synergy with clotrimazole) by screening 120,000 molecules from the NIH Molecular Libraries Small Molecule Repository [154]. The underlying mechanism of action of these small molecules is not known. We have recently demonstrated a novel antifungal small molecule that works against *Candida* biofilms [155].

CONCLUSIONS

Biofilm formation is a major virulence attribute for mucosal and systemic *Candida* infections. *Candida* biofilms are highly resistant to current antifungal agents and directly related to the therapeutic failure. Therefore, there is an urgent medical need to unravel novel antifungal strategies against the biofilms of this recalcitrant pathogen. Successful development of an effective anti-biofilm treatment could bring enormous benefits to the patient population suffering from ubiquitous *Candida* infections world over.

ACKNOWLEDGEMENTS

Some of the studies mentioned in this chapter were funded by the Health and Medical and Research Fund (HMRF), Hong Kong, and National Medical Research Council (NMRC), Singapore. Some of the material of this chapter has been republished from Seneviratne CJ, Jin L, Samaranayake LP. Biofilm lifestyle of *Candida*: A mini review. *Oral Dis*. 2008;14(7):582–90 and Wong SS, Samaranayake LP, Seneviratne CJ. In pursuit of the ideal antifungal agent for *Candida* infections: High-throughput screening of small molecules. *Drug Discov Today*. 2014;19(11):1721–30 with permission from John Wiley & Sons, and Elsevier Publishers. The work presented in Dr. Seneviratne's PhD thesis is also acknowledged.

CORRESPONDING AUTHOR

Chaminda Jayampath Seneviratne
Discipline of Oral Sciences
Faculty of Dentistry
National University of Singapore
Singapore
jaya@nus.edu.sg

REFERENCES

1. Samaranayake LP, MacFarlane TW. *Oral candidosis*. London: Wright-Butterworth; 1990.
2. Mayer FL, Wilson D, Hube B. *Candida albicans* pathogenicity mechanisms. *Virulence*. 2013;4(2):119–28.
3. Segal E. *Candida*, still number one: What do we know and where are we going from there? *Mycoses*. 2005;48(Suppl 1):3–11.
4. Polke M, Hube B, Jacobsen ID. *Candida* survival strategies. *Adv Appl Microbiol*. 2015;91:139–235.
5. Concia E, Azzini AM, Conti M. Epidemiology, incidence and risk factors for invasive candidiasis in high-risk patients. *Drugs*. 2009;69(Suppl 1):5–14.
6. Kojic EM, Darouiche RO. *Candida* infections of medical devices. *Clin Microbiol Rev*. 2004;17(2):255–67.
7. Zaoutis TE, Argon J, Chu J, Berlin JA, Walsh TJ, Feudtner C. The epidemiology and attributable outcomes of candidemia in adults and children hospitalized in the United States: A propensity analysis. *Clin Infect Dis*. 2005;41(9):1232–9.
8. Banerjee SN, Emori TG, Culver DH, Gaynes RP, Jarvis WR, Horan T, Edwards JR, Tolson J, Henderson T, Martone WJ. (1991). Secular trends in nosocomial primary blood-stream infections in the United-States, 1980–1989. *Am J Med*. 1991;91:S86–9.

9. Edmond MB, Wallace SE, McClish DK, Pfaller MA, Jones RN, Wenzel RP. Nosocomial bloodstream infections in United States hospitals: A three-year analysis. *Clin Infect Dis.* 1999;29:239–44.

10. Odds FC. *Candida* and *candidosis*. London: Baillière Tindall; 1998.

11. Samaranayake LP, Fidel PL, Naglik JR, Sweet SP, Teanpaisan R, Coogan MM, Blignaut E, Wanzala P. Fungal infections associated with HIV infection. *Oral Dis.* 2002;8:151–60.

12. Hagerty JA, Ortiz J, Reich D, Manzarbeitia C. Fungal infections in solid organ transplant patients. *Surg Infect*(Larchmt). 2003;4(3):263–71.

13. Patterson TF. Approaches to fungal diagnosis in transplantation. *Transpl Infect Dis.* 1999;1(4):262–72.

14. Becksague CM, Jarvis WR. Secular trends in the epidemiology of nosocomial fungal-infections in the United-States, 1980–1990. *J Infect Dis.* 1993;167(5):1247–51.

15. Pfaller MA, Diekema DJ. Twelve years of fluconazole in clinical practice: Global trends in species distribution and fluconazole susceptibility of bloodstream isolates of *Candida*. *Clin Microbiol Infect.* 2004;10(Suppl 1):11–23.

16. Pfaller MA, Jones RN, Doern GV, Sader HS, Messer SA, Houston A et al. Bloodstream infections due to *Candida* species: SENTRY antimicrobial surveillance program in North America and Latin America, 1997–1998. *Antimicrob Agents Chemother.* 2000;44(3):747–51.

17. Seneviratne CJ, Wong SS, Yuen KY, Meurman JH, Parnanen P, Vaara M et al. Antifungal susceptibility and virulence attributes of bloodstream isolates of *Candida* from Hong Kong and Finland. *Mycopathologia.* 2011;172(5):389–95.

18. Mariette C, Tavernier E, Hocquet D, Huynh A, Isnard F, Legrand F et al. Epidemiology of invasive fungal infections during induction therapy in adults with acute lymphoblastic leukemia: A GRAALL-2005 study. *Leuk Lymphoma.* 2016:1–8.

19. Sutcu M, Salman N, Akturk H, Dalgic N, Turel O, Kuzdan C et al. Epidemiologic and microbiologic evaluation of nosocomial infections associated with *Candida* spp. in children: A multicenter study from Istanbul, Turkey. *Am J Infect Control.* 2016;44(10):1139–43.

20. Li L, Redding S, Dongari-Bagtzoglou A. *Candida glabrata*: An emerging oral opportunistic pathogen. *J Dent Res.* 2007;86(3):204–15.

21. Redding SW, Dahiya MC, Kirkpatrick WR, Coco BJ, Patterson TF, Fothergill AW et al. *Candida glabrata* is an emerging cause of oropharyngeal candidiasis in patients receiving radiation for head and neck cancer. *Oral Surg Oral Med Oral Pathol Oral Radiol Endod.* 2004;97(1):47–52.

22. Quindos G. Epidemiology of candidaemia and invasive candidiasis. A changing face. *Rev Iberoam Micol.* 2014;31(1):42–8.

23. Muadcheingka T, Tantivitayakul P. Distribution of *Candida albicans* and non-albicans *Candida* species in oral candidiasis patients: Correlation between cell surface hydrophobicity and biofilm forming activities. *Arch Oral Biol.* 2015;60(6):894–901.

24. Berrouane YF, Herwaldt LA, Pfaller MA. Trends in antifungal use and epidemiology of nosocomial yeast infections in a university hospital. *J Clin Microbiol.* 1999;37(3):531–7.

25. Fidel PL Jr, Vazquez JA, Sobel JD. Candida glabrata: Review of epidemiology, pathogenesis, and clinical disease with comparison to *C. albicans*. *Clin Microbiol Rev.* 1999;12(1):80–96.

26. Kaur R, Domergue R, Zupancic ML, Cormack BP. A yeast by any other name: *Candida glabrata* and its interaction with the host. *Curr Opin Microbiol.* 2005;8(4):378–84.

27. Richardson MD. Changing patterns and trends in systemic fungal infections. *J Antimicrob Chemother.* 2005;56(Suppl 1):i5–11.

28. Tortorano AM, Caspani L, Rigoni AL, Biraghi E, Sicignano A, Viviani MA. Candidosis in the intensive care unit: A 20–year survey. *J Hosp Infect.* 2004;57(1):8–13.

29. Vallabhaneni S, Cleveland AA, Farley MM, Harrison LH, Schaffner W, Beldavs ZG et al. Epidemiology and risk factors for echinocandin nonsusceptible *Candida glabrata* bloodstream infections: Data from a large multisite population-based candidemia surveillance program, 2008–2014. *Open Forum Infect Dis.* 2015;2(4):ofv163.
30. Glockner A, Cornely OA. *Candida glabrata*: Unique features and challenges in the clinical management of invasive infections. *Mycoses.* 2015;58(8):445–50.
31. Srinivasnakshatri VK, Subramani P, Venkateshwaraprasad KN, Varma P. A fatal case of fungal empyema due to *Candida krusei* and *Candida tropicalis*: A rare occurrence with an atypical presentation. *J Clin Diagn Res.* 2014;8(11):DD01–2.
32. Seneviratne CJ, Jin L, Samaranayake LP. Biofilm lifestyle of *Candida*: A mini review. *Oral Dis.* 2008;14(7):582–90.
33. Costerton JW, Lewandowski Z, Caldwell DE, Korber DR, Lappin-Scott HM. Microbial biofilms. *Annu Rev Microbiol.* 1995;49:711–45.
34. Ramage G, Martinez JP, Lopez-Ribot JL. *Candida* biofilms on implanted biomaterials: A clinically significant problem. *FEMS Yeast Res.* 2006;6(7):979–86.
35. Tunney MM, Keane PF, Jones DS, Gorman SP. Comparative assessment of ureteral stent biomaterial encrustation. *Biomaterials.* 1996;17(15):1541–6.
36. Samaranayake YH, Wu PC, Samaranayake LP, So M. Relationship between the cell surface hydrophobicity and adherence of *Candida krusei* and *Candida albicans* to epithelial and denture acrylic surfaces. *Apmis* 1995;103:707–13.
37. Samaranayake LP, MacFarlane TW. The adhesion of the yeast *Candida albicans* to epithelial cells of human origin in vitro. *Arch Oral Biol.* 1981;26:815–20.
38. Tronchin G, Pihet M, Lopes-Bezerra LM, Bouchara JP. Adherence mechanisms in human pathogenic fungi. *Med Mycol.* 2008;46(8):749–72.
39. ten Cate JM, Klis FM, Pereira-Cenci T, Crielaard W, de Groot PW. Molecular and cellular mechanisms that lead to *Candida* biofilm formation. *J Dent Res.* 2009;88(2):105–15.
40. Zhao X, Oh SH, Yeater KM, Hoyer LL. Analysis of the *Candida albicans* Als2p and Als4p adhesins suggests the potential for compensatory function within the Als family. *Microbiol Sgm.* 2005;151:1619–30.
41. Hoyer LL, Green CB, Oh SH, Zhao X. Discovering the secrets of the *Candida albicans* agglutinin-like sequence (ALS) gene family: A sticky pursuit. *Med Mycol.* 2008;46(1):1–15.
42. de Groot PW, Bader O, de Boer AD, Weig M, Chauhan N. Adhesins in human fungal pathogens: Glue with plenty of stick. *Eukaryot Cell.* 2013;12(4):470–81.
43. Modrzewska B, Kurnatowski P. Adherence of *Candida* sp. to host tissues and cells as one of its pathogenicity features. *Ann Parasitol.* 2015;61(1):3–9.
44. Granger BL. Insight into the antiadhesive effect of yeast wall protein 1 of *Candida albicans*. *Eukaryot Cell.* 2012;11(6):795–805.
45. Chandra J, Kuhn DM, Mukherjee PK, Hoyer LL, McCormick T, Ghannoum MA. Biofilm formation by the fungal pathogen *Candida albicans*: Development, architecture, and drug resistance. *J Bacteriol.* 2001;183(18):5385–94.
46. Andes D, Nett J, Oschel P, Albrecht R, Marchillo K, Pitula A. Development and characterization of an in vivo central venous catheter *Candida albicans* biofilm model. *Infect Immun.* 2004;72(10):6023–31.
47. Kuhn DM, Chandra J, Mukherjee PK, Ghannoum MA. Comparison of biofilms formed by *Candida albicans* and *Candida parapsilosis* on bioprosthetic surfaces. *Infect Immun.* 2002;70(2):878–88.
48. Ramage G, Vande Walle K, Wickes BL, Lopez-Ribot JL. Biofilm formation by *Candida dubliniensis*. *J Clin Microbiol.* 2001;39(9):3234–40.
49. Hnisz D, Bardet AF, Nobile CJ, Petryshyn A, Glaser W, Schock U et al. A histone deacetylase adjusts transcription kinetics at coding sequences during *Candida albicans* morphogenesis. *PLoS Genet.* 2012;8(12):e1003118.

50. Uppuluri P, Pierce CG, Thomas DP, Bubeck SS, Saville SP, Lopez-Ribot JL. The transcriptional regulator Nrg1p controls *Candida albicans* biofilm formation and dispersion. *Eukaryot Cell*. 2010;9(10):1531–7.

51. Moran GP, MacCallum DM, Spiering MJ, Coleman DC, Sullivan DJ. Differential regulation of the transcriptional repressor NRG1 accounts for altered host-cell interactions in *Candida albicans* and *Candida dubliniensis*. *Mol Microbiol*. 2007;66(4):915–29.

52. Hnisz D, Majer O, Frohner IE, Komnenovic V, Kuchler K. The Set3/Hos2 histone deacetylase complex attenuates cAMP/PKA signaling to regulate morphogenesis and virulence of *Candida albicans*. *PLoS Pathog*. 2010;6(5):e1000889.

53. Nobile CJ, Fox EP, Hartooni N, Mitchell KF, Hnisz D, Andes DR et al. A histone deacetylase complex mediates biofilm dispersal and drug resistance in *Candida albicans*. *mBio*. 2014;5(3):e01201–14.

54. Murad AM, Leng P, Straffon M, Wishart J, Macaskill S, MacCallum D et al. NRG1 represses yeast-hypha morphogenesis and hypha-specific gene expression in *Candida albicans*. *EMBO J*. 2001;20(17):4742–52.

55. Seneviratne CJ, Rajan S, Wong SS, Tsang DN, Lai CK, Samaranayake LP et al. Antifungal susceptibility in serum and virulence determinants of *Candida* bloodstream isolates from Hong Kong. *Front Microbiol*. 2016;7:216.

56. Marcos-Zambrano LJ, Escribano P, Bouza E, Guinea J. Production of biofilm by *Candida* and non-*Candida* spp. isolates causing fungemia: Comparison of biomass production and metabolic activity and development of cut-off points. *Int J Med Microbiol*. 2014;304(8):1192–8.

57. Hawser SP, Douglas LJ. Biofilm formation by *Candida* species on the surface of catheter materials in vitro. *Infect Immun*. 1994;62(3):915–21.

58. Jin Y, Yip HK, Samaranayake YH, Yau JY, Samaranayake LP. Biofilm-forming ability of *Candida albicans* is unlikely to contribute to high levels of oral yeast carriage in cases of human immunodeficiency virus infection. *J Clin Microbiol*. 2003;41(7):2961–7.

59. Thein ZM, Samaranayake YH, Samaranayake LP. In vitro biofilm formation of *Candida albicans* and non-*albicans* species under dynamic and anaerobic conditions. *Arch Oral Biol*. 2007;52(8):761–7.

60. Thein ZM, Seneviratne CJ, Samaranayake YH, Samaranayake LP. Community lifestyle of *Candida* in mixed biofilms: A mini review. *Mycoses*. 2009;52(6):467–75.

61. Nobile CJ, Johnson AD. *Candida albicans* biofilms and human disease. *Annu Rev Microbiol*. 2015;69:71–92.

62. Seneviratne CJ, Jin LJ, Samaranayake YH, Samaranayake LP. Cell density and cell aging as factors modulating antifungal resistance of *Candida albicans* biofilms. *Antimicrob Agents Chemother*. 2008;52(9):3259–66.

63. Seneviratne CJ, Silva WJ, Jin LJ, Samaranayake YH, Samaranayake LP. Architectural analysis, viability assessment and growth kinetics of *Candida albicans* and *Candida glabrata* biofilms. *Arch Oral Biol*. 2009;54(11):1052–60.

64. Seneviratne CJ, Wang Y, Jin L, Abiko Y, Samaranayake LP. *Candida albicans* biofilm formation is associated with increased anti-oxidative capacities. *Proteomics*. 2008;8(14):2936–47.

65. Kuhn DM, George T, Chandra J, Mukherjee PK, Ghannoum MA. Antifungal susceptibility of *Candida* biofilms: Unique efficacy of amphotericin B lipid formulations and echinocandins. *Antimicrob Agents Chemother*. 2002;46(6):1773–80.

66. Honraet K, Goetghebeur E, Nelis HJ. Comparison of three assays for the quantification of *Candida* biomass in suspension and CDC reactor grown biofilms. *J Microbiol Methods*. 2005;63(3):287–95.

67. Peeters E, Nelis HJ, Coenye T. Comparison of multiple methods for quantification of microbial biofilms grown in microtiter plates. *J Microbiol Methods*. 2008;72(2):157–65.

68. Hawser SP, Douglas LJ. Resistance of *Candida albicans* biofilms to antifungal agents in vitro. *Antimicrob Agents Chemother.* 1995;39(9):2128–31.

69. Henriques M, Azeredo J, Oliveira R. *Candida albicans* and *Candida dubliniensis*: Comparison of biofilm formation in terms of biomass and activity. *Br J Biomed Sci.* 2006;63(1):5–11.

70. Ramage G, Vande Walle K, Wickes BL, Lopez-Ribot JL. Standardized method for in vitro antifungal susceptibility testing of *Candida albicans* biofilms. *Antimicrob Agents Chemother.* 2001;45(9):2475–9.

71. Kuhn DM, Balkis M, Chandra J, Mukherjee PK, Ghannoum MA. Uses and limitations of the XTT assay in studies of *Candida* growth and metabolism. *J Clin Microbiol.* 2003;41(1):506–8.

72. Tellier R, Krajden M, Grigoriew GA, Campbell I. Innovative endpoint determination system for antifungal susceptibility testing of yeasts. *Antimicrob Agents Chemother.* 1992;36(8):1619–25.

73. Nikawa H, Hamada T, Yamamoto T, Kumagai H. Effects of salivary or serum pellicles on the *Candida albicans* growth and biofilm formation on soft lining materials in vitro. *J Oral Rehabil.* 1997;24(8):594–604.

74. Nikawa H, Nishimura H, Hamada T, Makihira S, Samaranayake LP. Relationship between thigmotropism and *Candida* biofilm formation in vitro. *Mycopathologia.* 1998;144(3):125–9.

75. Jin Y, Samaranayake LP, Samaranayake Y, Yip HK. Biofilm formation of *Candida albicans* is variably affected by saliva and dietary sugars. *Arch Oral Biol.* 2004;49(10):789–98.

76. Hansen SK, Rainey PB, Haagensen JA, Molin S. Evolution of species interactions in a biofilm community. *Nature.* 2007;445(7127):533–6.

77. Heydorn A, Nielsen AT, Hentzer M, Sternberg C, Givskov M, Ersboll BK et al. Quantification of biofilm structures by the novel computer program COMSTAT. *Microbiology.* 2000;146 (Pt 10):2395–407.

78. Schindelin J, Arganda-Carreras I, Frise E, Kaynig V, Longair M, Pietzsch T et al. Fiji: An open-source platform for biological-image analysis. *Nat Methods.* 2012;9(7):676–82.

79. Seneviratne CJ, Zeng G, Truong T, Sze S, Wong W, Samaranayake L et al. New "haploid biofilm model" unravels IRA2 as a novel regulator of *Candida albicans* biofilm formation. *Sci Rep.* 2015;5:12433.

80. Chavez de Paz LE. Image analysis software based on color segmentation for characterization of viability and physiological activity of biofilms. *Appl Environ Microbiol.* 2009;75(6):1734–9.

81. Stewart PS, Costerton JW. Antibiotic resistance of bacteria in biofilms. *Lancet.* 2001;358(9276):135–8.

82. Seneviratne CJ, Zhang T, Fang HH, Jin LJ, Samaranayake LP. Distribution coefficients of dietary sugars in artificial *Candida* biofilms. *Mycopathologia.* 2009;167(6):325–31.

83. Al Fattani MA, Douglas LJ. Penetration of *Candida* biofilms by antifungal agents. *Antimicrob Agents Chemother.* 2004;48(10):3291–7.

84. Samaranayake YH, Ye J, Yau JYY, Cheung BPK, Samaranayake LP. In vitro method to study antifungal perfusion in *Candida* biofilms. *J Clin Microbiol.* 2005;43(2):818–25.

85. Douglas LJ. Penetration of antifungal agents through *Candida* biofilms. *Methods Mol Biol.* 2009;499:37–44.

86. Galitski T, Saldanha AJ, Styles CA, Lander ES, Fink GR. Ploidy regulation of gene expression. *Science.* 1999;285(5425):251–4.

87. Botstein D, Fink GR. Yeast: An experimental organism for 21st century biology. *Genetics.* 2011;189(3):695–704.

88. Jones T, Federspiel NA, Chibana H, Dungan J, Kalman S, Magee BB et al. The diploid genome sequence of *Candida albicans*. *Proc Natl Acad Sci U S A.* 2004;101(19):7329–34.

89. Noble SM, Johnson AD. Genetics of *Candida albicans*, a diploid human fungal pathogen. *Annu Rev Genet.* 2007;41:193–211.
90. Kelly R, Miller SM, Kurtz MB, Kirsch DR. Directed mutagenesis in *Candida albicans*: One-step gene disruption to isolate ura3 mutants. *Mol Cell Biol.* 1987;7(1): 199–208.
91. Kurtz MB, Marrinan J. Isolation of hem3 mutants from *Candida albicans* by sequential gene disruption. *Mol Gen Genet.* 1989;217(1):47–52.
92. Kakar SN, Magee PT. Genetic analysis of *Candida albicans*: Identification of different isoleucine-valine, methionine, and arginine alleles by complementation. *J Bacteriol.* 1982;151(3):1247–52.
93. Whelan WL, Magee PT. Natural heterozygosity in *Candida albicans*. *J Bacteriol.* 1981;145(2):896–903.
94. Bougnoux ME, Pujol C, Diogo D, Bouchier C, Soll DR, d'Enfert C. Mating is rare within as well as between clades of the human pathogen *Candida albicans*. *Fungal Genet Biol.* 2008;45(3):221–31.
95. Stark GR, Gudkov AV. Forward genetics in mammalian cells: Functional approaches to gene discovery. *Hum Mol Genet.* 1999;8(10):1925–38.
96. Hickman MA, Zeng G, Forche A, Hirakawa MP, Abbey D, Harrison BD et al. The 'obligate diploid' *Candida albicans* forms mating-competent haploids. *Nature.* 2013;494(7435):55–9.
97. Tanaka K, Nakafuku M, Tamanoi F, Kaziro Y, Matsumoto K, Toh-e A. IRA2, a second gene of *Saccharomyces cerevisiae* that encodes a protein with a domain homologous to mammalian ras GTPase-activating protein. *Mol Cell Biol.* 1990;10(8): 4303–13.
98. Mathe L, Van Dijck P. Recent insights into *Candida albicans* biofilm resistance mechanisms. *Curr Genet.* 2013;59(4):251–64.
99. LaFleur MD, Kumamoto CA, Lewis K. *Candida albicans* biofilms produce antifungal-tolerant persister cells. *Antimicrob Agents Chemother.* 2006;50(11):3839–46.
100. Chandra J, Kuhn DM, Mukherjee PK, Hoyer LL, McCormick T, Ghannoum MA. Biofilm formation by the fungal pathogen *Candida albicans*: Development, architecture, and drug resistance. *J Bacteriol.* 2001;183(18):5385–94.
101. Vanden Bossche H, Marichal P, Odds FC. Molecular mechanisms of drug resistance in fungi. *Trends Microbiol.* 1994;2(10):393–400.
102. Ellis D. Amphotericin B: Spectrum and resistance. *J Antimicrob Chemother.* 2002;49(Suppl 1):7–10.
103. LeBrun M, Grenier L, Bergeron MG, Thibault L, Labrecque G, Beauchamp D. Effect of fasting on temporal variation in the nephrotoxicity of amphotericin B in rats. *Antimicrob Agents Chemother.* 1999;43(3):520–4.
104. Olson JA, Adler-Moore JP, Jensen GM, Schwartz J, Dignani MC, Proffitt RT. Comparison of the physicochemical, antifungal, and toxic properties of two liposomal amphotericin B products. *Antimicrob Agents Chemother.* 2008;52(1):259–68.
105. Wasan KM, Conklin JS. Evaluation of renal toxicity and antifungal activity of free and liposomal amphotericin B following a single intravenous dose to diabetic rats with systemic candidiasis. *Antimicrob Agents Chemother.* 1996;40(8):1806–10.
106. Ellepola AN, Samaranayake LP. Oral candidal infections and antimycotics. *Crit Rev Oral Biol Med.* 2000;11(2):172–98.
107. Lewis RE. Pharmacodynamic implications for use of antifungal agents. *Curr Opin Pharmacol.* 2007;7(5):491–7.
108. Cappelletty D, Eiselstein-McKitrick K. The echinocandins. *Pharmacotherapy.* 2007;27(3):369–88.
109. Aguilar-Zapata D, Petraitiene R, Petraitis V. Echinocandins: The expanding antifungal armamentarium. *Clin Infect Dis.* 2015;61(Suppl 6):S604–11.

110. Wong SS, Samaranayake LP, Seneviratne CJ. In pursuit of the ideal antifungal agent for *Candida* infections: High-throughput screening of small molecules. *Drug Discov Today.* 2014;19(11):1721–30.

111. Potera C. Forging a link between biofilms and disease. *Science.* 1999;283(5409):1837, 9.

112. Chandra J, Mukherjee PK, Leidich SD, Faddoul FF, Hoyer LL, Douglas LJ et al. Antifungal resistance of candidal biofilms formed on denture acrylic in vitro. *J Dent Res.* 2001;80(3):903–8.

113. Bachmann SP, VandeWalle K, Ramage G, Patterson TF, Wickes BL, Graybill JR et al. In vitro activity of caspofungin against *Candida albicans* biofilms. *Antimicrob Agents Chemother.* 2002;46(11):3591–6.

114. Watamoto T, Samaranayake LP, Jayatilake JA, Egusa H, Yatani H, Seneviratne CJ. Effect of filamentation and mode of growth on antifungal susceptibility of *Candida albicans. Int J Antimicrob Agents.* 2009;34(4):333–9.

115. Chandra J, Mukherjee PK, Ghannoum MA. In vitro growth and analysis of *Candida* biofilms. *Nat Protoc.* 2008;3(12):1909–24.

116. Pierce CG, Uppuluri P, Tristan AR, Wormley FL, Jr., Mowat E, Ramage G et al. A simple and reproducible 96-well plate-based method for the formation of fungal biofilms and its application to antifungal susceptibility testing. *Nat Protoc.* 2008;3(9):1494–500.

117. Hawser S. Comparisons of the susceptibilities of planktonic and adherent *Candida albicans* to antifungal agents: A modified XTT tetrazolium assay using synchronised *C. albicans* cells. *J Med Vet Mycol.* 1996;34(2):149–52.

118. Baillie GS, Douglas LJ. Effect of growth rate on resistance of *Candida albicans* biofilms to antifungal agents. *Antimicrob Agents Chemother.* 1998;42(8):1900–5.

119. Kumamoto CA. *Candida* biofilms. *Curr Opin Microbiol.* 2002;5(6):608–11.

120. Zarnowski R, Westler WM, Lacmbouh GA, Marita JM, Bothe JR, Bernhardt J et al. Novel entries in a fungal biofilm matrix encyclopedia. *mBio.* 2014;5(4):e01333–14.

121. Nobile CJ, Nett JE, Hernday AD, Homann OR, Deneault JS, Nantel A et al. Biofilm matrix regulation by *Candida albicans* Zap1. *PLoS Biol.* 2009;7(6):e1000133.

122. Al Fattani MA, Douglas LJ. Biofilm matrix of *Candida albicans* and *Candida tropicalis*: Chemical composition and role in drug resistance. *J Med Microbiol.* 2006;55(8):999–1008.

123. Baillie GS, Douglas LJ. *Candida* biofilms and their susceptibility to antifungal agents. *Methods Enzymol.* 1999;310:644–56.

124. Baillie GS, Douglas LJ. Matrix polymers of *Candida* biofilms and their possible role in biofilm resistance to antifungal agents. *J Antimicrob Chemother.* 2000;46(3):397–403.

125. Lopez-Ribot JL. Large-scale biochemical profiling of the *Candida albicans* biofilm matrix: New compositional, structural, and functional insights. *mBio.* 2014;5(5):e01781–14.

126. Nett J, Lincoln L, Marchillo K, Massey R, Holoyda K, Hoff B et al. Putative role of beta-1,3 glucans in *Candida albicans* biofilm resistance. *Antimicrob Agents Chemother.* 2007;51(2):510–20.

127. Mukherjee PK, Chandra J, Kuhn DA, Ghannoum MA. Mechanism of fluconazole resistance in *Candida albicans* biofilms: Phase-specific role of efflux pumps and membrane sterols. *Infect Immun.* 2003;71(8):4333–40.

128. Garcia-Sanchez S, Aubert S, Iraqui I, Janbon G, Ghigo JM, d'Enfert C. *Candida albicans* biofilms: A developmental state associated with specific and stable gene expression patterns. *Eukaryot Cell.* 2004;3(2):536–45.

129. Keren I, Kaldalu N, Spoering A, Wang YP, Lewis K. Persister cells and tolerance to antimicrobials. *FEMS Microbiol Lett.* 2004;230(1):13–8.

130. Li P, Seneviratne CJ, Alpi E, Vizcaino JA, Jin L. Delicate metabolic control and coordinated stress response critically determine antifungal tolerance of *Candida albicans* biofilm persisters. *Antimicrob Agents Chemother.* 2015;59(10):6101–12.

131. LaFleur MD, Kumamoto CA, Lewis K. *Candida albicans* biofilms produce antifungal-tolerant persister cells. *AntimicrobAgents Chemother.* 2006;50(11):3839–46.
132. Payne DJ, Gwynn MN, Holmes DJ, Pompliano DL. Drugs for bad bugs: Confronting the challenges of antibacterial discovery. *Nat Rev Drug Discov.* 2007;6(1):29–40.
133. Brown D, Superti-Furga G. Rediscovering the sweet spot in drug discovery. *Drug Discov Today.* 2003;8(23):1067–77.
134. Seneviratne CJ, Rosa EA. Editorial. Antifungal drug discovery: New theories and new therapies. *Front Microbiol.* 2016;7:728.
135. Monteiro DR, Negri M, Silva S, Gorup LF, de Camargo ER, Oliveira R et al. Adhesion of *Candida* biofilm cells to human epithelial cells and polystyrene after treatment with silver nanoparticles. *Colloids Surf B Biointerfaces.* 2014;114:410–2.
136. Percival SL, Bowler PG, Russell D. Bacterial resistance to silver in wound care. *J Hosp Infect.* 2005;60(1):1–7.
137. de Lima R, Seabra AB, Duran N. Silver nanoparticles: A brief review of cytotoxicity and genotoxicity of chemically and biogenically synthesized nanoparticles. *J Appl Toxicol.* 2012;32(11):867–79.
138. Li Z, Sun J, Lan J, Qi Q. Effect of a denture base acrylic resin containing silver nanoparticles on *Candida albicans* adhesion and biofilm formation. *Gerodontology.* 2016;33(2):209–16.
139. Li J, Hirota K, Goto T, Yumoto H, Miyake Y, Ichikawa T. Biofilm formation of *Candida albicans* on implant overdenture materials and its removal. *J Dent.* 2012;40(8):686–92.
140. Monteiro DR, Gorup LF, Silva S, Negri M, de Camargo ER, Oliveira R et al. Silver colloidal nanoparticles: antifungal effect against adhered cells and biofilms of *Candida albicans* and *Candida glabrata*. *Biofouling.* 2011;27(7):711–9.
141. Lipinski CA, Lombardo F, Dominy BW, Feeney PJ. Experimental and computational approaches to estimate solubility and permeability in drug discovery and development settings. *Adv Drug Deliv Rev.* 2001;46(1–3):3–26.
142. Cong F, Cheung AK, Huang SM. Chemical genetics-based target identification in drug discovery. *Annu Rev Pharmacol Toxicol.* 2011;52:57–78.
143. Jeffery DA, Bogyo M. Chemical proteomics and its application to drug discovery. *Curr Opin Biotechnol.* 2003;14(1):87–95.
144. Spring DR. Chemical genetics to chemical genomics: Small molecules offer big insights. *Chem Soc Rev.* 2005;34(6):472–82.
145. Ward GE, Carey KL, Westwood NJ. Using small molecules to study big questions in cellular microbiology. *Cell Microbiol.* 2002;4(8):471–82.
146. Workman P, Collins I. Probing the probes: Fitness factors for small molecule tools. *Chem Biol.* 2010;17(6):561–77.
147. Lazo JS, Brady LS, Dingledine R. Building a pharmacological lexicon: Small molecule discovery in academia. *Mol Pharmacol.* 2007;72(1):1–7.
148. Wang Y, Xiao J, Suzek TO, Zhang J, Wang J, Bryant SH. PubChem: A public information system for analyzing bioactivities of small molecules. *Nucleic Acids Res.* 2009;37(Web Server issue):W623–33.
149. Chen J, Swamidass SJ, Dou Y, Bruand J, Baldi P. ChemDB: A public database of small molecules and related chemoinformatics resources. *Bioinformatics.* 2005;21(22):4133–9.
150. Ohlmeyer M, Zhou MM. Integration of small-molecule discovery in academic biomedical research. *Mt Sinai J Med* (New York). 2010;77(4):350–7.
151. Hopkins AL, Groom CR. The druggable genome. *Nat Rev Drug Discov.* 2002; 1(9):727–30.
152. Drews J. Drug discovery: A historical perspective. *Science.* 2000;287(5460):1960–4.
153. Edwards PJ, Gardner M, Klute W, Smith GF, Terrett NK. Applications of combinatorial chemistry to drug design and development. *Curr Opin Drug Discov Dev.* 1999;2(4):321–31.

154. LaFleur MD, Lucumi E, Napper AD, Diamond SL, Lewis K. Novel high-throughput screen against *Candida albicans* identifies antifungal potentiators and agents effective against biofilms. *J Antimicrob Chemother.* 2011;66(4):820–6.

155. Wong SS, Kao RY, Yuen KY, Wang Y, Yang D, Samaranayake LP et al. In vitro and in vivo activity of a novel antifungal small molecule against *Candida* infections. *PLoS ONE.* 2014;9(1):e85836.

6 Proteomics Approaches to Uncover the Drug Resistance Mechanisms of Microbial Biofilms

*Chaminda Jayampath Seneviratne,
Tanujaa Suriyanarayanan, Lin Qingsong
and Juan Antonio Vizcaíno*

CONTENTS

INTRODUCTION

The various properties of microbial biofilms and some of the techniques employed to study them have been described in the previous chapters. The focus of the current chapter is to enumerate the potential of proteomics in understanding the drug resistance mechanisms of microbial biofilms. One of the most important and intriguing properties of microbial biofilms is their increased resistance to challenging environmental conditions. For instance, microbial biofilms are more resistant to antimicrobial agents than their free-floating planktonic counterparts [1,2]. Hence, the minimum concentration of an antimicrobial drug required to eliminate a biofilm far exceeds the concentration required to eliminate planktonic organisms. In fact, at times, the high drug concentrations needed to treat biofilms as part of a given therapeutic regimen may not be tolerated by the human host. Both bacterial and fungal biofilms have been shown to be highly resistant to antibiotics and antifungals, respectively. The drug resistance mechanisms in biofilms usually proceed either via specialised drug efflux mechanisms that can pump out the drugs toxic to the microorganisms or through their extracellular matrix (ECM) components, which create barriers to the penetration of the drugs. Study of resistance mechanisms in biofilms therefore requires an approach that can comprehensively analyse the changes occurring in the microbial system on treatment with drugs. Surveillance of the proteome or metabolome profile of biofilms generally provides the best possible information in such scenarios. Correspondingly, in this chapter, we discuss the proteomics approaches that are commonly employed to uncover the drug resistance mechanisms of microbial biofilms.

Microorganisms are capable of efficiently sensing harmful environmental conditions and adjusting their protein expression accordingly to obviate the challenges faced [3]. Although general stress response pathways are well conserved among many bacterial species, there are also species-specific, stimuli-specific and lifestyle-specific protein expression patterns. Traditionally, researchers used to examine the functionality of a single gene or a protein to study the activity of an antimicrobial agent on microorganisms. However, the advent of omics approaches such as transcriptomics, proteomics and metabolomics, coupled with bioinformatics, heralded a new dawn in drug discovery allowing researchers to look into the 'big picture' of the microbial response to drug treatment. Transcriptomics, proteomics and metabolomics refer to the global analysis of gene, protein and metabolite expression, respectively. These approaches can be applied, for instance, in cells, tissues and organisms under defined conditions.

The term *proteome* was coined by Marc Wilkins to describe the 'protein complement of the genome' [4]. It represents the entire set of proteins expressed by an organism at a given point of time under a defined set of conditions [5]. Proteomics includes both qualitative and quantitative measurements of the proteome. It facilitates the accurate analysis of changes in cells/entire systems during growth, development and exposure to environmental factors. Post-translational modifications (PTMs), which are key events in defining the functions of proteins, can also be studied by proteomics techniques. Most importantly, gene expression profiles do not necessarily correlate with the gene products generated or with protein expression patterns [6]. Therefore, when suitably employed, proteomics can confer numerous advantages in obtaining the 'big picture' of the functionality of the organism.

Since the beginning of the twenty-first century, high-throughput proteomics studies have provided an unprecedented wealth of information [7]. Proteomics has gradually become an indispensable tool in microbiology, especially in understanding phenotypic behaviors, diagnostics and host–pathogen interactions [8–14]. An overview of the studies that have explored the biofilm proteome of medically important microorganisms to generate a better understanding of the resistance trait exhibited in the biofilm mode of growth is provided in this chapter (Table 6.1). In addition, studies

TABLE 6.1
Studies of Microbial Biofilm Proteome

Organism	Trait under Investigation	Technique Employed	Technical Details	Reference
Acinetobacter baumannii	Planktonic vs. biofilm	Gel-based and gel-free	DIGE/ iTRAQ, LC-MS/MS	Cabral et al., 2011 [15]
Acinetobacter baumannii	Planktonic vs. biofilm	Gel-based	Coomassie	Shin et al., 2009 [16]
Actinomyces naeslundii	Planktonic vs. biofilm	Gel-based	Colloidal Coomassie	Paddick et al., 2006 [17]
Aeromonas hydrophila	Drug-treated biofilms	Gel-free	TMT-labelling, LC-MS/MS analysis	Li et al., 2016 [18]
Aspergillus niger	Planktonic vs. biofilm (intracellular proteome)	Gel-based	Silver staining	Villena et al., 2009 [19]
Aspergillus fumigates	Planktonic vs. biofilm	Gel-based	DIGE	Bruns et al., 2010 [20]
Bacillus cereus	Planktonic vs. biofilm	Gel-based	Coomassie Blue	Oosthuizen et al., 2002 [21]
Bacillus subtilis	Planktonic vs. biofilm (membrane)	Gel-based	Coomassie Brilliant Blue	Morikawa et al., 2006 [22]
Bordetella pertussis	Planktonic vs. biofilm	Gel-based	Silver/colloidal Coomassie	Serra et al., 2008 [23]
Candida albicans	Planktonic vs. biofilm	Gel-based	DIGE	Mukherjee et al., 2006 [24]
C. albicans	Planktonic vs. biofilm	Gel-based	Coomassie/silver staining	Vediyappan and Chaffin, 2006 [25]
C. albicans	Planktonic vs. biofilm	Gel-based	SYPRO Ruby	Thomas et al., 2006 [26]
C. albicans	Planktonic vs. biofilm	Gel-based	Silver staining	Seneviratne et al., 2008 [27]
C. albicans	Planktonic, biofilms and EPS	Gel-based	DIGE	Martinez-Gomariz et al., 2009 [28]
Candida glabrata	Planktonic vs. biofilm	Gel-based	DIGE	Seneviratne et al., 2010 [29]
Campylobacter jejuni	Planktonic vs. biofilm	Gel-based	Silver stain	Dykes et al., 2003 [30]
C. jejuni	Planktonic vs. biofilm	Gel-based	Sypro Ruby	Kalmokoff et al., 2006 [31]

(Continued)

TABLE 6.1 (CONTINUED)
Studies of Microbial Biofilm Proteome

Organism	Trait under Investigation	Technique Employed	Technical Details	Author (References)
Cryptococcus neoformans	Planktonic vs. biofilm	Gel-free	Shotgun proteomics, LC-MS/MS analysis	Santi et al., 2014 [32]
Escherichia coli	Planktonic vs. biofilm	Gel-free	iTRAQ, QStar XL Hybrid ESI	Mukherjee et al., 2011 [33]
E. coli	Planktonic vs. biofilm	Gel-based	Silver staining	Collet et al., 2007 [34]; Orme et al., 2006 [35]; Kim et al., 2006 [36]; Tremoulet, 2002 [37]
Enterococcus faecalis	Biofilms	Gel-based	2D gel electrophoresis and MALDI-TOF identification	Qayyum et al., 2016 [38]
Haemophilus influenza	Extra cellular matrix (EPS)	Gel-based	SDS-PAGE and LC-MS/MS	Gallaher et al., 2006 [39]
Lactobacillus plantarum	Planktonic vs. biofilm	Gel-based	DIGE, MALDI-TOF identification	De Angelis et al., 2015 [40]
Listeria monocytogenes	Planktonic vs. biofilm (carbon starvation)	Gel-based	Radioactive labelling/ autoradiography	Helloin et al., 2003 [41]
Listeria monocytogenes	Planktonic vs. biofilm	Gel-based	Coomassie/silver staining	Tremoulet, 2002 [37]
L. monocytogenes	Planktonic vs. biofilm	Gel-based	SYPRO Ruby	Hefford et al., 2005 [42]
L. monocytogenes	Drug-treated planktonic vs. planktonic and drug-treated biofilm vs. biofilm	Gel-based	2D gel electrophoresis and LC-MS/MS analysis	Gómez et al., 2013 [43]
Mycobacterium semegmatis	Biofilms	Gel-based	Silver staining	Mukherjee and Chatterji, 2008 [12]
Neisseria meningitides	Planktonic vs. biofilm	Gel-based	Colloidal Coomassie	van Alen et al., 2010 [44]
Neisseria gonorrhoeae	Planktonic vs. biofilm	Gel-free	SILAC, LC-MS/MS analysis	Phillips et al., 2012 [45]
Porphyromonas gingivalis	Multi-species biofilm	Gel-free	LTQ MS, label-free	Kuboniwa et al., 2009 [46]

(Continued)

TABLE 6.1 (CONTINUED)
Studies of Microbial Biofilm Proteome

Organism	Trait under Investigation	Technique Employed	Technical Details	Author (References)
P. gingivalis	Planktonic vs. biofilm (cell envelope)	Gel-based and gel-free	$^{16}O/^{18}O$ proteolytic labelling	Ang et al., 2008 [47]
Proteus mirabilis	Planktonic vs. biofilm (WT and Δ*pst* mutant)	Gel-based	Silver staining	O'May et al., 2009 [11]
Pseudomonas aeruginosa	Planktonic vs. biofilm (lipidome)	Gel-free	ESI-MS/linear quadruple ion trap	Benamara et al., 2011 [48]
P. aeruginosa	Planktonic vs. biofilm	Gel-based	Silver staining	Steyn et al., 2001 [49]
P. aeruginosa	Planktonic, biofilm and gel-entrapped growth	Gel-based	Silver staining	Vilain et al., 2004 [50]
P. aeruginosa	Planktonic vs. biofilm (phosphoproteome)	Gel-based and gel-free	Phospho-(Ser/Thr) Phe antibodies/ ICAT	Petrova et al., 2009 [51]
P. aeruginosa	Planktonic vs. biofilm (development stages)	Gel-based	Silver staining	Southey-Pillig et al., 2005 [52]
P. aeruginosa	Planktonic vs. biofilm (strains/Ca²⁺)	Gel-based	Colloidal Coomassie	Patrauchan et al., 2007 [53]
P. aeruginosa	Planktonic vs. biofilm	Gel-free	LC-MS/MS analysis	Park et al., 2014 [54]
P. aeruginosa	Planktonic vs. biofilm	Gel-free	Label-free LC-MS/ MS analysis	Park et al., 2015 [55]
P. aeruginosa	Extracellular matrix of biofilms	Gel-free	iTRAQ, LC-MS/ MS analysis	Zhang et al., 2015 [56]
P. aeruginosa	Drug-treated biofilms	Gel-free	Pulsed SILAC, LC-MS/MS analysis	Chua et al., 2016 [57]
P. aeruginosa and *C. albicans*	Secretome of single and mixed-species biofilms	Gel-free	MALDI-TOF MS/ MS analysis	Purschke et al., 2012 [58]
Salmonella enteric	Biofilm adapted to benzalkonium chloride vs. untreated biofilms	Gel-based	Silver staining	Mangalappalli-Illathu and Kober, 2006 [59]
S. enteric	Planktonic vs. biofilm (benzalkonium chloride exposure)	Gel-based	Silver staining	Mangalappalli-Illathu et al., 2008 [60]

(Continued)

TABLE 6.1 (CONTINUED)
Studies of Microbial Biofilm Proteome

Organism	Trait under Investigation	Technique Employed	Technical Details	Author (References)
S. enteric	Biofilm under high-flow and low-flow	Gel-based	Silver staining	Mangalappalli-Illathu et al., 2008 [61]
Staphylococcus aureus	Planktonic vs. biofilm	Gel-based	Silver staining	Resch et al., 2006 [62]
S. aureus	Planktonic vs. biofilm (exoproteome)	Gel-free	iTRAQ	Muthukrishnan et al., 2011 [63]
S. aureus	Biofilms	Gel-free	Nano-LC-ESI-MS/MS	Islam et al., 2014 [64]
Staphylococcus xylosus	Planktonic vs. biofilm (EPS)	Gel-based	Colloidal Coomassie	Planchon et al., 2008 [65]
Streptococcus equi ssp. *zooepidemicus* (SEZ)	Planktonic vs. biofilm	Gel-based	2D gel electrophoresis and MALDI-TOF identification	Yi et al., 2014 [66]
Streptococcus mutans	Planktonic vs. biofilm	Gel-based	DIGE	Rathsam et al., 2005 [67]
S. mutans	Planktonic vs. biofilm	Gel-based	Sypro Ruby	Rathsam et al., 2005 [67]
S. mutans	Planktonic vs. biofilm	Gel-based	^{14}C labelling/ autoradiography	Svensater et al., 2001 [68]
S. mutans	Planktonic vs. mature biofilm (acid tolerance)	Gel-based	^{14}C labelling/ autoradiography	Welin et al., 2003 [69]
S. mutans	Planktonic vs. early adhesion of biofilm	Gel-based	Silver staining/^{14}C labelling	Welin et al., 2004 [70]
S. mutans	Planktonic vs. biofilm (reactivity with IgA)	Gel-based	Coomassie/silver staining	Sanui and Gregory, 2009 [71]
S. mutans	Planktonic vs. biofilm (effect of model/strain)	Gel-based	DIGE	Luppens and ten Cate, 2005 [72]
S. mutans	Drug-treated planktonic vs. planktonic and drug-treated biofilm vs. biofilm	Gel-based	2D gel electrophoresis and MALDI-TOF identification	Li et al., 2013 [73]
S. mutans	Biofilms	Gel-based	2D gel electrophoresis and LC-MS/MS analysis	Yoshida et al., 2015 [74]

(Continued)

TABLE 6.1 (CONTINUED)
Studies of Microbial Biofilm Proteome

Organism	Trait under Investigation	Technique Employed	Technical Details	Author (References)
Streptococcus suis	Planktonic vs. biofilm	Gel-based	2D gel electrophoresis and MALDI-TOF identification	Wang et al., 2012 [75]
S. suis	Drug-treated biofilms vs. biofilms	Gel-free	iTRAQ, ESI tandem MS/MS analysis by Q Exactive™	Zhao et al., 2015 [76]
Tannerella forsythia	Planktonic vs. biofilm	Gel-free	iTRAQ, ESI qTOF	Pham et al., 2010 [77]
Vibrio parahaemolyticus	Planktonic vs. biofilm	Gel-free	2D LC-MS/MS analysis	Dharmaprakash et al., 2014 [78]
Clinical samples	Dental plaque biofilm on enamel surface	Gel-based	Silver staining	Paes Leme et al., 2008 [79]

Note: DIGE, difference gel electrophoresis; ESI, electron spray ionisation; iTRAQ, isobaric tags for relative and absolute quantification; LC-MS: liquid chromatography–mass spectrometry; MALDI-TOF, matrix-assisted laser desorption/ionization time of flight; MS, mass spectrometry; SDS-PAGE, sodium dodecyl sulfate–polyacrylamide gel electrophoresis; qTOF, quadrupole time of flight.

that have provided important insights about proteins involved in biofilm formation, without directly examining the biofilm proteome, are also mentioned. However, a discussion of proteomics studies of biofilms formed on plants and natural ecosystems such as acid mine drainage systems are not within the scope of this chapter and readers are referred to some excellent reviews elsewhere [80–82].

SAMPLE PREPARATION FOR BIOFILM PROTEOMICS STUDIES

Efficient and reproducible methods of protein extraction play an important role in the success of any proteomics experiment. It should be noted that there is no 'universal' protocol or technique that can be followed for any biological question under consideration. Similarly, it is not possible to have a fixed sample preparation method for all the microbial biofilm samples, as there can be considerable diversity in protein quantity, molecular weight, charge, hydrophobicity, PTMs and interaction with other molecules, among others [83]. Consequently, one must carefully customise available proteomics resources for each study, rather than following a common protocol. The choice of an optimum protocol would minimise potential protein losses during processing, enrich the recovery of proteins and avoid contamination issues. In general, two major strategies are used to extract proteins from biological samples that are compatible for downstream mass spectrometry (MS)-based identification [84].

The first method involves the use of detergents to solubilise proteins and separate them by sodium dodecyl sulphate–polyacrylamide gel electrophoresis (SDS-PAGE) followed by in-gel trypsin digestion. The second is a more broadly used detergent-free method, where strong chaotropic reagents such as urea and thiourea are used for protein extraction followed by protein precipitation and digestion under in-solution denaturing conditions. Some of the recent studies have developed more generalised and efficient sample preparation methods. For instance, Matthias Mann's group has introduced a filter-aided sample preparation (FASP) method, which combines the advantages of in-gel and in-solution digestion approaches [84]. Also, a recent protocol published in the area of plant proteomics has suggested a possible universal protocol for total protein extraction involving trichloroacetic acid (TCA)/acetone precipitation followed by SDS and phenol extraction [85].

Certain studies have employed a combination of different protocols to obtain a better proteome coverage. They rely on improving the separation of peptides after the protein digestion and before they are analysed in the mass spectrometer. For instance, in a proteomics study on *Vibrio parahaemolyticus*, a bacterial pathogen associated with foodborne infections, two protocols that differ in their detergent concentrations and cell lysis methods were used to extract total proteins from 12-, 24- and 48-h planktonic cultures and 24- and 48-h biofilm cultures [78]. This resulted in the identification of a total of 2,199 proteins using LC-MS/MS [liquid chromatography–tandem MS] providing 45.5% total coverage of the proteome of the microorganism.

Various prefractionation techniques can also be used to study the sub-proteomes of microorganisms in the planktonic as well as biofilm modes. For instance, subcellular compartments, such as bacterial outer membrane (OM), have been successfully isolated using different prefractionation approaches [35,86–89]. Similarly, extracellular components, such as outer membrane vesicles [OMVs], which are associated with bacterial survival and virulence, have also been isolated from planktonic and biofilm cultures of the bacteria and subjected to proteomics analysis [55]. One such study by Park and colleagues analysed the differential proteomic expression of biofilm versus planktonic OMVs in *Pseudomonas aeruginosa,* which showed an increase in the expression of porins such as OprD and OprE, and of the peptidoglycan binding proteins OprI and OprF in the biofilm proteome. The quantitative study revealed that drug-binding cytoplasmic proteins and porins are shuttled into the OMVs from the whole cells, resulting in antibiotic resistance, thereby improving our understanding of biofilm-specific OMVs.

In another study, Rathsam and colleagues studied the sub-proteomes of *Streptococcus mutans* biofilms. *S. mutans* is a bacterium associated with dental decay [67]. The study utilised prefractionation techniques that had been previously used in planktonic cells to obtain 'wall', 'cytoplasmic' and 'membrane' fractions and observed that fractionation, and the subsequent recombination of the 'cellular' and 'wall' fractions, were able to significantly increase the number of proteins obtained, compared to the whole-cell preparation method. Prefractionation approaches have also been used to obtain the cell envelope proteome of planktonic and biofilm *Porphyromonas gingivalis* [47] and the sub-proteomes of mixed-species biofilms consisting of *P. gingivalis, Streptococcus gordonii* and *Fusobacterium nucleatum* [46]. These techniques can be successfully employed in fungal proteomics studies also. Subcellular organelles such as the cell wall, plasma membrane, mitochondria, Golgi apparatus, nucleus and peroxisome in the fungal species *Saccharamoyces cerevisiae* and *Candida albicans* have been successfully isolated and prefractionated for downstream proteomics identification [90–93]. Therefore, when used appropriately, prefractionation can improve the yield and the coverage of the biofilm proteome under investigation, compared to direct extraction of the whole-cell proteome methods.

PROTEOMIC APPROACHES IN BIOFILM PROTEOMICS STUDIES

Proteomics studies are usually carried out using either gel-based or gel-free techniques. The gel-based techniques are the traditional methods of proteomics analysis and are based on one- or two-dimensional gel electrophoresis, while gel-free proteomics analysis techniques are more recent, resulting from technological advancements in the field of mass spectrometry. It is noteworthy that according to PubMed, more than half of the published proteomics studies from 2000 to 2010 have used gel-based techniques [94]. However, in recent years, the trend has clearly moved towards gel-free approaches because of their simpler sample preparation steps. MS-based gel-free proteomics are now widely used for investigations such as protein sequencing, identification of PTMs and protein–protein interactions [95]. The terms gel-based and gel-free are used throughout this chapter in discussing studies on biofilm proteomics.

GEL-BASED PROTEOMICS

Two-dimensional gel electrophoresis (2-DE) was first developed by O'Farell in the 1970s and has been the cornerstone of proteomics until the advent of gel-free proteomics [96,97]. Traditionally, in gel-based approaches, proteins are first separated using a gel and then the extracted spots are digested with a protease, most commonly trypsin [98]. Following 2-DE, various staining methods such as Silver stain, Coomassie Blue and fluorescent dyes are used to visualise the gel (Figure 6.1a). In fact, one of the advantages of gel-based proteomics techniques is that they provide a visual representation in the gel of the proteome under investigation, containing valuable information about the relative size, isoelectric point and abundance of the proteins. Gel-based techniques can separate thousands of proteins and the currently used protocols can produce 2,000–3,000 detectable proteins spots. The differential expression profile of the proteins can be analysed using appropriate software such as ImageMaster (Amersham Biosciences), Progenesis (Nonlinear Dynamics), Decyder (GE Healthcare Life Sciences), PDQuest (BioRad), Melanie (Geneva Bioinformatics), ELISE and HERMes. It should be noted that the analytical methods and algorithms used in different software tools vary considerably [99].

Significant advances in gel-based proteomics were made in the 1990s with the introduction of the 2D-difference gel electrophoresis (2D-DIGE) technique by Unlu's research group. In 2D-DIGE, complex protein mixtures are labelled with fluorescent dyes (e.g. Cy2, Cy4 and Cy5), before 2-DE [100,101]. There are two

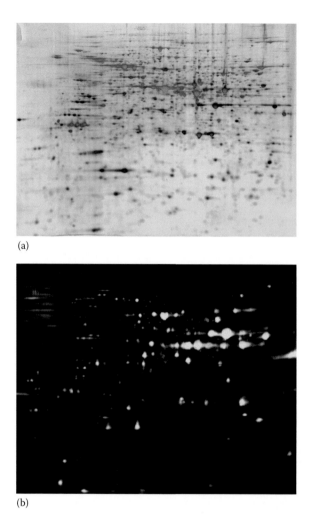

(a)

(b)

FIGURE 6.1 (a) Examples of classical gel-based proteomics using two-dimensional gel electrophoresis followed by silver staining. (b) Gel-based proteomics using 2D-DIGE.

major advantages of 2D-DIGE over traditional 2-DE methods. First, as many as three samples can be run in a single gel, thereby reducing experimental variations and making protein quantification more accurate. Second, gel-to-gel variations can be resolved by introducing an internal control. DIGE has been successfully applied in both bacterial and fungal biofilm studies (Figure 6.1b) [20,40,102,103]. However, gel-based approaches are limited by several technical hurdles, such as in the case of resolving hydrophobic proteins and low-abundance proteins. In particular, the first-dimension isoelectric focusing in conventional 2-DE platforms is not compatible enough with hydrophobic proteins and proteins with extreme isoelectric points. The second-dimension and/or the different staining techniques are not sufficiently sensitive to recover low molecular weight and low-abundance proteins. Other drawbacks are the limited detection of membrane proteins caused by their poor solubility and the limited dynamic range. Overall, lack of reproducibility, co-migration of proteins in spots and limited dynamic range are some of the major problems in gel-based proteomics [104,105]. In addition, these methods are labor-intensive, time-consuming and difficult to automate. Therefore, as previously mentioned, most researchers have already moved to gel-free platforms for proteomics analysis.

GEL-FREE MS-BASED PROTEOMICS APPROACHES

Recent advances in MS have rendered gel-free proteomics techniques increasingly popular and widely applied [106,107]. MS-based techniques allow a larger number of proteins to be identified and quantified in a relatively shorter time and can also detect, to a certain extent, difficult protein fractions such as membrane and low-abundance proteins.

Classically there are two major approaches in gel-free proteomics: bottom-up and top-down [98,108]. Top-down proteomics involves the analysis of intact proteins, whereas bottom-up proteomics approach represents the analysis of a complex peptide mixture after proteolysis with an enzyme, most commonly trypsin. Currently, the bottom-up (also known as shotgun) proteomics approach is more popular and more commonly employed because of its wider spectrum of applications and existing instrumentation. In the bottom-up approach, proteins are first digested to obtain peptides, which are subsequently subjected to MS-based analysis. Some studies have combined top-down and bottom-up proteomics approaches for better interpretation of results [109].

MS-based proteomics analysis can be either qualitative or quantitative. Quantitative MS-based analysis of proteins in samples can be carried out using two main approaches. Differentially expressed proteins can be quantified by either isotopic-labelling or label-free MS analysis. Differential isotopic labelling methods such as isobaric Tags for Relative and Absolute Quantitation (iTRAQ), Isotope-Coded Affinity Tags (ICAT), Stable-Isotope Labelling by Amino acids in Cell culture (SILAC) and Tandem Mass Tag (TMT), among others, can be used for relative quantification, including those studies related to biofilm proteomics [15,77,110,111].

EXAMPLES OF GEL-FREE PROTEOMICS APPROACHES IN MICROBIAL BIOFILM STUDIES

Gel-free proteomics techniques are now being widely used in the analysis of microbial populations and biofilms. Many of the recent microbial studies have employed quantitative gel-free proteomics methods for evaluating protein expression differences. For instance, Philips and colleagues conducted a proteome profiling of planktonic and biofilm *Neisseria gonorrhoeae* using SILAC labelling approach [45]. Proteins were extracted from ^{13}C-labelled planktonic cells and unlabelled biofilms. The heavy and light protein extracts were mixed and analysed by LC-MS/MS. A total of 757 proteins were identified, including 152 unique proteins that have a significant differential expression. The overexpressed proteins were mostly involved in energy metabolism and located in the cell envelope. The low-expressed proteins were mostly involved in protein synthesis. This study suggested a shift of gonococcal biofilms to anaerobic state. Other such isotopic-labelling based studies include analysis of the differential protein expression of biofilms of antibiotic-sensitive and -resistant strains of *Aeromonas hydrophila* by TMT labelling and iTRAQ-based analysis of *Candida* biofilm samples (Figure 6.2) [18].

Label-free strategies based on counting unique spectra or peak intensities constitute the second main group of quantification approaches. These techniques have been used in bacterial as well as fungal biofilm studies [46,112–118]. *Aggregatibacter actinomycetemcomitans* is an oral bacterial pathogen residing in the subgingival biofilms and associated with rapidly progressing 'gum disease' called aggressive periodontitis. Periodontitis, commonly known as gum disease, results from chronic inflammatory destruction of the tooth supporting structure or 'periodontium' due to aberrant host response to the pathogenic dental plaque biofilm [119]. Label-free quantitative proteomics techniques were employed to examine the interactions between *A. actinomycetemcomitans* and other oral bacterial species in a mixed-species biofilm environment [114]. This study found that 483 of the 728 quantified bacterial proteins excluding those of *A. actinomycetemcomitans* were differentially expressed. Interestingly, all quantified proteins from *Prevotella intermedia*, an oral bacterium, seemed to be overexpressed while most quantified proteins from *Campylobacter rectus*, *Streptococcus anginosus* and *P. gingivalis* were expressed in a lower level in the presence of *A. actinomycetemcomitans*.

There are only a few studies which have examined the host–biofilm interaction. Proteins secreted by the biofilm-challenged gingival epithelium are key signalling molecules for the initiation and propagation of the early host innate immune responses [120]. Bostanci and colleagues used label-free quantitative to screen for the host proteins secreted in a coculture of multilayered gingival epithelium with a 10-species subgingival biofilm model [113]. They identified a significant role of the 'red-complex' bacterial species in the observed effects. Bacterial response to prolonged desiccation conditions was examined using both iTRAQ and label-free proteomics of the clinical strain *Acinetobacter baumannii* [117]. With prolonged desiccation, *A. baumannii* tends to form biofilms on surfaces and transforms to a dormant 'persister' population. The resultant proteome was reflective of the changes observed, that is, lower expression of proteins involved in transcription and translation and increased expression of previously known persister-associated proteins. Interestingly, antioxidant proteins such as glutathione peroxidase, catalase H or superoxide dismutase were present in the persister proteome. Hence, it was proposed that formation of persister cells may be a mechanism that the bacterium uses to survive stress conditions such as lack of nutrients found in intensive care units (ICUs), causing consistent infections in the patients. Another study examined the physiological consequences of amyloid-mediated biofilm formation in *P. aeruginosa* PAO1 using label-free approaches [116]. The presence of functional amyloid heavily impacted the *P. aeruginosa* proteome. There was an increase in the alginate and pyoverdine synthesis machinery, which turned *P. aeruginosa* PAO1 into an unexpected mucoid phenotype.

In fungal studies, label-free proteomics approaches have been utilised to decipher the mechanism of persister population in *C. albicans* biofilms [118]. There are several unique advantages to both labelled and label-free quantitative methods and some studies have advocated the use of a combined strategy to improve the protein coverage [121].

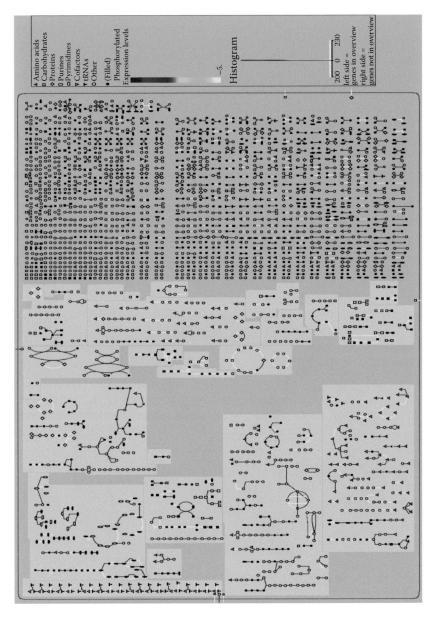
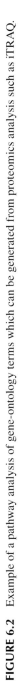

FIGURE 6.2 Example of a pathway analysis of gene-ontology terms which can be generated from proteomics analysis such as iTRAQ.

PROTEOMICS STRATEGIES TO UNCOVER DRUG RESISTANCE OF MICROBIAL BIOFILMS

Both genomics and proteomics studies have suggested that genes and proteins in biofilms are expressed differently from those in planktonic state [122,123]. These findings suggest that microorganisms have a separate 'biofilm phenotype' with a unique expression profile of genes and proteins. The most intriguing and elusive phenotypic feature of microbial biofilms is their increased resistance to harsh environmental conditions including antimicrobial challenges, compared to planktonic cells [1,2,124]. Though several hypotheses related to this phenomenon have been proposed, the exact mechanism of resistance has not yet been fully elucidated (Figure 6.3). Some of the possible resistance mechanisms include an altered metabolic state, the presence of extracellular matrix, oxidative stress response, differential gene or protein expression or the presence of a highly drug-tolerant 'persisters' population [124–127]. Proteomics studies on microbial biofilms have indeed provided a significant leap in our understanding of this phenomenon. A brief account of these studies, their major findings and implications are given in the text that follows.

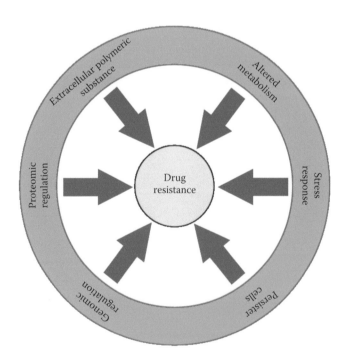

FIGURE 6.3 Factors that may contribute to the higher drug resistance in microbial biofilms. (Reproduced from Seneviratne CJ et al. *Proteomics*, 2012. With permission.)

BIOFILM PROTEOMICS STUDIES ON ALTERED METABOLIC RATE

Biofilms are composed of a heterogeneous collection of cells with different metabolic activities. It has been suggested that the upper layers are metabolically active, whereas the lower layers are in a state of quiescence [2,124,128]. The slower rates of growth, protein synthesis and metabolic activity could be attributed to the increased resistance of microbial biofilms. There are several studies that support as well as contradict this theory. Among studies corroborating this notion, a shotgun proteomics study on *E. coli* biofilms showed that major energy-generating events such as glycolysis and the pentose phosphate pathways are expressed at lower levels in biofilms [110]. This lower expression of the glycolysis pathway has also been shown in *S. mutans* biofilms, compared to the planktonic proteome [67]. A study on fungal biofilms, using *Candida glabrata*, demonstrated the lower expression of carbohydrate metabolism related proteins in biofilms when compared to the planktonic state [103]. In a more recent study of *Staphylococcus aureus* biofilms, the effects of different fluid shear rates on biofilms were evaluated by a global proteomics analysis using nano-LC-ESI-MS/MS [64]. The biofilms were grown in flow cells under four different fluid shear rates to identify their effect on biofilm-associated proteins and the proteins were extracted from the membrane and cytosolic fractions. Sixteen proteins in the membrane fraction and eight proteins in the cytosolic fraction showed significant changes in their expression profile under increased shear conditions. The altered proteins were related to metabolic functions such as glycolysis and the tricarboxylic acid (TCA) pathways, protein synthesis and stress tolerance. However, fibronectin-binding and collagen-binding protein levels were unchanged. The study demonstrated that the general metabolic functions of the bacterium are reduced under high-shear conditions, but without changes in their binding capacity.

On the other hand, other proteomics studies of *S. aureus* biofilms have shown that cells may be metabolically active in the later stages of biofilm development, as glycolysis-associated proteins were found to be overexpressed [62]. In addition, one study on *S. mutans* biofilms also showed overexpression of the glycolysis pathway in the biofilm proteome [71]. Moreover, a comparative proteomics study of the planktonic and the biofilm states of *V. parahaemolyticus* revealed that pathways such as glycolysis, citrate cycle, purine metabolism and pyruvate metabolism function similarly between planktonic and biofilms modes [78]. It is thus possible that reduced metabolic activity might not be the only reason for the increased antimicrobial resistance in biofilms. However, it is important to highlight that variations in methodology, microorganisms, stages of biofilm development and the spatio-temporal organisation of biofilms in the aforementioned biofilm proteomics studies could also be the reasons behind the contradictory reports of metabolic response in biofilms.

The age of biofilms can also affect the resistance phenomena observed. Mature biofilms are normally more resistant than younger biofilms. The analysis of biofilms using a time-course experiment would be an ideal way to capture the dynamic changes occurring during the biofilm development. One such study was performed in *Streptococcus pneumoniae*, a bacterial pathogen that accounts for a significant global burden of morbidity and mortality. Comparative iTRAQ analysis was performed on a planktonic log-phase culture and on one-day and seven-day biofilms in a *S. pneumoniae* clinical serotype 14 strain [93]. Overall, 244 proteins were identified, of which more than 80% were differentially expressed during biofilm development. Compared to the planktonic proteome, the one-day-old nascent biofilm exhibited less expression of proteins associated with glycolysis, which is consistent with other reports demonstrating the lower expression of glycolytic proteins. Proteins involved in translation, transcription and virulence were also expressed at lower levels at this stage. In contrast, proteins with roles in pyruvate, carbohydrate and arginine metabolism were significantly increased in mature biofilms. This suggests an initial slowdown of metabolic processes to adapt to the biofilm lifestyle followed by an increased metabolic activity in later stages. Interestingly, seven-day-old biofilms showed that metabolic activity returned to levels comparable to those of log-phase planktonic cells. In another time-course study of *P. aeruginosa*, the profiles showed an increased antibiotic resistance and decreased metabolic activity in the biofilm mode [54]. Hence, more time-course proteomics studies of microbial biofilms are needed to gain a better understanding of the metabolic responses elicited.

BIOFILM PROTEOMICS STUDIES ON EXTRACELLULAR POLYMERIC SUBSTANCES

The formation of biofilms involves the production of EPS by microorganisms, which constitutes a unique feature of the microbial biofilms. EPS consists of polysaccharides, proteins, nucleic acids and lipids [129]. It forms a gel-like, highly hydrated and locally charged three-dimensional scaffold encompassing the biofilm community and acts as a barrier to the diffusion of antimicrobial agents, providing an increased drug resistance to the microbial community. There are numerous studies which have examined the nature and function of EPS in microbial biofilms [127,130,131]. It has been proposed that targeting EPS could be an efficient strategy to limit biofilm formation [132]. In fact, the examination of the biofilm matrix may reveal potential candidates that could be used as drug targets and provide some insight into drug resistance. Although most EPS studies have focused on their polysaccharide components, some studies have specifically focused on their protein components. It is important to note that the study of the polysaccharide components of EPS would be better suited to metabolomics, as described in Chapter 7 [133–135].

The study of EPS proteins poses some significant challenges, especially in relation to obtaining a successful and reproducible protein extraction step, as the EPS is protected by several components which greatly complicate the process of protein recovery. We think that EPS extraction protocols used for environmental biofilms formed on wastewater treatment reactors could serve as guidelines for other biofilm studies [136]. In fact, physical and chemical extraction methods as well as a combination of both have been used to extract EPS. Physical extraction methods detach EPS from the cells using mechanical forces while chemical methods disrupt the binding interactions between the EPS and the cells to accelerate the solution of EPS. The nature of EPS and hence the difficulty of extraction varies from study to study. Hence, optimisation of extraction methodology should be performed before the start of the experiment to obtain the most efficient protein recovery. Some proteomics studies that have explored EPS proteins are described in the text that follows.

Gallaher and colleagues studied the EPS proteins of non-typeable *H. influenza* and identified 265 proteins, including UspA, a universal stress response protein, which has previously been shown to be important for biofilm formation [39]. Another recent study used two clinical *S. aureus* strains including a methicillin-resistant *S. aureus* (MRSA) and a methicillin sensitive clinical strain, to examine the exoproteomes of exopolysaccharide-based and protein-based biofilm matrices [137]. A total of 33 extracellular proteins were detected. More notably, 28 of the 33 proteins had been previously identified in the biofilm exoproteome of *S. aureus* strain D30, isolated from a persistent nasal carrier [63]. Hence, this study demonstrated that the biofilm mode of *S. aureus* contained many more immuno-evasive proteins than the cells in the planktonic mode. Another study by Gil and colleagues showed that a common core of secreted proteins was contained in the exoproteomes of both methicillin-resistant and non-methicillin-resistant strains [137]. The EPS contained many proteins involved in pathogenesis, such as toxins like leukocidin, EsaA and truncated beta-hemolysin, and immunomodulatory proteins like lipoprotein, immunodominant antigen B, immunodominant antigen A and IgG-binding protein. In addition, a markedly large number of proteins involved in carbohydrate metabolism such as phosphoglycerate mutase, triosephosphate isomerase, enolase, glyceraldehyde-3-phosphate dehydrogenase, glucose-6-phosphate isomerase and alcohol dehydrogenase were also found in the biofilm matrix. Follow-up studies using biofilm matrix exoprotein extracts were able to induce a humoral immune response and elicit the production of interleukin-10 (IL-10) and IL-17 in mice. Interestingly, when mice were immunised with biofilm-matrix extracts, bacterial counts of the *in vivo* biofilms declined significantly. Hence, this proteomics study was instrumental in demonstrating that an extract containing biofilm matrix exoproteins could induce a protective immune response against *S. aureus* biofilm-related infections [98]. In another study, EPS proteins obtained from *P. aeruginosa* biofilms at different stages were examined using iTRAQ to elucidate the functions of ECM proteins in the biofilm structure [56]. Matrix-associated proteins were extracted from 12-, 24-, 48- and 96-h biofilms of *P. aeruginosa*. The analysis identified 389 proteins and observed an increase in the levels of stress resistance and nutrient-metabolism proteins over the period of the biofilm growth. Furthermore, putative effectors of the type III secretion system were also identified in the matrix. The study suggested that ECM proteins may play a role in stress resistance, nutrient acquisition and pathogenesis. There are other proteomics studies that have explored different aspects of EPS in various bacterial biofilms [21,23].

Recently, a comprehensive study on *C. albicans* EPS was performed by Zarnowski and colleagues [138]. The authors were able to carefully extract the EPS component from *C. albicans* without any cell wall contamination. Interestingly, contrary to the common belief, they reported that proteins represented the main component, far exceeding the polysaccharide content. A total of 565 proteins were identified in the *C. albicans* biofilm matrix. Subsequently, 458 different functions of the proteins spanning 16 metabolic pathways were discerned using the Kyoto Encyclopaedia of Genes and Genomes (KEGG) database. The most abundantly represented pathways were related to carbohydrate metabolism, which had 177 functional proteins. Eight of the identified matrix proteins, that is, Xog1, Exg1, Bgl2, Pmt1, Pmt2, Pmt4, Pmt6 and Hsp70, had previously been reported to impact biofilm formation. However, proteomics technologies have not yet been fully exploited to unravel the essential information about EPS proteins of microbial biofilms. Future research in this field should make use of the novel technologies available to dig the important protein regulators in the EPS gold mine of microbial biofilm, which can aid in the development of novel anti-biofilm strategies.

BIOFILM PROTEOMICS STUDIES OF OXIDATIVE STRESS RESPONSE (INCREASED ANTI-OXIDATIVE ACTIVITY)

Activation of oxidative stress response pathways in biofilms is another hypothesis that has been proposed to account for the increased drug resistance of microbial biofilms. This hypothesis has gained considerable attention in recent years because of the strong evidence generated from studies of bacterial and fungal biofilms. Implications of these findings in relation to higher drug resistance observed in microbial biofilms are discussed in the text that follows.

One study examined the role of periplasmic oxidative defence proteins, copper–zinc superoxide dismutase (SodC) and thiol peroxidase (Tpx) from Shiga toxin–producing *E. coli* O157:H7 (STEC) biofilms [36]. Proteomics analyses showed significantly higher expression levels of elements of both periplasmic antioxidant systems (SodC and Tpx) when STEC cells were grown in the biofilm mode than when grown in the planktonic mode. These findings were further confirmed by the observation that *sodC* and *tpx* mutants were more susceptible to hydrogen peroxide than the STEC wild-type. STEC mutans also displayed significant reductions in their capability to adhere to epithelial cells and abiotic surfaces. Therefore, for the first time, it was revealed that *sodC* and *tpx* gene products contributed to the formation of *E. coli* biofilms.

Neisseria meningitidis is a commensal bacterium that resides in the human nasopharynx but which, under certain conditions, can cause invasive diseases such as meningitis. Comparative proteomics analysis of planktonic and biofilm cultures of *N. meningitidis* showed that the oxidative defence system–related proteins MntC and SodC were expressed in higher levels in the biofilm mode of growth [44]. MntC and SodC are well-known components of the oxidative defence system. Subsequently, *MntC* knock-out mutants showed more susceptibility to Paraquat, an agent that induces the production of intracellular reactive oxygen species (ROS). Interestingly, biofilm formation of *MntC* mutants was completely abrogated. However, this phenotype could be compensated by complementation of *mntC in trans*. Hence, *MntC* seems to protect the bacterium against ROS in the biofilm mode of growth, but not in the planktonic mode. In another study, a considerable number of stress response proteins including antioxidants were found to be expressed in high amounts in the *Actinomyces naeslundii* biofilm, when compared to the planktonic proteome [17]. These proteins included Fe/Mn superoxide dismutase, thioredoxin, general stress protein 14, co-chaperone GrpE HSP10 and HSP70. Superoxide dismutase has been shown to be expressed in higher levels in the biofilm modes compared to the planktonic modes of bacteria such as *Listeria monocytogenes* and *Salmonella enterica* [37,60]. The higher expression of alkyl hydroperoxide reductase and catalase–hydroperoxidase II observed in the comparative proteomics study on the planktonic and biofilm mode of *Acinetobacter baumannii* indicates higher antioxidative capacities in the biofilm mode of growth [15]. Comparative proteomics studies on planktonic versus biofilm modes of bacterial pathogens such as *Campylobacter* jejuni and *H. influenzae* have further corroborated that alkyl-hydroperoxide reductase is an important antioxidant expressed at higher levels in the biofilm mode compared to the planktonic mode [31,39]. Hence, the aforementioned findings provide evidence for the role of antioxidant defence system in the drug resistance of microbial biofilms. The biofilm proteome of another bacterium, *Tanerella forsythia*, which is associated with periodontal disease, when compared with the planktonic proteome also demonstrated higher expression levels of oxidative stress–related proteins – for example, Dps, AhpC and Hsp20 [77]. *T. forsythia* biofilm cells were more resistant to oxidative stress than planktonic cells. The proteome of *P. aeruginosa* also exhibited increased levels of antioxidant proteins in the biofilm mode of growth [53].

In a recent study, the biofilm formation determinants of *Enterococcus faecalis* were characterised using a traditional proteomics approach [38]. Interestingly, they selected one biofilm-efficient strain, which formed stronger and denser biofilm and one biofilm-deficient strain, which formed meagre biofilm, and examined them together with *Enterococcus faecalis* wild-type MTCC 2729. The proteins extracted from *E. faecalis* biofilms were subjected to 2-DE gel electrophoresis followed by Coomassie Brilliant Blue staining, in-gel digestion and matrix-assisted laser desorption/ionization–time of flight (MALDI-TOF) MS analysis. The study identified a total of 13 proteins, with the majority of the differentially expressed proteins belonging to the translation elongation machinery. This study also proposed that deficient biofilm formation of the strain is due to the underexpression of the osmotically inducible protein C, which is an OsmC/Ohr family oxidative stress protein. Somewhat similar observations were made in a label-free proteomics study on *L. monocytogenes* biofilm, which also employed both strong and weak biofilm formers, and compared their proteomics profiles [139]. The study suggested that the biofilm mode of growth is associated with an abundance of stress-defence proteins, which is related to the more chemically resistant phenotype compared to the planktonic mode. The strong biofilm former showed a higher level of resilience and had overall more stress tolerance than the weak biofilm former. Moreover, in a recent study, the proteins required for *Streptococcus mutans* biofilm formation in a competitive environment were analysed by a gel-based 2-DE proteomics approach. Proteins were extracted from the biofilms of *S. mutans* grown in the presence and the absence of *S. gordonii*, a competitive coloniser of the tooth surface [74]. The analysis identified that the peroxide-resistant protein Dpr is increased in the biofilms of *S. mutans* grown in the presence of *S. gordonii*. This shows that Dpr might be essential for the survival of *S. mutans* on teeth surfaces in the presence of other colonising oral streptococci.

Studies on fungal biofilms agree with the hypothesis of increased antioxidative capacities as a mechanism for the higher antifungal resistance in biofilms. Elevated expression of antioxidant proteins such as Sod1, Tsa1 and Ahp1 have been observed in biofilms of *C. albicans* [27,28,103]. Evidence that oxidative stress could play a pivotal role in the biofilm mode of growth also comes from community proteomic studies on microbial biofilms from acid-mine drains [80]. However, one major question related to this hypothesis remains to be determined: whether the elevated antimicrobial oxidative stress response is a primary or secondary trait of the biofilm phenotype. One may argue that limited nutrition supply, increased cell density and lack of efficient waste disposal may contribute to the increased oxidative stress in microbial biofilms. As a result of expression of oxidative defence system proteins with high antioxidative capacities, increased antimicrobial resistance may follow as a secondary trait. The benefit of this adaptive response to biofilms is a 'bonus' trait, because many antimicrobials, as well as the human immune system, use the generation of ROS as a strategy to overcome microbial colonisation. Further research is needed to explore the oxidative stress response as a mechanism for increased antimicrobial resistance in microbial biofilms.

FUNGAL BIOFILM PROTEOMICS

A substantial number of fungal genomes have been sequenced and many more are in progress [140]. In parallel, appropriate databases have been set up allowing researchers to embark on fungal proteomics studies with genomics support [141]. The *C. albicans* genome was sequenced by the Stanford Genome Technology Center (SGTC), and the Assembly 19 of the sequence was published in 2004 [142,143]. CandidaDB (http://genolist.pasteur.fr/CandidaDB) [144] is a database that provides annotation of the Assembly 19 carried out by the European Galar Fungail consortium. The *Saccharomyces* Genome Database (SGD; www.yeastgenome.org) has long been the keeper of the original eukaryotic reference genome sequence and supported numerous fungal proteomics works [145,146].

Fungal proteomics differs from bacterial proteomics in certain aspects. One of the challenges in fungal proteomics sample preparation is the layered cell wall of the fungus. It is reported that the cell wall makes up close to 30% of the cell dry weight of the fungus, of which 80–90% represents polysaccharides [147,148]. *Candida* species have cell wall proteins covalently linked to polysaccharides such as beta-1,6-glucan forming glycoprotein complexes, which cause two major disadvantages. First, the presence of phosphodiester bridges or uronic acids or pyruvylation results in the large negative charges of *N*- or *O*-linked carbohydrate side chains. Because of this, a 2-DE analysis of the protein lysate will provide glycoforms with different isoelectric points [140]. Second, because of these variations on the length of *N*- or *O*-linked carbohydrate side chains of glycoproteins, numerous glycoforms ranging widely in mass can also appear in the gels. Therefore, fungal glycoproteins produce multiple fuzzy spots complicating PMF and quantitation, lowering the resolution and sensitivity of the results [140]. Therefore, some studies have recommended conducting fractionations before proteomics studies of *C. albicans*. For instance, cell wall fractions have been separated from the cytosolic fractions and studied separately for the proteomics expression both in the planktonic and the biofilms modes of the organism [149].

Candida species, which are the major fungal pathogens of humans and responsible for both mucosal and systemic mycoses, have been the centre of fungal proteomics studies. More details of these organisms and their biofilms are described in the fungal biofilms in Chapter 5. Compared to bacterial proteomics, only a small number of studies are available for *Candida* biofilms [24–28,118,138,149,150]. Mukherjee et al. (2006) showed that the alcohol dehydrogenase [Adh1p] is significantly expressed at a lower level in *Candida* biofilms compared with planktonic cells, and Adh1p restricts the ability of *Candida* to form biofilms [24]. Thus, disruption of ADH significantly enhances the biofilm-forming ability of *Candida in vitro*. This observation was confirmed by an engineered human oral mucosa model and an *in vivo* rat model. Other studies have shown that *Candida* biofilms possess enhanced antioxidative capacities that could contribute to an increased drug resistance. Comparative proteomics analysis of both *C. albicans* and *C. glabrata* has shown that antioxidant proteins such as Ahp1p and Trx1p are expressed at higher levels in the biofilm mode compared to the planktonic mode [27,103]. Such findings are similar to those from studies performed on bacterial biofilms.

Mixed *Candida* and bacterial biofilms have also been studied [58]. In a recent study, the secretome of *P. aeruginosa* and *C. albicans* mixed biofilms was studied by MALDI-TOF MS/MS analysis [58]. A total of 247 proteins were identified from the analysis, with 170 belonging to *P. aeruginosa* and 77 to *C. albicans*. In the mixed species biofilms, 131 proteins were identified, with 92 belonging to *P. aeruginosa* and 39 to *C. albicans*. In the single species biofilms, the observed diversity of proteins was higher in both the organisms, with 73 proteins found in *C. albicans* and 154 proteins in *P. aeruginosa* secretome. In the mixed-species biofilms, *P. aeruginosa* had significantly higher amounts of 16 proteins, including exotoxin A and iron acquisition proteins. The study indicated that iron sequestering is increased in *P. aeruginosa* when present in mixed-species biofilms, whereas in *C. albicans* the metabolism was significantly reduced along with iron acquisition proteins.

Biofilms of other fungal species such as *Aspergillus* and *Cryptococcus* have been studied in very few proteomics studies so far [32,151]. In a recent study of *Cryptococcus neoformans*, a pathogenic yeast in immunocompromised patients, differences in protein expression between planktonic and biofilm cells were studied by shotgun proteomics [152]. The differentially expressed proteins in *C. neoformans* were related to metabolism, protein turnover and global stress responses. Biofilms had increased levels of proteins related to oxidation–reduction, proteolysis and response to stress and reduced levels of proteins related to metabolic processes, transport and translation. Proteomics and transcriptomics studies of *A. fumigatus* biofilms have shown that the metabolic activity of the biofilm mode decreases as the biofilm matures: the enzymes of glycolysis, the TCA cycle and ATP synthesis were expressed at a lower level, while proteins related to sulfur metabolism and oxidative stress were overexpressed [20]. However, proteins involved in the biosynthesis of secondary metabolites such as gliotoxin (a mycotoxin) were significantly overexpressed, which may confer protection from the host immune system and enable its survival and persistence in chronic lung infections. Although the intracellular proteome of *A. niger* biofilms and submerged cultures have been studied, most of the proteins identified were hypothetical proteins [19]. This highlights some of the limitations faced by proteomics researchers.

DRUG-RESPONSE PROTEOMICS OF BIOFILMS

To gain a better understanding of the drug resistance mechanisms observed in microbial biofilms, it is essential to study the dynamic changes occurring in biofilms on drug treatment. Therefore, a large number of studies have been performed to examine the factors that account for a higher drug resistance in microbial biofilms. These studies have shown that the drug resistance is not dependent on the number of cells [153]. Some groups have proposed that the higher drug resistance of biofilms is due to the polysaccharide matrix secreted by the biofilms, while other groups have disagreed. For instance, a study compared the proteomic expression of *S. enterica* under different flow conditions [61]. Despite apparent changes occurring in the biofilm structure and EPS composition, no major shift in whole-cell protein expression patterns was seen between 168-h old low-flow and high-flow biofilms. This is in agreement with the fact that the resistance of biofilms may not be directly linked with their structure [154]. Hence, EPS may not be the sole reason behind the drug resistance of the biofilms. In recent years, to understand the mechanistic aspect of this phenomenon, greater attention has been paid to decipher the drug induced proteomics changes in the microbial biofilms.

Another reason for the increased drug resistance could be due to the presence of 'persister' cells in biofilms. 'Persisters' are a subpopulation of biofilms that are highly resistant to repeated exposure of drugs at high concentrations. Some of the recent proteomics studies have attempted to study this process. Colistin is a last-resort polymyxin antibiotic available for the treatment of infections caused by drug-resistant Gram-negative bacteria such as *P. aeruginosa*. The antibiotic tolerance of the *P. aeruginosa* biofilm subpopulation was investigated by a pulsed stable isotope labelling with amino acids (SILAC) approach [57]. *P. aeruginosa* biofilms were grown under a flow cell setup and then treated with colistin to kill the antibiotic sensitive population. The treated biofilms were then labelled with ^{13}Clysine for 48 h to identify the proteins produced in the antibiotic-tolerant subpopulation. The study identified proteins required for type IV pili assembly and quorum sensing (QS) regulated proteins such as LasB, chitinase and phenazine/pycocyanin synthesis proteins to be highly expressed in the antibiotic-tolerant subpopulation. The study suggested that type IV pili help the antibiotic-tolerant cells to migrate to the top layer of biofilms whereas QS helps in establishing new antibiotic-tolerant subpopulations. Hence, the study proposed that incorporation of QS and motility inhibitors with the traditional antibiotics could prevent persistent infections in affected patient populations.

Another proteomics study has been performed on the biofilms of susceptible and resistant *A. hydrophila* strains that were subjected to chlortetracycline treatment to induce stress [18]. The analysis identified an increase of fatty acid biosynthesis proteins in the resistant strains. The study demonstrated that increase in fatty acid biosynthesis may play an important role in antibiotic resistance of *A. hydrophila*. Hence the study suggested that a cocktail of chlortetracycline and triclosan may be a more effective therapy for *A. hydrophila* biofilm infections. A proteomics study was performed on the inhibitory effects of carolacton, a secondary metabolite isolated from the myxobacterium *Sorangium cellulosum*, exhibiting strong destructive effects on *S. mutans* biofilms using a 2-DE gel-based approach [73]. In this study, the proteome profile of drug-treated planktonic versus untreated planktonic *S. mutans* and drug-treated biofilm versus untreated biofilm *S. mutans* were compared. Proteins from the cytoplasmic and extracellular fractions of *S. mutans* were analysed, with a total of 239 protein spots, of which 192 were cytoplasmic proteins. The study demonstrated that in both planktonic and biofilm cells, the inhibitory effects of carolacton were exerted by disturbing peptidoglycan biosynthesis and degradation. This suggested that damage to cell wall integrity leads to cell death on treatment with carolacton.

STUDY OF POST-TRANSLATIONAL MODIFICATIONS IN BIOFILMS

Post-translational modifications (PTMs) such as phosphorylation, glycosylation, lipidation, methylation and ubiquitination often take place in proteins after translation, to either activate or suppress their functions. The study of such PTMs of biofilm proteins can help in capturing the accurate snapshot of reactions occurring within a biological system on a particular stimulus. Traditionally, PTMs such as protein phosphorylation, glycosylation and nitrosylation have been investigated for a single or a few proteins. In the past, most of the PTMs were examined by gel-based approaches, although this trend has considerably changed recently, as mentioned earlier. In gel-based analyses, the proteome fractions under investigation such as glycoproteins and/ or phosphoproteins are enriched using glycol-beads or phospho-beads, respectively. Following the 2-DE, Pro-Q Diamond and Pro-Q Emerald can be used to specifically stain the glycoprotein and phosphoprotein fractions, respectively.

In recent years, a considerable number of glycoproteomics studies have been performed [155]. Glycoproteomics is gaining popularity for the study of prokaryotic organisms, as glycosylation contributes to the virulence of many bacterial pathogens [156]. This type of study has been performed on some fungi as well [157].

Phosphorylation is one of the most widespread PTMs of living systems, including prokaryotic organisms as well. Five types of phosphorylation modifications could occur in prokaryotes, namely the addition of phosphate moieties to serine, threonine, tyrosine, histidine and aspartate. Until quite recently, prokaryotic protein phosphorylation was known to occur predominantly on histidine and aspartate, whereas phosphorylation on serine, threonine and tyrosine was attributed to eukaryotic systems. One of the preliminary studies that demonstrated the possibility of serine, threonine and/or tyrosine phosphorylation in prokaryotic systems was the identification of reversible phosphorylation of a serine residue in the isocitrate dehydrogenase of *E. coli* [158]. Several subsequent studies have led to the identification of numerous other bacterial proteins phosphorylated on serine, threonine and tyrosine, regulating various functions such as gene expression, transport, metabolic processes and virulence, as well as their corresponding serine, threonine and/or tyrosine protein kinases [159]. In the past decade, a tremendous wealth of information regarding the global occurrence of protein phosphorylation in prokaryotic systems has been generated, mostly on the proteome-wide occurrence of serine/threonine/tyrosine phosphorylation. This is because histidine and aspartate phosphorylation are more transient and hence difficult to capture. More recently, several high-throughput phosphoproteomics studies have clearly shown that phosphorylated Ser/Thr/Tyr residues are a ubiquitous presence in prokaryotic systems, possibly regulating several fundamental biological processes [160]. One such pioneering phosphoproteomics study is the global, gel-free and site-specific analysis of the *B. subtilis* phosphoproteome by Mann's group. The study characterised 103 unique phosphopeptides from 78 *B. subtilis* proteins and determined 78 phosphorylation sites: 54 on serine, 16 on threonine and 8 on tyrosine. Phosphorylation sites were present on almost all glycolysis and TCA cycle enzymes, several kinases and members of the phosphoenolpyruvate-dependent phosphotransferase system. Another study, performed on *E. coli*, investigated the phosphorylation of ribosomal proteins [161]. However, these pioneering studies are mostly on the planktonic state of microbes and there are only a few existing studies that have specifically mapped the phosphoproteome of microbial biofilms. For instance, the phosphoproteome of *P. aeruginosa* was investigated during the course of biofilm development [51]. It was revealed that biofilm development and maturation were regulated by three previously undescribed two-component systems: BfiSR harboring an RpoD-like domain, an OmpR-like BfmSR and MifSR belonging to the family of NtrC-like transcriptional regulators. These regulatory systems were sequentially phosphorylated during the development of *P. aeruginosa* biofilms and inactivation of bfiS, bfmR and mifR stopped the biofilm formation at a specific early stage of development. Similarly, suppression of bfiS, bfmR and mifR expression in established biofilms prompted the biofilm to collapse. The inactivation of these systems had no influence on the planktonic mode of growth. The study demonstrated that these two-component systems have unique signalling roles in the development and maintenance of the normal biofilm architecture, without any effect on planktonic cells. Such preliminary studies on the phosphoproteome of microbial biofilms have generated a large amount of interest in this field, holding significant promise for the future of biofilm phosphoproteomics.

METAPROTEOMICS STUDIES OF BIOFILMS

Most of the existing studies on microbial biofilms have been performed under *in vitro* conditions simulating *in vivo* biofilms. Notwithstanding the insight gained from *in vitro* studies, it is obvious that *in vitro* biofilms are not equivalent to their *in vivo* counterparts. Therefore, it is worth looking into the data derived from *in vivo* or clinical study samples. The introduction of metaproteomics has made such studies possible. Metaproteomics can be defined as the large-scale characterisation of the entire protein complement of environmental microbiota at a given point in time. It has been used to study complex samples derived from clinical settings, and natural ecosystems such as wastewaters, or acid mine drainage, among many other applications [82,162]. Metaproteomics tools have facilitated the study of microbial communities both at a functional biomolecular and a whole-community level [163,164].

In this context, metaproteomics approaches have been successfully applied to decipher the complex environment of biofilms which could be of vital importance in clinical settings [80]. This approach could help in investigating clinical samples such as dental plaque biofilms and gut microbiota, including drug resistance in microbial biofilms. A detailed discussion of the techniques and implications of metaproteomics is beyond the scope of this chapter and readers are referred to some excellent reviews on the topic [81,82,165].

CONCLUDING REMARKS

The mechanism of drug resistance in microbial biofilms is one of the 'holy grails' that modern scientists are struggling to find. The natural complexity of biofilms, the confounding nature of protein interactions and the dynamic changes of this system have long hindered our understanding of biofilms. Study of such complex systems would therefore be better aided by breaking down the numerous biological questions into several smaller parts and structuring the type of analyses required to answer each of the parts. The consolidation of these smaller pieces of information can help us in providing the final perspective of this system. Rapid advancements in technology and an increasing repertoire of proteomics strategies have brought forward significant strides towards the achievement of this goal. The availability of genomes of microbial species and supporting computational tools are also rapidly expanding, and therefore the possibility of the identification of the 'complete proteome' of an organism is nearing realisation. Furthermore, the use of proteomics with simultaneous application of transcriptomics and other multidimensional technologies may also provide clinically relevant solutions in the near future.

CORRESPONDING AUTHOR

Chaminda Jayampath Seneviratne
Discipline of Oral Sciences
Faculty of Dentistry
National University of Singapore
Singapore
jaya@nus.edu.sg

REFERENCES

1. Hoiby N, Bjarnsholt T, Givskov M, Molin S, Ciofu O. Antibiotic resistance of bacterial biofilms. *Int J Antimicrob Agents.* 2010;35(4):322–32.
2. Fux CA, Costerton JW, Stewart PS, Stoodley P. Survival strategies of infectious biofilms. *Trends Microbiol.* 2005;13(1):34–40.
3. Armitage JP, Dorman CJ, Hellingwerf K, Schmitt R, Summers D, Holland B. Thinking and decision making, bacterial style: Bacterial Neural Networks, Obernai, France, 7th–12th June 2002. *Mol Microbiol.* 2003;47(2):583–93.
4. Wilkins MR, Sanchez JC, Gooley AA, Appel RD, Humphery-Smith I, Hochstrasser DF et al. Progress with proteome projects: Why all proteins expressed by a genome should be identified and how to do it. *Biotechnol Genet Eng Rev.* 1996;13:19–50.
5. Tyers M, Mann M. From genomics to proteomics. *Nature.* 2003;422(6928):193–7.
6. Pradet-Balade B, Boulme F, Beug H, Mullner EW, Garcia-Sanz JA. Translation control: Bridging the gap between genomics and proteomics? *Trends Biochem Sci.* 2001;26(4):225–9.
7. Pandey A, Mann M. Proteomics to study genes and genomes. *Nature.* 2000; 405(6788):837–46.

8. Phillips CI, Bogyo M. Proteomics meets microbiology: Technical advances in the global mapping of protein expression and function. *Cell Microbiol.* 2005;7(8):1061–76.
9. Zhang CG, Chromy BA, McCutchen-Maloney SL. Host-pathogen interactions: A proteomic view. *Expert Rev Proteomics.* 2005;2(2):187–202.
10. Zhang W, Li F, Nie L. Integrating multiple 'omics' analysis for microbial biology: Application and methodologies. *Microbiology.* 2010;156(Pt 2):287–301.
11. O'May GA, Jacobsen SM, Longwell M, Stoodley P, Mobley HL, Shirtliff ME. The high-affinity phosphate transporter Pst in *Proteus mirabilis* HI4320 and its importance in biofilm formation. *Microbiology.* 2009;155(Pt 5):1523–35.
12. Mukherjee R, Chatterji D. Proteomics and mass spectrometric studies reveal planktonic growth of *Mycobacterium smegmatis* in biofilm cultures in the absence of rpoZ. *J Chromatogr B Analyt Technol Biomed Life Sci.* 2008;861(2):196–202.
13. Ruiz L, Hidalgo C, Blanco-Miguez A, Lourenco A, Sanchez B, Margolles A. Tackling probiotic and gut microbiota functionality through proteomics. *J Proteomics.* 2016; 147:28–39.
14. Cheng K, Chui H, Domish L, Hernandez D, Wang G. Recent development of mass spectrometry and proteomics applications in identification and typing of bacteria. *Proteomics Clin Appl.* 2016;10(4):346–57.
15. Cabral MP, Soares NC, Aranda J, Parreira JR, Rumbo C, Poza M et al. Proteomic and functional analyses reveal a unique lifestyle for *Acinetobacter baumannii* biofilms and a key role for histidine metabolism. *J Proteome Res.* 2011;10:3399–3417.
16. Shin JH, Lee HW, Kim SM, Kim J. Proteomic analysis of *Acinetobacter baumannii* in biofilm and planktonic growth mode. *J. Microbiol.* 2009;47(6):728–35.
17. Paddick JS, Brailsford SR, Rao S, Soares RF, Kidd EA, Beighton D et al. Effect of biofilm growth on expression of surface proteins of *Actinomyces naeslundii* genospecies 2. *Appl Environ Microbiol.* 2006;72(5):3774–9.
18. Li W, Yao Z, Sun L, Hu W, Cao J, Lin W et al. Proteomics analysis reveals a potential antibiotic cocktail therapy strategy for *Aeromonas hydrophila* infection in biofilm. *J Proteome Res.* 2016;15(6):1810–20.
19. Villena GK, Venkatesh L, Yamazaki A, Tsuyumu S. Initial intracellular proteome profile of *Aspergillus niger* biofilms. *Rev Peru Biol.* 2009;16(1):101–8.
20. Bruns S, Seidler M, Albrecht D, Salvenmoser S, Remme N, Hertweck C et al. Functional genomic profiling of *Aspergillus fumigatus* biofilm reveals enhanced production of the mycotoxin gliotoxin. *Proteomics.* 2010;10(17):3097–107.
21. Oosthuizen MC, Steyn B, Theron J, Cosette P, Lindsay D, Von Holy A et al. Proteomic analysis reveals differential protein expression by *Bacillus cereus* during biofilm formation. *Appl Environ Microbiol.* 2002;68(6):2770–80.
22. Morikawa M, Kagihiro S, Haruki M, Takano K, Branda S, Kolter R, Kanaya S. Biofilm formation by a *Bacillus subtilis* strain that produces gamma-polyglutamate. *Microbiology.* 2006;152(9):2801–7.
23. Serra DO, Lucking G, Weiland F, Schulz S, Gorg A, Yantorno OM et al. Proteome approaches combined with Fourier transform infrared spectroscopy revealed a distinctive biofilm physiology in *Bordetella pertussis*. *Proteomics.* 2008;8(23–24):4995–5010.
24. Mukherjee PK, Mohamed S, Chandra J, Kuhn D, Liu S, Antar OS et al. Alcohol dehydrogenase restricts the ability of the pathogen *Candida albicans* to form a biofilm on catheter surfaces through an ethanol-based mechanism. *Infect Immun.* 2006;74(7):3804–16.
25. Vediyappan G, Chaffin WL. Non-glucan attached proteins of *Candida albicans* biofilm formed on various surfaces. *Mycopathologia.* 2006;161(1):3–10.
26. Thomas DP, Bachmann SP, Lopez-Ribot JL. Proteomics for the analysis of the *Candida albicans* biofilm lifestyle. *Proteomics.* 2006;6(21):5795–804.

27. Seneviratne CJ, Wang Y, Jin L, Abiko Y, Samaranayake LP. *Candida albicans* biofilm formation is associated with increased anti-oxidative capacities. *Proteomics.* 2008; 8(14):2936–47.

28. Martinez-Gomariz M, Perumal P, Mekala S, Nombela C, Chaffin WL, Gil C. Proteomic analysis of cytoplasmic and surface proteins from yeast cells, hyphae, and biofilms of *Candida albicans. Proteomics.* 2009;9(8):2230–52.

29. Seneviratne, CJ, Wang Y, Jin L, Abiko Y, Samaranayake LP. Proteomics of drug resistance in *Candida glabrata* biofilms. *Proteomics.* 2010;10(7):1444–54.

30. Dykes GA, Sampathkumar B, Korber DR. Planktonic or biofilm growth affects survival, hydrophobicity and protein expression patterns of a pathogenic *Campylobacter jejuni* strain. *Int. J. Food Microbiol.* 2003;89(1):1–10.

31. Kalmokoff M, Lanthier P, Tremblay TL, Foss M, Lau PC, Sanders G et al. Proteomic analysis of *Campylobacter jejuni* 11168 biofilms reveals a role for the motility complex in biofilm formation. *J Bacteriol.* 2006;188(12):4312–20.

32. Santi L, Beys-da-Silva WO, Berger M, Calzolari D, Guimaraes JA, Moresco JJ et al. Proteomic profile of *Cryptococcus neoformans* biofilm reveals changes in metabolic processes. *J Proteome Res.* 2014;13(3):1545–59.

33. Mukherjee J, Ow SY, Noirel J, Biggs CA. Quantitative protein expression and cell surface characteristics of *Escherichia coli* MG1655 biofilms. *Proteomics.* 2011;11(3):339–51.

34. Collet A, Vilain S, Cosette P, Junter GA, Jouenne T, Phillips RS et al. Protein expression in *Escherichia coli* S17–1 biofilms: Impact of indole. *Antonie Van Leeuwenhoek.* 2007;91(1):71–85.

35. Orme R, Douglas CW, Rimmer S, Webb M. Proteomic analysis of *Escherichia coli* biofilms reveals the overexpression of the outer membrane protein OmpA. *Proteomics.* 2006;6(15):4269–77.

36. Kim YH, Lee Y, Kim S, Yeom J, Yeom S, Seok Kim B et al. The role of periplasmic antioxidant enzymes (superoxide dismutase and thiol peroxidase) of the Shiga toxin-producing *Escherichia coli* O157:H7 in the formation of biofilms. *Proteomics.* 2006;6(23):6181–93.

37. Tremoulet F, Duche O, Namane A, Martinie B, Labadie JC. Comparison of protein patterns of *Listeria monocytogenes* grown in biofilm or in planktonic mode by proteomic analysis. *FEMS Microbiol Lett.* 2002;210(1):25–31.

38. Qayyum S, Sharma D, Bisht D, Khan AU. Protein translation machinery holds a key for transition of planktonic cells to biofilm state in *Enterococcus faecalis*: A proteomic approach. *Biochem Biophys Res Commun.* 2016;474(4):652–9.

39. Gallaher TK, Wu S, Webster P, Aguilera R. Identification of biofilm proteins in non-typeable *Haemophilus Influenzae. BMC Microbiol.* 2006;6:65.

40. De Angelis M, Siragusa S, Campanella D, Di Cagno R, Gobbetti M. Comparative proteomic analysis of biofilm and planktonic cells of *Lactobacillus plantarum* DB200. *Proteomics.* 2015;15(13):2244–57.

41. Helloin E, Jansch L, Phan-Thanh L. Carbon starvation survival of *Listeria monocytogenes* in planktonic state and in biofilm: A proteomic study. *Proteomics.* 2003;3(10): 2052–64.

42. Hefford MA, D'Aoust S, Cyr TD, Austin JW, Sanders G, Kheradpir E, Kalmokoff ML. Proteomic and microscopic analysis of biofilms formed by *Listeria monocytogenes* 568. *Can J Microbiol.* 2005;51(3):197–208.

43. Gómez NC, Abriouel H, Ennahar S, Gálvez A. Comparative proteomic analysis of *Listeria monocytogenes* exposed to enterocin AS-48 in planktonic and sessile states. *Int J Food Microbiol.* 2013;167(2):202–7.

44. van Alen T, Claus H, Zahedi RP, Groh J, Blazyca H, Lappann M et al. Comparative proteomic analysis of biofilm and planktonic cells of *Neisseria meningitidis. Proteomics.* 2010;10(24):4512–21.

45. Phillips NJ, Steichen CT, Schilling B, Post DM, Niles RK, Bair TB et al. Proteomic analysis of *Neisseria gonorrhoeae* biofilms shows shift to anaerobic respiration and changes in nutrient transport and outermembrane proteins. *PLoS ONE*. 2012;7(6):e38303.

46. Kuboniwa M, Hendrickson EL, Xia Q, Wang T, Xie H, Hackett M et al. Proteomics of *Porphyromonas gingivalis* within a model oral microbial community. *BMC Microbiol*. 2009;9:98.

47. Ang CS, Veith PD, Dashper SG, Reynolds EC. Application of 16O/18O reverse proteolytic labeling to determine the effect of biofilm culture on the cell envelope proteome of *Porphyromonas gingivalis* W50. *Proteomics*. 2008;8(8):1645–60.

48. Benamara H, Rihouey C, Jouenne T, Alexandre S. Impact of the biofilm mode of growth on the inner membrane phospholipid composition and lipid domains in *Pseudomonas aeruginosa*. *Biochim. Biophys. Acta*. 2011;1808(1):98–105.

49. Steyn B, Oosthuizen MC, MacDonald R, Theron J, Brozel VS. The use of glass wool as an attachment surface for studying phenotypic changes in *Pseudomonas aeruginosa* biofilms by two-dimensional gel electrophoresis. *Proteomics*. 2001;1(7):871–9.

50. Vilain S, Cosette P, Hubert M, Lange C, Junter GA, Jouenne T. Comparative proteomic analysis of planktonic and immobilized *Pseudomonas aeruginosa* cells: A multivariate statistical approach. *Anal. Biochem*. 2004;329(1):120–30.

51. Petrova OE, Sauer K. A novel signaling network essential for regulating *Pseudomonas aeruginosa* biofilm development. *PLoS Pathog*. 2009;5(11):e1000668.

52. Southey-Pillig CJ, Davies DG, Sauer K. Characterization of temporal protein production in *Pseudomonas aeruginosa* biofilms. *J. Bacteriol*. 2005;187(23):8114–26.

53. Patrauchan MA, Sarkisova SA, Franklin MJ. Strain-specific proteome responses of *Pseudomonas aeruginosa* to biofilm-associated growth and to calcium. *Microbiology*. 2007;153(Pt 11):3838–51.

54. Park AJ, Murphy K, Krieger JR, Brewer D, Taylor P, Habash M et al. A temporal examination of the planktonic and biofilm proteome of whole cell *Pseudomonas aeruginosa* PAO1 using quantitative mass spectrometry. *Mol Cell Proteomics*. 2014; 13(4):1095–105.

55. Park AJ, Murphy K, Surette MD, Bandoro C, Krieger JR, Taylor P et al. Tracking the dynamic relationship between cellular systems and extracellular subproteomes in *Pseudomonas aeruginosa* biofilms. *J Proteome Res*. 2015;14(11):4524–37.

56. Zhang W, Sun J, Ding W, Lin J, Tian R, Lu L et al. Extracellular matrix-associated proteins form an integral and dynamic system during *Pseudomonas aeruginosa* biofilm development. *Front Cell Infect Microbiol*. 2015;5.

57. Chua SL, Yam JKH, Hao P, Adav SS, Salido MM, Liu Y et al. Selective labelling and eradication of antibiotic-tolerant bacterial populations in *Pseudomonas aeruginosa* biofilms. *Nat Commun*. 2016;7.

58. Purschke FG, Hiller E, Trick I, Rupp S. Flexible survival strategies of *Pseudomonas aeruginosa* in biofilms result in increased fitness compared with *Candida albicans*. *Mol Cell Proteomics*. 2012;11(12):1652–69.

59. Mangalappalli-Illathu AK, Korber DR. Adaptive resistance and differential protein expression of *Salmonella enterica* serovar *Enteritidis* biofilms exposed to benzalkonium chloride. *Antimicrob. Agents Chemother*. 2006;50(11):3588–96.

60. Mangalappalli-Illathu AK, Vidovic S, Korber DR. Differential adaptive response and survival of *Salmonella enterica* serovar enteritidis planktonic and biofilm cells exposed to benzalkonium chloride. *Antimicrob Agents Chemother*. 2008;52(10): 3669–80.

61. Mangalappalli-Illathu AK, Lawrence JR, Swerhone GD, Korber DR. Architectural adaptation and protein expression patterns of Salmonella enterica serovar Enteritidis biofilms under laminar flow conditions. *Int. J. Food Microbiol*. 2008;123:109–120.

62. Resch A, Leicht S, Saric M, Pasztor L, Jakob A, Gotz F et al. Comparative proteome analysis of *Staphylococcus aureus* biofilm and planktonic cells and correlation with transcriptome profiling. *Proteomics*. 2006;6(6):1867–77.

63. Muthukrishnan G, Quinn GA, Lamers RP, Diaz C, Cole AL, Chen S et al. Exoproteome of *Staphylococcus aureus* reveals putative determinants of nasal carriage. *J Proteome Res*. 2011;10(4):2064–78.

64. Islam N, Kim Y, Ross JM, Marten MR. Proteomic analysis of *Staphylococcus aureus* biofilm cells grown under physiologically relevant fluid shear stress conditions. *Proteome Sci*. 2014;12(1):1.

65. Planchon S, Desvaux M, Chafsey I, Chambon C, Leroy S, Hebraud M et al. Comparative subproteome analyses of planktonic and sessile *Staphylococcus xylosus* C2a: New insight in cell physiology of a coagulase-negative Staphylococcus in biofilm. *J. Proteome Res*. 2009;8(4):1797–1809.

66. Yi L, Wang Y, Ma Z, Zhang H, Li Y, Zheng J-x, Yang Y-c, Fan H-j, Lu C-p . Biofilm formation of *Streptococcus equi* ssp. *zooepidemicus* and comparative proteomic analysis of biofilm and planktonic cells. *Curr Microbiol*. 2014;69(3):227–33.

67. Rathsam C, Eaton RE, Simpson CL, Browne GV, Berg T, Harty DW et al. Up-regulation of competence- but not stress-responsive proteins accompanies an altered metabolic phenotype in *Streptococcus mutans* biofilms. *Microbiology*. 2005;151(Pt 6):1823–37.

68. Svensäter G, Welin J, Wilkins JC, Beighton D, Hamilton IR. Protein expression by planktonic and biofilm cells of *Streptococcus mutans*. *FEMS Microbiol Lett*. 2001;205(1):139–46.

69. Welin J, Wilkins JC, Beighton D, Wrzesinski K, Fey SJ, Mose-Larsen P et al. Effect of acid shock on protein expression by biofilm cells of *Streptococcus mutans*. *FEMS Microbiol. Lett*. 2003;227:287–93.

70. Welin J, Wilkins JC, Beighton D, Svensater G. Protein expression by *Streptococcus mutans* during initial stage of biofilm formation. *Appl. Environ. Microbiol*. 2004;70(6): 3736–41.

71. Sanui T, Gregory RL. Analysis of *Streptococcus mutans* biofilm proteins recognized by salivary immunoglobulin A. *Oral Microbiol Immunol*. 2009;24(5):361–8.

72. Luppens SB, ten Cate JM. Effect of biofilm model, mode of growth, and strain on *Streptococcus mutans* protein expression as determined by two-dimensional difference gel electrophoresis. *J. Proteome Res*. 2005;4(2):232–7.

73. Li J, Wang W, Wang Y, Zeng AP. Two-dimensional gel-based proteomic of the caries causative bacterium *Streptococcus mutans* UA159 and insight into the inhibitory effect of carolacton. *Proteomics*. 2013;13(23–24):3470–7.

74. Yoshida A, Niki M, Yamamoto Y, Yasunaga A, Ansai T. Proteome analysis identifies the Dpr protein of *Streptococcus mutans* as an important factor in the presence of early streptococcal colonizers of tooth surfaces. *PLoS ONE*. 2015;10(3):e0121176.

75. Wang Y, Yi L, Wu Z, Shao J, Liu G, Fan H, Zhang W, Lu C. Comparative proteomic analysis of *Streptococcus suis* biofilms and planktonic cells that identified biofilm infection-related immunogenic proteins. *PLoS One*. 2012;7(4):e33371.

76. Zhao Y-L, Zhou Y-H, Chen J-Q, Huang Q-Y, Han Q, Liu B, Cheng G-D, Li Y-H. Quantitative proteomic analysis of sub-MIC erythromycin inhibiting biofilm formation of S. suis in vitro. *J Proteomics*. 2015;116:1–14.

77. Pham TK, Roy S, Noirel J, Douglas I, Wright PC, Stafford GP. A quantitative proteomic analysis of biofilm adaptation by the periodontal pathogen *Tannerella forsythia*. *Proteomics*. 2010;10(17):3130–41.

78. Dharmaprakash A, Mutt E, Jaleel A, Ramanathan S, Thomas S. Proteome profile of a pandemic *Vibrio parahaemolyticus* SC192 strain in the planktonic and biofilm condition. *Biofouling*. 2014;30(6):729–39.

79. Paes Leme AF, Bellato CM, Bedi G, Cury AA, Koo H, Cury JA. Effects of sucrose on the extracellular matrix of plaque-like biofilm formed in vivo, studied by proteomic analysis. *Caries Res.* 2008;42(6):435–43.

80. Ram RJ, Verberkmoes NC, Thelen MP, Tyson GW, Baker BJ, Blake RC 2nd et al. Community proteomics of a natural microbial biofilm. *Science.* 2005;308(5730):1915–20.

81. VerBerkmoes NC, Denef VJ, Hettich RL, Banfield JF. Systems biology: Functional analysis of natural microbial consortia using community proteomics. *Nat Rev Microbiol.* 2009;7(3):196–205.

82. Schneider T, Riedel K. Environmental proteomics: Analysis of structure and function of microbial communities. *Proteomics.* 2010;10(4):785–98.

83. Bhadauria V, Zhao WS, Wang LX, Zhang Y, Liu JH, Yang J et al. Advances in fungal proteomics. *Microbiol Res.* 2007;162(3):193–200.

84. Wisniewski JR, Zougman A, Nagaraj N, Mann M. Universal sample preparation method for proteome analysis. *Nat Methods.* 2009;6(5):359–62.

85. Wu X, Xiong E, Wang W, Scali M, Cresti M. Universal sample preparation method integrating trichloroacetic acid/acetone precipitation with phenol extraction for crop proteomic analysis. *Nat Protoc.* 2014;9(2):362–74.

86. Rhomberg TA, Karlberg O, Mini T, Zimny-Arndt U, Wickenberg U, Rottgen M et al. Proteomic analysis of the sarcosine-insoluble outer membrane fraction of the bacterial pathogen *Bartonella henselae*. *Proteomics.* 2004;4(10):3021–33.

87. Thein M, Sauer G, Paramasivam N, Grin I, Linke D. Efficient subfractionation of gram-negative bacteria for proteomics studies. *J Proteome Res.* 2010;9(12):6135–47.

88. Brinkworth AJ, Hammer CH, Olano LR, Kobayashi SD, Chen L, Kreiswirth BN et al. Identification of outer membrane and exoproteins of carbapenem-resistant multilocus sequence type 258 *Klebsiella pneumoniae*. *PloS ONE.* 2015;10(4):e0123219.

89. Martorana AM, Motta S, Di Silvestre D, Falchi F, Deho G, Mauri P et al. Dissecting *Escherichia coli* outer membrane biogenesis using differential proteomics. *PloS ONE.* 2014;9(6):e100941.

90. Wiederhold E, Veenhoff LM, Poolman B, Slotboom DJ. Proteomics of *Saccharomyces cerevisiae* organelles. *Mol Cell Proteomics.* 2010;9(3):431–45.

91. Premsler T, Zahedi RP, Lewandrowski U, Sickmann A. Recent advances in yeast organelle and membrane proteomics. *Proteomics.* 2009;9(20):4731–43.

92. Reales-Calderon JA, Martinez-Solano L, Martinez-Gomariz M, Nombela C, Molero G, Gil C. Sub-proteomic study on macrophage response to *Candida albicans* unravels new proteins involved in the host defense against the fungus. *J Proteomics.* 2012;75(15):4734–46.

93. Allan RN, Morgan S, Brito-Mutunayagam S, Skipp P, Feelisch M, Hayes SM et al. Low concentrations of nitric oxide modulate *Streptococcus pneumoniae* biofilm metabolism and antibiotic tolerance. *Antimicrob Agents Chemother.* 2016;60(4):2456–66.

94. Oliveira BM, Coorssen JR, Martins-de-Souza D. 2DE: The phoenix of proteomics. *J Proteomics.* 2014;104:140–50.

95. Aebersold R, Mann M. Mass spectrometry-based proteomics. *Nature.* 2003;422(6928):198–207.

96. Gorg A, Weiss W, Dunn MJ. Current two-dimensional electrophoresis technology for proteomics. *Proteomics.* 2004;4(12):3665–85.

97. Rabilloud T, Chevallet M, Luche S, Lelong C. Two-dimensional gel electrophoresis in proteomics: Past, present and future. *J Proteomics.* 2010;73(11):2064–77.

98. Gregorich ZR, Chang YH, Ge Y. Proteomics in heart failure: Top-down or bottom-up? *Pflugers Arch: Eur J Physiol.* 2014;466(6):1199–209.

99. Appel RD, Palagi PM, Walther D, Vargas JR, Sanchez JC, Ravier F et al. Melanie II: A third-generation software package for analysis of two-dimensional electrophoresis images: I. Features and user interface. *Electrophoresis.* 1997;18(15):2724–34.

100. Patton WF, Beechem JM. Rainbow's end: The quest for multiplexed fluorescence quantitative analysis in proteomics. *Curr Opin Chem Biol.* 2002;6(1):63–9.

101. Unlu M, Morgan ME, Minden JS. Difference gel electrophoresis: A single gel method for detecting changes in protein extracts. *Electrophoresis.* 1997;18(11):2071–7.

102. Rathsam C, Eaton RE, Simpson CL, Browne GV, Valova VA, Harty DW et al. Two-dimensional fluorescence difference gel electrophoretic analysis of *Streptococcus mutans* biofilms. *J Proteome Res.* 2005;4(6):2161–73.

103. Seneviratne CJ, Wang Y, Jin L, Abiko Y, Samaranayake LP. Proteomics of drug resistance in *Candida glabrata* biofilms. *Proteomics.* 2010;10(7):1444–54.

104. Hamdan M, Righetti PG. Assessment of protein expression by means of 2-D gel electrophoresis with and without mass spectrometry. *Mass Spectrom Rev.* 2003;22(4): 272–84.

105. Bunai K, Yamane K. Effectiveness and limitation of two-dimensional gel electrophoresis in bacterial membrane protein proteomics and perspectives. *J Chromatogr B Analyt Technol Biomed Life Sci.* 2005;815(1–2):227–36.

106. Armirotti A, Damonte G. Achievements and perspectives of top-down proteomics. *Proteomics.* 2010;10(20):3566–76.

107. Soufi Y, Soufi B. Mass Spectrometry-based bacterial proteomics: Focus on dermatologic microbial pathogens. *Front Microbiol.* 2016;7:181.

108. Moradian A, Kalli A, Sweredoski MJ, Hess S. The top-down, middle-down, and bottom-up mass spectrometry approaches for characterization of histone variants and their post-translational modifications. *Proteomics.* 2014;14(4–5):489–97.

109. Millea KM, Krull IS, Cohen SA, Gebler JC, Berger SJ. Integration of multidimensional chromatographic protein separations with a combined 'top-down' and 'bottom-up' proteomic strategy. *J Proteome Res.* 2006;5(1):135–46.

110. Mukherjee J, Ow SY, Noirel J, Biggs CA. Quantitative protein expression and cell surface characteristics of *Escherichia coli* MG1655 biofilms. *Proteomics.* 2011;11(3):339–51.

111. Chua SL, Yam JK, Hao P, Adav SS, Salido MM, Liu Y et al. Selective labelling and eradication of antibiotic-tolerant bacterial populations in *Pseudomonas aeruginosa* biofilms. *Nat Commun.* 2016;7:10750.

112. Pan C, Banfield JF. Quantitative metaproteomics: Functional insights into microbial communities. *Methods Mol Biol.* 2014;1096:231–40.

113. Bostanci N, Bao K, Wahlander A, Grossmann J, Thurnheer T, Belibasakis GN. Secretome of gingival epithelium in response to subgingival biofilms. *Mol Oral Microbiol.* 2015;30(4):323–35.

114. Bao K, Bostanci N, Selevsek N, Thurnheer T, Belibasakis GN. Quantitative proteomics reveal distinct protein regulations caused by *Aggregatibacter actinomycetemcomitans* within subgingival biofilms. *PloS ONE.* 2015;10(3):e0119222.

115. Mata MM, da Silva WP, Wilson R, Lowe E, Bowman JP. Attached and planktonic *Listeria monocytogenes* global proteomic responses and associated influence of strain genetics and temperature. *J Proteome Res.* 2015;14(2):1161–73.

116. Herbst FA, Sondergaard MT, Kjeldal H, Stensballe A, Nielsen PH, Dueholm MS. Major proteomic changes associated with amyloid-induced biofilm formation in *Pseudomonas aeruginosa* PAO1. *J Proteome Res.* 2015;14(1):72–81.

117. Gayoso CM, Mateos J, Mendez JA, Fernandez-Puente P, Rumbo C, Tomas M et al. Molecular mechanisms involved in the response to desiccation stress and persistence in *Acinetobacter baumannii*. *J Proteome Res.* 2014;13(2):460–76.

118. Li P, Seneviratne CJ, Alpi E, Vizcaino JA, Jin L. Delicate Metabolic control and coordinated stress response critically determine antifungal tolerance of *Candida albicans* biofilm persisters. *Antimicrob Agents Chemother.* 2015;59(10):6101–12.

119. Seneviratne CJ, Zhang CF, Samaranayake LP. Dental plaque biofilm in oral health and disease. *Chin J Dent Res.* 2011;14(2):87–94.

120. Trindade F, Oppenheim FG, Helmerhorst EJ, Amado F, Gomes PS, Vitorino R. Uncovering the molecular networks in periodontitis. *Proteomics Clin Appl.* 2014;8(9–10):748–61.
121. Li Z, Adams RM, Chourey K, Hurst GB, Hettich RL, Pan C. Systematic comparison of label-free, metabolic labeling, and isobaric chemical labeling for quantitative proteomics on LTQ Orbitrap Velos. *J Proteome Res.* 2012;11(3):1582–90.
122. Hall-Stoodley L, Costerton JW, Stoodley P. Bacterial biofilms: From the natural environment to infectious diseases. *Nat Rev Microbiol.* 2004;2(2):95–108.
123. Sauer K. The genomics and proteomics of biofilm formation. *Genome Biol.* 2003;4(6):219.
124. Seneviratne CJ, Jin L, Samaranayake LP. Biofilm lifestyle of *Candida*: A mini review. Oral Dis. 2008;14(7):582–90.
125. Lewis K. Persister cells. *Annu Rev Microbiol.* 2010;64:357–72.
126. Costerton JW, Lewandowski Z, Caldwell DE, Korber DR, Lappin-Scott HM. Microbial biofilms. *Annu Rev Microbiol.* 1995;49:711–45.
127. Lopez D, Vlamakis H, Kolter R. Biofilms. *Cold Spring Harb Perspect Biol.* 2(7): a000398.
128. Donlan RM, Costerton JW. Biofilms: Survival mechanisms of clinically relevant microorganisms. *Clin Microbiol Rev.* 2002;15(2):167–93.
129. Flemming HC, Wingender J. The biofilm matrix. *Nat Rev Microbiol.* 8(9):623–33.
130. Branda SS, Vik S, Friedman L, Kolter R. Biofilms: The matrix revisited. *Trends Microbiol.* 2005;13(1):20–6.
131. Jabbouri S, Sadovskaya I. Characteristics of the biofilm matrix and its role as a possible target for the detection and eradication of *Staphylococcus epidermidis* associated with medical implant infections. *FEMS Immunol Med Microbiol.* 59(3):280–91.
132. Xavier JB, Picioreanu C, Rani SA, van Loosdrecht MC, Stewart PS. Biofilm-control strategies based on enzymic disruption of the extracellular polymeric substance matrix: A modelling study. *Microbiology.* 2005;151(Pt 12):3817–32.
133. Marvasi M, Visscher PT, Casillas Martinez L. Exopolymeric substances (EPS) from *Bacillus subtilis*: Polymers and genes encoding their synthesis. *FEMS Microbiol Lett.*313(1):1–9.
134. Vu B, Chen M, Crawford RJ, Ivanova EP. Bacterial extracellular polysaccharides involved in biofilm formation. *Molecules.* 2009;14(7):2535–54.
135. Latasa C, Solano C, Penades JR, Lasa I. Biofilm-associated proteins. *C R Biol.* 2006;329(11):849–57.
136. Sheng GP, Yu HQ, Li XY. Extracellular polymeric substances (EPS) of microbial aggregates in biological wastewater treatment systems: A review. *Biotechnol Adv.* 2010;28(6):882–94.
137. Gil C, Solano C, Burgui S, Latasa C, Garcia B, Toledo-Arana A et al. Biofilm matrix exoproteins induce a protective immune response against *Staphylococcus aureus* biofilm infection. *Infect Immun.* 2014;82(3):1017–29.
138. Zarnowski R, Westler WM, Lacmbouh GA, Marita JM, Bothe JR, Bernhardt J et al. Novel entries in a fungal biofilm matrix encyclopedia. *mBio.* 2014;5(4):e01333–14.
139. Mata MM, da Silva WP, Wilson R, Lowe E, Bowman JP. Attached and planktonic *Listeria monocytogenes* global proteomic responses and associated influence of strain genetics and temperature. *J Proteome Res.* 2015;14(2):1161–73.
140. Aguilar-Pontes MV, de Vries RP, Zhou M. (Post-)genomics approaches in fungal research. *Brief Funct Genomics.* 2014;13(6):424–39.
141. Martin T, Sherman DJ, Durrens P. The Genolevures database. *C R Biol.* 2011;334(8–9):585–9.
142. Skrzypek MS, Binkley J, Sherlock G. How to use the *Candida* Genome Database. *Methods Mol Biol.* 2016;1356:3–15.

143. Arnaud MB, Costanzo MC, Skrzypek MS, Binkley G, Lane C, Miyasato SR et al. The *Candida* Genome Database (CGD), a community resource for *Candida albicans* gene and protein information. *Nucleic Acids Res.* 2005;33(Database issue):D358–63.

144. d'Enfert C, Goyard S, Rodriguez-Arnaveilhe S, Frangeul L, Jones L, Tekaia F et al. CandidaDB: A genome database for *Candida albicans* pathogenomics. *Nucleic Acids Res.* 2005;33(Database issue):D353–7.

145. Engel SR, Weng S, Binkley G, Paskov K, Song G, Cherry JM. From one to many: Expanding the *Saccharomyces cerevisiae* reference genome panel. *Database: J Biol databases Curat.* 2016;2016:baw020, doi:10.1093/database/baw020.

146. Cherry JM. The *Saccharomyces* Genome Database: A tool for discovery. *Cold Spring Harbor Protoc.* 2015;2015(12):pdb.top083840, doi:10.1101/pdb.top083840.

147. Castillo L, Calvo E, Martinez AI, Ruiz-Herrera J, Valentin E, Lopez JA et al. A study of the *Candida albicans* cell wall proteome. *Proteomics.* 2008;8(18):3871–81.

148. Chaffin WL. *Candida albicans* cell wall proteins. *Microbiol Mol Biol Rev: MMBR.* 2008;72(3):495–544.

149. Vialas V, Perumal P, Gutierrez D, Ximenez-Embun P, Nombela C, Gil C et al. Cell surface shaving of *Candida albicans* biofilms, hyphae, and yeast form cells. *Proteomics.* 2012;12(14):2331–9.

150. Seneviratne CJ, Wang Y, Jin L, Abiko Y, Samaranayake LP. Proteomics of drug resistance in *Candida glabrata* biofilms. *Proteomics.* 2010;10(7):1444–54.

151. Muszkieta L, Beauvais A, Pahtz V, Gibbons JG, Anton Leberre V, Beau R et al. Investigation of *Aspergillus fumigatus* biofilm formation by various "omics" approaches. *Front Microbiol.* 2013;4:13.

152. Santi L, Beys-da-Silva WO, Berger M, Calzolari D, Guimarães JA, Moresco JJ et al. Proteomic profile of *Cryptococcus neoformans* biofilm reveals changes in metabolic processes. *J Proteome Res.* 2014;13(3):1545–59.

153. Seneviratne CJ, Jin LJ, Samaranayake YH, Samaranayake LP. Cell density and cell aging as factors modulating antifungal resistance of *Candida albicans* biofilms. *Antimicrob Agents Chemother.* 2008;52(9):3259–66.

154. Baillie GS, Douglas LJ. Matrix polymers of *Candida* biofilms and their possible role in biofilm resistance to antifungal agents. *J. Antimicrob. Chemother.* 2000;46(3):397–403.

155. Hitchen PG, Twigger K, Valiente E, Langdon RH, Wren BW, Dell A. Glycoproteomics: A powerful tool for characterizing the diverse glycoforms of bacterial pilins and flagellins. *Biochem Soc Trans.* 2010;38(5):1307–13.

156. Hitchen PG, Dell A. Bacterial glycoproteomics. *Microbiology.* 2006;152(Pt 6):1575–80.

157. Yin QY, de Groot PW, de Koster CG, Klis FM. Mass spectrometry-based proteomics of fungal wall glycoproteins. *Trends Microbiol.* 2008;16(1):20–6.

158. Borthwick AC, Holms WH, Nimmo HG. The phosphorylation of *Escherichia coli* isocitrate dehydrogenase in intact cells. *Biochem J.* 1984;222(3):797–804.

159. Deutscher J, Saier MH. Ser/Thr/Tyr protein phosphorylation in bacteria - for long time neglected, now well established. *J Mol Microbiol Biotechnol.* 2005;9(3–4):125–31.

160. Macek B, Mijakovic I, Olsen JV, Gnad F, Kumar C, Jensen PR et al. The serine/threonine/tyrosine phosphoproteome of the model bacterium *Bacillus subtilis*. *Mol Cell Proteomics.* 2007;6(4):697–707.

161. Soung GY, Miller JL, Koc H, Koc EC. Comprehensive analysis of phosphorylated proteins of *Escherichia coli* ribosomes. *J Proteome Res.* 2009;8(7):3390–402.

162. Denef VJ, Kalnejais LH, Mueller RS, Wilmes P, Baker BJ, Thomas BC et al. Proteogenomic basis for ecological divergence of closely related bacteria in natural acidophilic microbial communities. *Proc Natl Acad Sci U S A.* 2010;107(6):2383–90.

163. Mueller RS, Denef VJ, Kalnejais LH, Suttle KB, Thomas BC, Wilmes P et al. Ecological distribution and population physiology defined by proteomics in a natural microbial community. *Mol Syst Biol.* 2010;6:374.

164. Lo I, Denef VJ, Verberkmoes NC, Shah MB, Goltsman D, DiBartolo G et al. Strain-resolved community proteomics reveals recombining genomes of acidophilic bacteria. *Nature*. 2007;446(7135):537–41.

165. Wilmes P, Bond PL. Microbial community proteomics: Elucidating the catalysts and metabolic mechanisms that drive the Earth's biogeochemical cycles. *Curr Opin Microbiol*. 2009;12(3):310–7.

7 Metabolomics of Microbial Biofilms

Current Status and Future Directions

Tanujaa Suriyanarayanan,
Chaminda Jayampath Seneviratne, Wei Ling Ng,
Shruti Pavagadhi and Sanjay Swarup

CONTENTS

INTRODUCTION

Biofilms are matrix-enclosed microbial communities that form at interfaces of phases, such as liquid, solid and air and are the preferred mode of life in most natural conditions. They provide advantage to microorganisms to survive under diverse stress conditions such as nutrient deprivation, antibiotic treatment or other harsh environments. Physiology, growth and behaviour of microbes in the biofilm mode of life differ vastly from those of their free-living or planktonic mode of life [1]. Greater insights into the biofilm lifestyle of microorganisms can lead to effective strategies for controlling clinical and environmental biofilms. Hence, the characterisation of biofilms has emerged as one of the leading tools for drug discovery, treatment of infections, control of environmental biofilms, among other applications [2].

Several approaches, ranging from genetic to phenotypic characterisation of microbes, have been employed for understanding the nature of biofilms, critical factors governing their formation and the development of drug resistance mechanisms in biofilms. As the extent of changes occurring in this mode are quite large, systems level 'omics' approaches are especially suited to elucidate the reprogramming of microbial functions in this lifestyle. Genomics, proteomics and transcriptomics are some of the common omics approaches adopted for the analysis of microbial biofilms. Recently, attempts have also been made to study the attachment pattern of different bacteria to surfaces and integrate the data set with genomics and proteomics [3,4]. Despite significant leaps in our knowledge of biofilms, the aforementioned omics approaches present a major caveat, that is, they do not usually reveal the end-physiological state of a microbe. The biological flow of information is from genes to proteins to metabolites. Thus, metabolites are the final end-products resulting from all the changes occurring within a system [5]. Hence, profiling all the metabolites in a system can provide the much needed final biochemical or physiological phenotype of the cellular response. However, metabolic pathways are complex with a large amount of internetworking and are sensitive to even minor changes in the system, thereby posing significant challenges in providing an overall metabolite fingerprint. Recent technological advancements have helped in significantly overcoming this bottleneck and have led to the emergence of metabolomics as an invaluable tool in the field of microbial biofilms [6–12].

Metabolites are low molecular weight intermediates or end-products of enzyme-catalysed reactions in a cell. These molecules perform important structural and functional roles either within the cells or after secretion from the cells. Accordingly, metabolites can be classified as either primary or secondary metabolites. Molecules that are produced actively during growth phase and are essential for growth and development are known as primary or central metabolites. Examples of primary metabolites include alcohols such as ethanol and amino acids. Molecules that are not vital for growth and development but having specialised functions in the overall survivability and adaptability of the organism are known as secondary metabolites. Examples of secondary metabolites include antibiotics, pigments and second-messenger signalling molecules. Some of the secondary metabolites, such as antibiotics, help in competitive survival of the microorganism. These molecules can be used as defence mechanisms against other microbes. Some secondary metabolites also signal for the dormancy state of microbes under unfavourable conditions to promote survival and subsequent release from dormancy on favourable conditions. These metabolites are typically produced during stationary phase in planktonic growth conditions, or in biofilms, and may serve ecological functions [13].

The collection of all metabolites found in an organism is defined as a metabolome. The comprehensive detection, identification and quantification of the metabolome of a biological system is called metabolomics. As metabolites are representative of the end-states of biochemical activity, they are directly correlated with the observed phenotype, whereas genes and proteins undergo various epigenetic or post-translational modifications; hence, they are loosely correlated with the biochemical phenotype. Moreover, gene or protein expression changes can result in amplified changes in metabolism even when no phenotypic changes are observed. Thus, metabolomics can serve as an end-point monitoring tool. But, the types of metabolites observed in different organisms can be quite different, making the technology more organism-specific than generic [5,6].

Similar to gene expression profile, key primary and secondary metabolites also have a significant influence on biofilm formation. Thereby, metabolic profiling along with modelling of complex biological systems can help in the identification of pathways involved in biofilm formation, thus providing strategies for controlling biofilm development. Furthermore, metabolomics provides a valuable tool for investigating antibiotic resistance in biofilms [14]. The flux of metabolites observed during antibiotic resistance can be used to identify the key molecules and mechanisms of drug resistance. This, in turn, can lead to the development of drugs specific for the identified molecules. Metabolomics approaches have been used in the identification of antibiotic resistance mechanisms in bacteria such as *Staphylococcus aureus* [15]. Similarly, monitoring metabolite changes have been used to investigate the effects of various environmental stimuli on biofilm formation [16]. Apart from exploring antibiotic resistance, drug-discovery studies benefit significantly from metabolomics studies. This arises from the fact that certain molecules such as autoinducers have indispensable roles in biofilm formation. Molecules that mimic or inhibit the activity of autoinducers have been proposed as promising new approaches to mitigate biofilms and can be screened using metabolomics [17]. Similarly, the identification of other inter- or intracellular small molecules associated with biofilm attachment and development using metabolomics can be potential drug targets [8].

Biofilms consist of spatially organised collection of heterogeneous cells existing in varying states of metabolic activities to maximise survival. To gain a better understanding of the nature and behaviour of biofilms, it is essential to analyse comprehensively all the metabolic states occurring within their intricate community structure. Metabolomics, thereby, provides a systematic platform to examine the complex biofilm community [8].

METABOLOMICS APPROACHES FOR BIOFILM CHARACTERISATION

Metabolomics can be used to study changes in specific and predetermined biological pathways of interest, or to observie organism-wide changes in the metabolite profile. Hence, metabolomics approaches can broadly be classified into two categories, namely, targeted and untargeted approaches. Accordingly, metabolomics characterisation of biofilms can be performed either through global (non-specific) or targeted (specific) metabolite analysis [18,19]. Selecting an appropriate metabolomics approach is determined by the overall goal of the study and the number of metabolites to be captured. The targeted approach is driven by a hypothesis or a specific biological question in mind. For instance, the targeted approach is suitable in cases where the aim is to quantify specific extracellular polysaccharides involved in biofilm matrix formation. As this approach focuses on a specific central pathway of interest, it provides a direct answer to the biological question under consideration. However, in a discovery-based study, untargeted or profiling based metabolomics is more appropriate. The aim of this approach is to capture as many metabolites as possible in the samples under comparison without any bias. Unlike targeted metabolomics, which is driven by a specific hypothesis, untargeted metabolomics aims to generate hypotheses. The data set generated from an untargeted metabolomics experiment is also of significant complexity, presenting a major hurdle to the interpretation of meaningful data from the metabolic profiling. Manual inspection of the data is difficult, necessitating the development of specific software for data analysis. Freeware such as MetDAT, XCMS, Mzmine, MetaboAnalyst, MetAlign, MathDAMP, MetExplore and datPAV as well as mass spectrometry manufacturers' proprietary software such as Mass Profiler Professional (MPP), Sieve, Mass Hunter and Progenesis are some of the currently available software products for data preprocessing and analysis [20–26]. These software products have made a huge contribution towards the elucidation of significant metabolomics patterns during data assimilation. However, further validation tools are still required for successful interpretation of biological data derived from untargeted metabolomics [27]. Nevertheless, untargeted metabolomics profiling can serve as a valuable tool both in drug discovery and identification of heretofore unidentified pathways involved in biofilm formation [18,28].

OVERALL WORKFLOW OF METABOLOMICS

Metabolomics experiments usually encompass several steps starting from sample collection/extraction, sample analysis by either mass spectrometry (MS) or nuclear magnetic resonance (NMR) instrumentation, followed by data analysis, interpretation and database curation. A sequence of possible workflows that can be followed in a metabolomics experiment is shown in Figure 7.1.

SAMPLE PREPARATION FOR METABOLOMICS ANALYSIS

One of the most crucial steps in ensuring the success of a metabolomics experiment is the sample preparation process. The quality and credibility of metabolomics

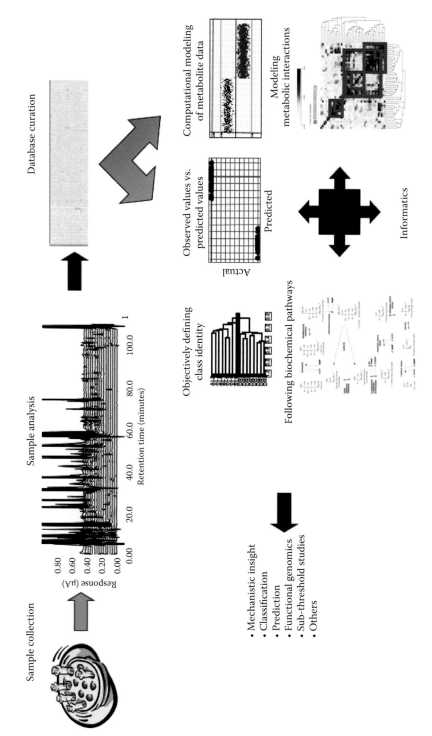

FIGURE 7.1 Possible workflows in metabolomics experiments.

data will invariably depend on sample harvesting and subsequent treatment procedures. The choice of an appropriate sample extraction platform affects the extent and depth of metabolite coverage and further biological interpretation. Sampling and extraction procedures are often dependent on the type of intended analysis, that is, targeted or profiling based metabolomics. For instance, sample preparation for untargeted/profiling based metabolomics should ideally be non-selective, have minimal metabolite loss/degradation/leakage and be reproducible [29,30]. Some of the important considerations for efficient sample preparation are highlighted in review reports from metabolomics consortium [19]. Good practices of sample preparation begin with quenching of the biological reactions occurring within the biofilm, prior to metabolites extraction. Metabolites such as pyruvate, fumarate, oxoglutarate, phosphoenolpyruvate and fructose-6-phosphate have turnover rates in ranging from milliseconds to tens of seconds [31,32]. Therefore, an effective way to quench all biological activities rapidly is necessary to obtain a reliable 'snapshot' of the metabolome. Without proper quenching, sample-to-sample variability and other types of data complexity will be introduced into the analysis. Proper care should be taken to avoid the induction of stress responses or cellular death mechanisms during quenching. One of the efficient quenching approaches involves reducing temperature of the samples by immersing in prechilled organic solution to halt metabolic activities within biofilm cells. Prechilled methanol (–20°C) is a commonly used extraction solvent for quenching. It is ideally suited for quenching because of its minimal toxicity and low freezing point compared to other organic solvents [33]. However, the percentage of methanol which allows for minimal leakage of metabolites varies from study to study and different sample types [30,34]. For example, one study showed that 40% methanol was the most optimal for quenching of *Penicillium chrysogenum*, while another study showed that 6% methanol was best suited for the quenching of *S. aureus* biofilms [12,35].

Sample handling steps also have a major influence on the data quality. The methods employed for extraction and quenching as well as the sample storage conditions can result in metabolite structure modifications. This, in turn, can increase the complexity of data sets and introduce a greater number of intersample variations [36]. Improper or incomplete removal of cell growth medium/washing results in erroneous data, as the cell growth medium is often supplemented with salts and nutrients, which might affect the column chemistry and resulting MS spectra. Centrifugation and fast-filtration methods are commonly employed to remove the cell growth medium before metabolites extraction. Centrifugation should be carried out in cold conditions. However, it usually takes a longer time, which may result in possible metabolite changes due to stress. Filtration is much faster and allows easy quenching of cells on a filter membrane. On the other hand, centrifugation is more consistent as the retrieval of cells from filter membrane varies considerably [8,37]. An NMR-based study on *S. aureus* showed that filtration followed by quenching provides the highest yield of metabolites [38]. Therefore, it is advisable to optimise the sample handling steps before the actual experiment to ensure that the sampling procedures are efficient and reliable.

Following the effective quenching and separation of medium from the cells, cell lysis and metabolite extraction can be performed either sequentially or simultaneously. Mechanical disruption methods such as glass beads/sonication or chemical disruption methods such as organic solvent-based methods are some of the commonly used cell lysis methodologies. Trichloroacetic acid has been traditionally used for lysing cells from filter paper. However, it generates significant background noise for metabolomics data. An optimal extraction buffer should be both non-selective and non-destructive [29]. One such commonly used extraction solvent is a 5:2:2 *v/v* mixture of methanol, chloroform and water [39]. In the case of metabolite extractions that include lipids, a modified Bligh and Dryer extraction method employing a 1:1 *v/v* mixture of methanol and chloroform, or water and chloroform is used [40]. Other extraction mixtures, such as 80% methanol or 50% methanol, are also commonly used, as they are simpler and more likely to be robust for high-throughput studies [39]. In some cases, acid, acetonitrile, or two-phase methanol/chloroform protocols are needed for separating polar and non-polar metabolites. For NMR analysis, metabolites are usually dissolved in a D_2O (heavy water, deuterium oxide) buffer or $CDCl_3$ (chloroform) [41]. Therefore, before considering any metabolomics analysis, an optimum extraction solvent should be developed, based on the nature and purpose of the study. This would often require evaluation of at least two or three extraction solvent protocols/systems in the trial phase of the study before commencing the final runs.

Sample preparation method is always governed by the nature of samples being analysed. In certain cases, where the study has to focus on metabolites that are released by the cells into the medium, the sample preparation is minimal, as cell lysis steps can be avoided. However, for analysis of metabolites within the cells, the preparation is more complex owing to the number of steps involved and the diverse range of metabolites found. In these cases, the washing step is absolutely essential as metabolites from the medium can affect the trend of intracellular metabolites observed. Hence, an ideal metabolomics experiment should carefully evaluate the nature of the organism and the type of analysis required before proceeding with the workflow. When analysing the metabolites profile of biofilms, the method of choice also depends on the way biofilms are cultivated. Biofilms can be studied under either static or continuous flow (washout) conditions. A number of studies have reported the use of microfluidic devices (flow cells) for cultivation of biofilms which are now commercially available (BioSurface Technologies [BST] Inc., www.biofilms.biz/flow-cells; Biocentrum-DTU 2005, DTU Systems Biology) [42]. These devices allow researchers to control the physical and chemical environment around the microorganisms, ensuring uniformity of fluid flow and homogeneity of biofilm formation. However, using such 'lab-on-a-chip'–based systems pose numerous challenges for metabolomics studies. The recovery of biofilm biomass from the chip/substrate and metabolite extraction are often more tedious and complicated than in other systems. Based on the type and arrangement of flow cells, the sampling procedures have to be tweaked and manipulated. This can be done by combining some of the sampling methods mentioned previously, along with scaling up of the number of flow cells to obtain an efficient recovery of biofilms from the flow cells, as well as a sufficient amount of metabolites for analysis [43].

The handling of large sample sets can introduce batch variations in metabolomics data. Ideal sampling and extraction strategies should therefore be efficient and reproducible, and should also have integrated quality control parameters to minimise batch effects. There are two ways to reduce and minimise the batch effects: (i) randomisation of samples from extraction step onwards and (ii) introduction of housekeeping compounds or internal quantitative controls in metabolite extracts. Isotopically labelled internal standards could be introduced either during the extraction process or just before injecting the samples into the MS machine. Addition of internal standards during the extraction process could also be used to evaluate the extraction efficiency and recovery when developing a new extraction procedure. These steps aid in data preprocessing, normalisation and MS peak alignment [44–46].

MODES OF METABOLOMICS ANALYSIS

Analysis of metabolomics data varies with each experimental setup and nature of biological question answered. The various modes of analysis include (a) metabolic fingerprinting, which generates a characteristic metabolic 'signature' for the samples, and differences in this pattern can be used to compare across different sample sets, but without any actual quantitation of metabolites [47,48]; (b) metabolic profiling, which proceeds via the quantitative analysis of all possible metabolites, both characterised and uncharacterised, according to their chemical nature and pathway association [49–51]; and (c) target isotope-based analysis, which selectively focuses on quantitation of metabolites that belong to a particular group or pathway using the most suitable analytical technique [52–54]. Metabolomics has to be paired with pattern recognition and bioinformatics approaches to detect metabolites and monitor their changes [55–57].

INSTRUMENTATION FOR METABOLOMICS STUDY

To date, the generation of metabolomics data has been performed mainly with NMR and MS approaches [58]. Liquid chromatography–mass spectrometry (LC-MS) is very commonly employed in MS-based metabolic profiling. Gas chromatography–mass spectrometry (GC-MS) is also used for quantitative metabolic profiling, but is largely limited to volatile compounds. MS determines the composition of molecules based on the mass-to-charge ratio (m/z) of charged particles, while NMR exploits the molecular behaviour in the magnetic field to allow for the identification of different nuclei based on their resonance frequency [59].

MS INSTRUMENTATION

Mass spectrometers result in the generation of charged metabolites through an ionisation process, followed by the analysis of the ions and fragment ions on the basis of their m/z. Many different combinations of ion sources and mass analysers result in different configurations of mass spectrometers that can be used for metabolite ionisation and ion analysis.

LC-MS

LC-MS, which combines the features of conventional liquid chromatography–based separation and mass spectrometry–based analysis is one of the predominantly used techniques for the analysis of biological and clinical samples. The high sensitivity of LC-MS, along with its capability to handle complex mixtures, makes it indispensable in the fields of biochemical genetics, drug discovery, *in vitro* and *in vivo* screening, high-throughput screening and several other clinical applications. As MS analysis is based on the conversion of analytes to ions, several ionisation techniques have been developed for application in LC-MS. The ionisation sources can be varied according to the nature of the analyte [60,61]. Some of the most commonly used ionisation sources for LC-MS are described in the text that follows.

LC-MS Ionisation Sources

Ionisation sources applied for LC-MS instruments include electrospray ionisation (ESI), atmospheric pressure chemical ionisation (APCI), and atmospheric pressure photoionisation (APPI). Although only a brief summary is provided below for biologist and clinician users, excellent reviews and books are available for more detailed handling of this vast topic [34,62,63].

ESI

ESI is a technique that produces ions through the use of electrospray, where a fine aerosol is generated by applying a high voltage to the liquid containing analytes. It works well with moderately polar metabolites, xenobiotics, and peptides. ESI is called a 'soft ionisation' technique, which is highly useful in producing ions from macromolecules, as it facilitates the ionisation of macromolecules without fragmentation. However, it can sometimes be useful to increase the 'in-source' fragmentation of ESI and this can be achieved by applying a series of increasing voltages to increase collisions with nitrogen molecules. This technique is useful in the identification of components with common structural features. As the ion formation process requires extensive solvent evaporation (desolvation) and decrease in initial droplet size, solvents used in ESI are typically prepared by mixing volatile organic compounds with water to increase conductivity. These can then provide a proton source for the ionisation process [64,65].

The analyte samples enter the mass spectrometer through a metal capillary that carries a potential difference of 3–5 kV and nebulised at the tip of the capillary to form a fine spray of charged droplets. Inert gases such as nitrogen can be used in large-flow electrosprays to allow additional nebulisation. On desolvation, the droplets become unstable and reach Rayleigh limit. At this point, the surface tension holding the droplets together is overcome by the electrostatic repulsion between the droplets [66]. The droplets then undergo Coulomb fission, whereby many smaller and more stable droplets are created by losing 1.0–2.3% of their mass together with 10–18% of their charge each time the fission process occurs. The ions generated from analyte samples are then subjected to analysis by transferring them into the high vacuum of a mass spectrometer via a series of small apertures and focussing voltages. The mass spectrometer can be operated in either positive or negative ion mode to detect positive or negative ions. The operational mode of the mass spectrometer can also be switched within a single run to facilitate analysis of both ions [67,68].

The major advantage of ESI over other atmospheric pressure ionisation processes is the production of multiply charged ions that can effectively span the analyser's mass range, thereby accommodating the wide kDa–MDa size range usually seen in protein and polypeptide molecules. Structural information can also be obtained by coupling ESI with tandem mass spectrometry (ESI-MS/MS). Moreover, ESI allows the retention of solution-phase information into gas phase. Although ESI is the most widely used ion source for biological molecules, neutral and low-polarity molecules, such as lipids, may not be efficiently ionised by this method [65]. Two alternative ionisation methods that can be applied for such analytes are described in the text that follows.

APCI

In APCI, the analyte liquid is pumped through a capillary and nebulised at the tip. A corona discharge located near the tip of the capillary is used to ionise the gas and solvent molecules present in the ion source. The analyte samples react with the ions generated and become ionised in turn by means of charge transfer. APCI is a particularly useful technique for ionising small thermally stable molecules that are not effectively ionised by ESI. Moderately polar metabolites, such as fatty acids and steroids, are suitable for ionisation through APCI mode. It has been reported that APCI mode is more sensitive than ESI mode for detection of phospholipids, especially phosphoethanolamines [69]. Another distinction from ESI is that multiple charging does not occur and so singly charged ions dominate [70].

APPI

In APPI, the analyte sample is subjected to ionisation by ultraviolet light instead of the corona discharge used in APCI. It is a relatively recent technique that predominantly generates singly charged ions to facilitate the analysis of neutral and less polar compounds, such as polycyclic aromatics. After nebulisation, photons are used to further excite and ionise the molecules. The photon energy is chosen so as to minimise the simultaneous ionisation of both solvents and ion source gases [71,72].

GC-MS AND GC/GC-MS

Gas chromatography coupled with mass spectrometer (GC-MS) is regarded as 'the gold standard' for the analysis of compounds such as environmental contaminants as well as for forensic science applications. The major advantage of GC-MS lies in its use of both retention time and mass spectrum to identify the species. Electron ionisation and chemical ionisation are the commonly used ionisation sources for GC-MS. As the fragmentation patterns of compounds are reproducible when ionised by a fixed electron voltage (usually −70 eV), the fragmentation spectra generated by GC-MS, unlike LC-MS, do not vary with different instruments, thereby facilitating database creation and data sharing among users. Additionally, there are standardised protocols for sample treatment and quantification using the appropriate standards available for measurement of single compounds or related sets of metabolites. The main limitation of GC-MS is that it can be used only for metabolites that are either volatile in nature, or can be made volatile through the derivatisation process. Furthermore, all non-volatile metabolites have to be removed through sample treatment before the sample can undergo analysis [73,74].

MS Mass Analysers

There are various types of mass analysers coupled to an ion source in MS instruments. These include quadrupole analysers, time-of-flight (TOF) analysers, ion trap analysers and hybrid analysers.

Quadrupole Analysers

Quadrupole analysers are made up of a set of four parallel metal rods, where a combination of constant and varying radio frequency voltages allows a narrow band of m/z values to be transmitted along the axis of the rods. Most quadrupole analysers can scan a range of m/z values up to 4,000 m/z, with scan speeds up to 1,000 m/z per second by means of varying the voltages with time. Because the analyser operates at unit mass resolution, the mass accuracy obtained is at best 0.1 m/z [75].

To improve the detection limits of targeted analytes, the quadrupoles can also be set to devote more detector time to monitor a number of specific m/z values by stepping the voltages. This can be carried out within a few milliseconds by allowing a panel of m/z values to be stepped through for detecting several analytes.

Quadrupole analysers can be used either singly, or in differential tandem mass spectrometer configuration to obtain increased specificity of mass analysis over that of single configuration. An example of a tandem MS with two or more stages of mass analysis is a particularly useful configuration known as a triple quadrupole mass spectrometer. It is made up of a collision cell placed between two quadrupole mass analysers. Ions can be induced to undergo fragmentation in the collision cell by means of collision with an inert gas such as nitrogen, in a process known as collision-induced dissociation (CID). The collision cell is composed of a quadrupole that specifically maintains the low pressure of the collision gas required for dissociation, and transmission of the fragment ions [76,77].

Targeted analysis of metabolites can be performed by selected reaction monitoring (SRM). Major ions produced during ESI and subsequent fragmented ions produced during CID can be specifically detected by SRM, where only analytes with the specific precursor/product ion combination will be monitored. In a biological sample, which is usually very complex, other components may likely produce precursor ions of similar or identical m/z values as that of the intended analyte. However, it is unlikely that the fragment product ions would also be of similar size. Therefore, SRM improves the specificity of the detection process [77]. The application of SRM to monitor several metabolites simultaneously is called multiple reaction monitoring (MRM), which is quite frequently used in LC-MS assays. In MRM, the first and third quadrupoles can be simultaneously set to scan a range of different m/z values to detect a large panel of analyte targets. Quadrupole analysers in single or triple quadrupole configuration find widespread applications in clinical biochemistry because of their ease of scanning and the generation of good quality quantitative data [78].

TOF Analysers

TOF-MS analysers measure the time taken by ions to travel from the beginning to the end of a field-free flight tube. The ions are accelerated through a pulsed high voltage to convert the output of the detector into a mass spectrum. The velocity of the ions is dependent on their m/z values. TOF analysers can acquire spectra quickly with high sensitivity and mass accuracy that allow determination of molecular formulas for small molecules [79]. They are largely employed in GC-MS systems. Though TOF-MS analysers facilitate fast data acquisition and analyte detection, the data acquired have only nominal mass resolution. However, their rapid detection of metabolites increases the throughput by reducing the analysis time. TOF analysers are often used in metabolomics studies, where a comprehensive two-dimensional chromatography is used to capture a wide range of metabolites (both polar and nonpolar) with a single injection [80].

Ion Trap Analysers

Ion trap analysers trap ions in three-dimensional space using static and radio frequency voltages generated by three hyberbolic electrodes. The trapped ions are then ejected sequentially based on their m/z values creating a mass spectrum. Specific ions can also be trapped by the application of a specific exciting voltage which allows other ions to be ejected. Inert gases such as helium can then be introduced into the trap to induce fragmentation. A particular feature of interest is known as the MS^n capability, which allows the fragmentation and isolation of ions several times in succession to obtain the final mass spectrum [81].

Orbitrap™ is an ion trap analyser that was introduced in 2000. It consists of an outer barrel-like electrode and a coaxial inner spindle-like electrode that trap ions in an orbital motion around the spindle [82]. Ions are trapped on elliptical trajectories around the inner electrode, by balancing their electrostatic attractions to the inner electrode with centrifugal forces. The frequency signal from the trapped ions are detected and converted to a mass spectrum using Fourier transformation. Orbitrap™ routinely provides a mass accuracy of 2–5 ppm, which is higher than that of most of the TOF analysers. Orbitrap™ is a formidable alternative to TOF mass analysers in terms of its mass accuracy and resolving power. It is currently being used extensively for targeted analysis, and has become a mainstream instrument in LC-MS–based metabolomics [69].

Hybrid Analysers

Tandem mass spectrometers using different combinations of mass analysers are now commonly employed. For example, the third quadrupole of a triple quadrupole MS can be replaced by a TOF analyser to produce a quadrupole TOF (QTOF) mass spectrometer. Although QTOFs are more limited in their scanning functions compared to triple quadrupole instruments, they are used extensively in the field of proteomics. This is because QTOF is able to provide a fingerprint of the compound structure by producing a full-scan MS/MS product ion spectrum. Yet another classic example of hybrid analyser is Orbitrap™ velos, which has an ion trap in the front and an orbitrap analyser in the rear end of the instrument. This setup introduces greater flexibility for metabolomics studies (both targeted and untargeted analysis) [83].

Another commonly used hybrid instrument is known as a linear ion trap or QTrap. In this configuration, the third quadrupole of a triple quadrupole MS operates in a different mode to allow trapping of ions and then sequentially separating them on the basis of their m/z values. To combine the useful features of both triple quadrupole and ion trap analysers, the operation of the third quadrupole can be switched between ion trap and conventional quadrupole modes. When the instrument is used in ion trap mode, its product ion scanning sensitivity is enhanced because of the additional stage of fragmentation and mass analysis (MS^3) [83].

LC-MS versus GC-MS

LC-MS technique provides high sensitivity and selectivity for the molecules identified. It is used in the case of non-volatile compounds, and in studies that are discovery based and involving large data sets. The technique has broader application as it can be used to separate a wide variety of organic compounds. LC-MS can also provide more comprehensive datasets encompassing molecular weight, structure, density, quantity and purity of samples. GC-MS is more limited to volatile compounds and has significant applications in forensic science. In terms of maintenance, GC-MS is both easier to operate as well as to maintain compared to LC-MS [84]. Certain analytes, such as essential oils, free fatty acids, sterols, carotenoids, phenolics, diglycerides, mono-, di- and trisaccharides and sugar alcohols are more compatible with GC-MS. GC-MS offers better separation for structurally similar compounds (e.g. free fatty acids) and is more suitable for less polar analytes. However, certain classes of analytes such as polyamines, nucleotides, ionic species and organic acids are compatible only with LC-MS [85]. Ideally, for untargeted analysis, both the platforms should be explored to obtain full metabolome coverage. For targeted metabolite analysis, the choice of platform would largely depend on the analyte chemistry.

NMR

NMR is the only spectroscopic technique from which a complete analysis and interpretation of the entire spectrum is normally expected [86]. Although a larger amount of sample is required for NMR compared to MS, it is a non-destructive technique. The concept of NMR is based on 'the phenomenon that occurs when the nuclei of certain atoms are immersed in a static magnetic field and exposed to a second oscillating magnetic field' [87,88]. Only nuclei that possess a spin can experience this phenomenon. This property is possessed by several atomic nuclei having either odd numbers of protons or neutrons or both. All isotopes that contain an odd number of protons, and/or of neutrons have an intrinsic magnetic moment and angular momentum. The most commonly studied nuclei are ^1H and ^{13}C. NMR is, therefore, dependent on the property of nuclear magnetism. It is a physical phenomenon in which nuclei in a magnetic field absorb and reemit electromagnetic radiation [8].

Applications of NMR are widely documented in the analysis of biofluids (urine, saliva, blood and serum samples) for identification of disease biomarkers, treatment monitoring and understanding disease pathogenesis [89]. Apart from biofluids, NMR also finds its applications in areas of environmental metabolomics. NMR has been employed to investigate the effects of environmental stressors associated with biofilm development of *S. epidermis* which indicated the central role of the tricarboxylic acid (TCA) cycle [90].

MS versus NMR

The major advantage conferred by MS is its sensitivity in the detection of analytes, even in the femto or attomolar range. This enables detection of a wide range of metabolites within a given sample set. While the detection is extremely sensitive, a problem with MS arises in the quantification aspect. The analytes in a MS study are affected by the sample preparation and environment. The use of internal standards can ensure accurate quantification, but is a limitation in discovery-driven studies. In NMR-based studies, the major strength is the accuracy of quantification, while the limitation is sensitivity, which is of the order 10 μM. NMR is advantageous for broad-based analysis, as its sensitivity is not influenced by metabolite pKa or hydrophobicity. MS, on the other hand, needs ESI to detect polar molecules, and APCI or APPI to detect non-polar molecules. Furthermore, NMR can provide highly quantitative and reproducible data for multivariate statistical methods that can in turn compensate for its limited sensitivity. However, NMR analysis on complex samples can generate a large number of peaks in a small chemical shift range that can overlap with each other in the spectrum. This results in potentially important compounds being overshadowed by larger peaks. MS, in contrast, permits highly specific identification of multiple metabolites at low concentrations. Though technological advancements are facilitating improved detection and quantification in both systems, the choice of instrumentation should again be determined based on the biological system and complexity [91].

DATA ANALYSIS AND INTERPRETATION

The post-success of any metabolomics experiment depends on the data handling methodology. The global metabolome of a biological sample would require hundreds or thousands of metabolites to be assessed simultaneously. To obtain meaningful information from the metabolites profile, statistical analysis and validation methods should be applied to the data set generated. Because ¹H-NMR or MS spectra generate hundreds of highly redundant signals from endogenous metabolites, it is necessary to reduce the data set to smaller subsets of about 100–500 spectral segments. The raw data obtained from the instrumental platform has to be preprocessed to minimise noise and artefacts, before the real biological variations can be captured. For MS-based metabolomics, preprocessing involves exploratory data analysis (EDA) of the raw data to check for any experimental errors. Following EDA, the raw data are cleaned up using other preprocessing steps such as baseline correction, filtering and noise removal and normalisation. These steps can be performed either on the MS manufacturer's software or freeware as discussed previously in the chapter. After normalisation, peak picking is performed by assigning molecular features after de-isotoping and de-adducting (removing adducts ions). After preprocessing, the reduced spectral datasets along with their respective signal intensities are entered into statistical programs for data analysis [19].

There are several sequential steps to be followed in metabolomics data analysis, which are represented in Figure 7.2. The first step of metabolomics data

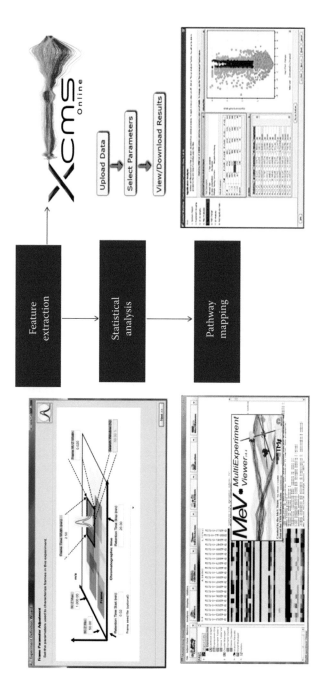

FIGURE 7.2 An example of a workflow of metabolomics data processing.

analysis enables pattern recognition, or clustering of groups such as normal versus mutant, or planktonic versus biofilm, based on differences in their spectral patterns. Interpretation of scores from this analysis provides information about the relationships/trends/groupings among samples as well as the presence of outliers. But the quantity and complexity of data arising from NMR and MS studies necessitate the use of computer-aided statistical interpretation in majority of metabolic profiling studies to obtain meaningful information from the complex raw data. Two major types of pattern recognition processes, unsupervised and supervised, are used in multivariate statistics of large data sets. Hierarchical cluster analysis and principal component analysis are examples of unsupervised approaches, which measure the innate variation in data sets; principal component regression and neural networks are examples of supervised approaches, which use prior information to generate pattern clusters [92]. Many other statistical approaches are also available, including spectral decomposition, linear discriminant analysis, Bayesian spectral decomposition and other chemometric methods [93]. Some of the common tools used for depicting metabolite profile differences after multivariate statistical analysis are shown in Figure 7.3.

On completion of multivariate statistical analysis, the spectral regions resulting in group clustering in step 1 are identified and then linked to specific metabolites on the basis of their NMR chemical shifts or MS spectrum. This kind of mapping is usually done with the help of a database search such as Human Metabolome Database (www .hmdb.ca). The third and final step of metabolomics data analysis involves quantitation and association of putative biomarkers to a particular characteristic or outcome. Statistical approaches used in this step can be either Student's t-test or ANOVA, depending on the number and size of groups [25,94].

Apart from developments in data analysis and interpretation approaches, initiatives have also been taken to share and verify the datasets obtained by metabolomics researchers globally. The Metabolomics Standards Initiative (MSI) was conceived in 2005 and is now coordinated by Data Standards Task Group of the Metabolomics Society. MSI aims to foster and coordinate efforts in enabling efficient storage, exchange and verification of metabolomics data sets (www.metabolomics-msi.org /home.html).

BIOFILM METABOLOMICS: PRACTICAL APPLICATIONS

The most common types of biofilm analysis include studying the differences between planktonic and biofilm states, understanding the metabolic changes occurring during biofilm formation and examining the nature and differences in the extracellular matrix composition encompassing biofilms. But this kind of study encounters many practical challenges, as highlighted in the previous sections. A cellular metabolome contains thousands of metabolites, with a magnitude range of picomoles to millimoles in concentrations. Therefore, it is generally not possible to analyse all the cellular metabolites in a single experiment. In addition, the composition of extracellular matrix is highly complex, making the correct separation and identification of its components difficult.

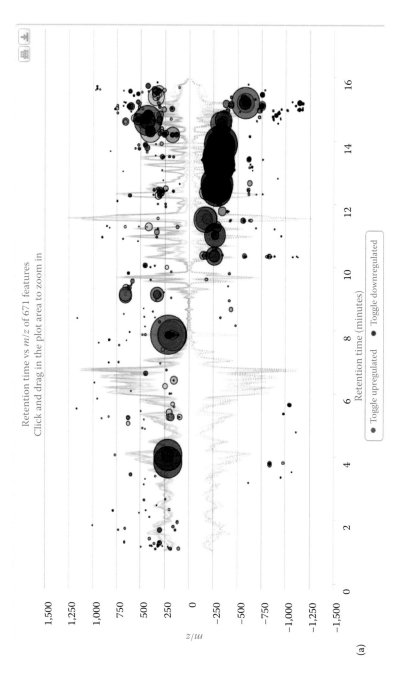

(a)

FIGURE 7.3 An example of up-regulated and down-regulated metabolic profiles of target with respect to control identified using (a) multivariate statistical analysis by TOGGLE (www.omictools.com). *(Continued)*

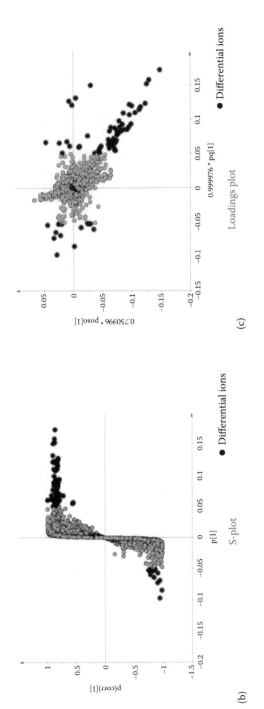

FIGURE 7.3 (CONTINUED) An example of up-regulated and down-regulated metabolic profiles of target with respect to control identified using (b) S-plots and (c) loadings plot.

EXTRACELLULAR POLYMERIC SUBSTANCES IN BIOFILMS

A typical biofilm consists of two extracellular components: the extracellular polymeric matrix in which the cells are embedded forming aggregates, and the interstitial voids and channels separating the microcolonies [95]. The matrix immobilising the biofilm cells facilitates cell–cell communication, co-ordination of responses and formation of microconsortia. It also confers protection against desiccation, antibiotics, biocides, ultraviolet radiation and host immune responses [96]. The extracellular matrix composed of polymeric substances provides elasticity to the biofilms, while the interstitial void constituted mainly by water provides the viscous part. The extracellular matrix is the dominant structural component of the biofilm and usually contains all major classes of macromolecules such as polysaccharides, proteins, nucleic acids, peptidoglycans and lipids. The composition and the abundance of extracellular polymeric substances (EPS) dictate the structural stability and elasticity of biofilms in most cases. Hence, to gain a better understanding of their role in biofilms, it is essential to analyse the EPS composition and differences in different scenarios and organisms [97].

A major portion of the EPS is composed of exopolysaccharides, which complicates the extraction as well as the analysis of EPS. Some of these exopolysaccharides are in the form of homopolysaccharides, while most of them are heteropolysaccharides composed of a mixture of neutral and charge residues. The most well-known exopolysaccharides present inside biofilms are alginate, cellulose and poly-N-acetyl glucosamine (PNAG). Alginate is an exopolysaccharide of relatively high molecular mass (104–106 g/mL) occurring in brown algae and certain bacterial strains. Its presence in bacteria *Azotobacter vinelandii* and *Pseudomonas aeruginosa* has been studied extensively. It consists of the uronic acid residues β-D-mannuronate (M) and its C-5 epimer, α-L-guluronate (G). The functional properties of alginate strongly correlate with its composition (M/G ratio) and with the uronic acid sequence. The mechanical properties of alginate gels can vary depending on the amount of guluronic acid present in the polymer. Alginate is involved both in microcolony formation in the early stages of biofilm development, and in providing mechanical stability to the biofilms [96,97].

Cellulose is the most abundant sugar polymer found in plants, animals, fungi and in bacteria such as *Salmonella*, *Escherichia coli*, *Acetobacter*, *Agrobacterium* and *Rhizobium*. It is produced as a crucial component of the extracellular matrix of *Salmonella* and *E. coli* biofilms. Cellulose consists of β-1-4–linked linear glucose and cellulose fibers formed by means of hydrogen bonds between the chains of glucose. The resultant sheets are highly stable, with their number varying based on the nature of the environment. Cellulose has a crystalline structure. It is liquid at room temperature, but forms a gel at temperatures above 50°C or below 10°C. On gelification, cellulose solutions remain stable in the gel state at room temperature. The mechanical properties of biofilms of bacterial species producing cellulose may be explained by the gel structure of cellulose [97].

PNAG is a polymer essential for adherence and biofilm formation of certain bacterial species. It was first described in *Staphylococcus* species and subsequently in *E. coli*. PNAG is a positively charged linear homoglycan composed of β-1,6-N-acetylglucosamine residues with approximately 20% deacetylated residues. It forms a protective matrix around biofilm cells, and mediates cell-to-cell interactions. It can also reinforce the matrix structure by interacting with extracellular DNA (eDNA) [97].

The other components of EPS such as lipids, proteins and eDNA, together with exopolysaccharides, span a wide range of functions in biofilm development and resistance, namely, in adhesion, aggregation, cohesion, water retention, providing a protective barrier, sorption of organic compounds and inorganic ions, exchange of genetic information and performing enzymatic functions. More information on the specific functions conferred by each of these EPS components can be found in some of the detailed reviews on EPS [96].

Challenges in EPS Extraction and Analysis

The analysis of EPS is quite challenging because of its complex nature and difficulty of extraction. Most of the common EPS extraction methodologies are suitable only for obtaining the soluble portion of the EPS. The insoluble portion of EPS is difficult to isolate, and very few methods are developed keeping this criterion in consideration [96]. The abundance of carbohydrate moieties in the EPS greatly complicates the extraction process. Most of these exopolysaccharides are insoluble and not easily separated from the cells, making the precise determination of their physical properties and chemical structures very difficult. Moreover, they can exist in either ordered or disordered forms [98]. The disordered forms are favoured by elevated temperatures and extremely low ionic concentrations. Based on the surrounding environment, biofilms can be exposed to a wide range of hydrodynamic conditions, which can greatly influence the matrix and structure of biofilms. The majority of the matrix exopolysaccharides are very long with linear or branched chains and a molecular mass of 500–2,000 kDa. They can be either homopolymers such as cellulose, curdlan or dextran, or heteropolymers such as alginate, emulsan, gellan or xanthan. They are generally constituted by monosaccharides and some non-carbohydrate substituents such as acetate, pyruvate, succinate and phosphate. The composition and conformation of the sugar monomers determine the properties of the exopolysaccharides and thus ultimately of the biofilm matrix. Mono-carbohydrate exopolysaccharides are often constituted by sugars such as D-glucose, D-galactose, D-mannose, L-fucose, L-rhamnose, L-arabinose, N-acetyl-D-glucose amine and N-acetyl-D-galactose amine as well as the uronic acids D-glucuronic acid, D-galacturonic acid, D-manuronic acid and L-guluronic acid. Some of the less frequently occurring sugar monomers are D-ribose, D-xylose, 3-keto-deoxy-D-mannooctulosonic acid and several hexoseamineuronic acids [96].

The presence of components such as lipids, proteins and DNA in the extracellular matrix also needs to be considered while developing an extraction method for EPS. Therefore, the extraction and analysis of EPS from biofilms usually requires a multimethod protocol capable of accommodating a wide spectrum of biological macromolecules [97].

EPS Extraction from Biofilms

The extraction of EPS from biofilms can be done using physical, chemical or enzymatic disruption methods. The nature of association of the EPS with the cell surface can be used to determine the appropriate extraction method. Some EPS are tightly associated with the cells through covalent interactions, whereas others are more easily dissociated.

The easily detachable ones can be subjected to physical disruption. Physical disruption includes methods such as high-speed centrifugation, dialysis, filtration, ion exchange and ultrasonication. Chemical methods of extractions are required for firmly associated EPS. For example, EPS cross-linked by divalent cations can be released from the biofilm matrix by the use of complexing agents such as ethylenediamine tetraacetic acid (EDTA), cation-exchange resins such as Dowex or formaldehyde treatment with or without sodium hydroxide. The chemical extraction methods can sometimes modify the composition of EPS, but greatly increase the efficiency of release of EPS from the biofilms. The yield of EPS from physical methods is usually lower than that from chemical methods. However, physical methods minimise the cross contamination of chemical reagents with samples. In some cases, a combination of physical and chemical methods provides a much higher yield [99,100].

PROFILING OF PLANKTONIC VERSUS BIOFILM CELLS

Many studies focus on the metabolites profile differences between the planktonic and biofilm state of microorganisms to gain a better perspective of the biofilm formation mechanism. Insights into the inherent differences between the two states can help in devising better strategies to curb biofilm formation, particularly of pathogenic microorganisms. Figure 7.4 shows the metabolite spectra for planktonic versus biofilm state of *P. aeruginosa*, where reverse-phase LC-MS was used to determine the composition of molecules on the basis of their mass to charge ratio. The resultant metabolite detection and quantification acquired in the form of a spectrum is shown in the figure. The polar metabolites would be eluted in the earlier part of the spectrum, while hydrophobic metabolites would be eluted in the latter part of the spectrum. It is evident from Figure 7.4 that there is significant increase in the amount of hydrophobic metabolites in biofilms when compared to planktonic cells. This is the expected trend as biofilms produce more EPS to encapsulate the cells and form the classical three-dimensional biofilm architecture.

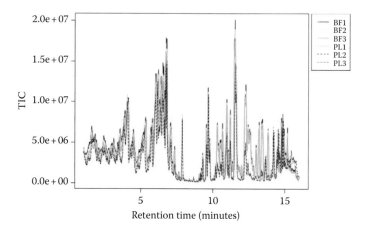

FIGURE 7.4 An example of metabolic spectra of planktonic and biofilm cells of *P. aeruginosa*. Total ion chromatogram. (Ng Weiling, Peter Benke, and Sanjay Swarup, unpublished work.)

BIOFILM METABOLOMICS: CASE STUDIES

Metabolome Analysis of Oral Biofilms Using a Combination of Capillary Electrophoresis and TOF MS

A recent study of human supragingivial plaque obtained before and after a glucose rinse revealed complex metabolite profile and effects of this treatment [101]. In oral biofilm studies, the usual factors analysed are microbiome composition, microenvironments and functions of microbial groups. This study evaluated changes occurring in metabolite profiles of central carbon metabolism of dental plaque and representative oral bacteria such as *Streptococcus mutans*, *S. sanguinis*, *Actinomyces oris*, and *A. naeslundii* on glucose rinse. The study identified differential regulation of metabolites such as glucose-6-phosphate, fructose-6-phosphate, fructose 1, 6-bisphosphate and phosphoenol pyruvate in both dental plaque and oral bacteria after glucose treatment.

In brief, dental plaque allowed to form overnight was collected from volunteers before and after glucose rinse. The plaque samples were immediately immersed in ice-cold methanol after collection, and metabolites extracted from samples were analysed by a combination of capillary electrophoresis and TOF MS (CE-MS). Similarly, metabolites were extracted from representative oral bacteria before and after glucose rinse. CE combined with TOF MS was used to separate and quantify metabolites involved in the central carbon metabolism, including the EMP pathway, pentose phosphate pathway and TCA cycle (Table 7.1). Detailed information on the workflow and data interpretation can be found in the paper [101,102]. CE is an excellent separator of ionised small molecules, such as metabolic intermediates, most

TABLE 7.1
Profile of Significantly Affected Metabolites of the Central Carbon Metabolism of Supragingivial Plaque on Glucose Rinse

Significantly Affected Metabolite in Plaque	Metabolic Pathway	Before Glucose Rinse (nmol/mg)	After Glucose Rinse (nmol/mg)
Glucose-6-phosphate	EMP pathway	0.133 ± 0.002	0.442 ± 0.087
Fructose-6-phosphate	EMP pathway	0.033 ± 0.006	0.108 ± 0.025
Dihydroxyacetone phosphate	EMP pathway	0.037 ± 0.004	0.074 ± 0.011
Pyruvate	EMP pathway	0.588 ± 0.461	4.236 ± 2.731
Ribulose-5-phosphate	Pentose phosphate pathway	0.029 ± 0.014	0.054 ± 0.021
Sedoheptulose-7-phosphate	Pentose phosphate pathway	0.058 ± 0.019	0.143 ± 0.041
Lactate	TCA cycle	1.737 ± 0.823	13.124 ± 12.712

Source: Adapted from Takahashi N, Washio J, Mayanagi G. Metabolomics of supragingival plaque and oral bacteria. *Journal of Dental Research*. 2010;89(12):1383–8; Takahashi N, Washio J, Mayanagi G. Metabolomic approach to oral biofilm characterization: A future direction of biofilm research. *Journal of Oral Biosciences*. 2012;54(3):138–43.

of which are polar and ionic small molecules, while MS is an excellent technique for analysis of molecular mass. Using this system, it was possible to identify and quantify most metabolic intermediates of the central carbon metabolism along with the changes occurring in the metabolites after glucose rinse. The comparison of supragingivial plaque and oral bacteria showed a similarity in the metabolite profiles of supragingivial plaque with both *Streptococcus* and *Actinomyces*, implying their cohabitation in plaque [101].

Metabolic Differentiation of Planktonic and Biofilm Modes of *S. aureus*

A recent study on the planktonic and biofilm modes of *S. aureus* revealed significant changes in the arginate biosynthesis pathway indicating their metabolically distinct nature and highlighted the use of metabolomics as a valuable tool for distinguishing between the two growth modes [12].

In brief, the study employed a novel bead beating method in a chloroform/methanol/water (1:3:1) extraction solvent for both sample extraction and quenching. The biofilms were grown in a 96-well plate under static conditions. Hydrophilic interaction liquid chromatography (HILIC)–mass spectrometry (LC-MS) coupled with Orbitrap™ was used for analysing the samples. Detailed information on the workflow and data interpretation can be found in Reference [12]. Five hundred and thirty metabolites were found to be significantly altered between planktonic and biofilm states, with 151 and 177 metabolites up-regulated with $\log_2$ fold changes ≥ 1 in planktonic and biofilm states respectively. Mapping of metabolites using the Kyoto Encyclopaedia of Genes and Genomes (KEGG) showed 129 pathways that were altered in at least two of their metabolites. The arginine biosynthesis pathway was the most significantly altered pathway between the two states (Table 7.2).

TABLE 7.2

Differentially Regulated Metabolites Profile of Arginine Biosynthesis Pathway between the Planktonic and Biofilm States of *S. aureus*

Arginine Biosynthesis Metabolite	$\log_2$ Fold Change between Planktonic and Biofilm States
Aspartate	1.577
Glutamate	1.0159
Citrulline	3.5413
N-Acetyl-L-glutamate	4.3654
N-Acetyl-L-citrulline	5.049
N-Acetyl-ornithine	1.068
Arginine	1.3781

Source: Adapted from Stipetic LH, Dalby MJ, Davies RL, Morton FR, Ramage G, Burgess KE. A novel metabolomic approach used for the comparison of *Staphylococcus aureus* planktonic cells and biofilm samples. *Metabolomics*. 2016;12(4):1–11.

FUTURE DIRECTIONS

The past decade has shown an explosive growth in the field of metabolomics. Numerous methods and tools for data analysis, interpretation and representation have made the use of this technology much easier in scope and application. Metabolomics methods are now providing a platform for extensive screening of drug targets and biomarker discovery studies. The use of metabolomics until now has been more predominant in mammalian, plant and planktonic microbial systems, whereas the global perspective of microbial biofilms has been limited because of complications in sample preparation [19,103]. However, with the development of new biofilm models and efficient extraction methods for extracellular polysaccharides, this field holds much promise in providing an in-depth view of biofilm lifestyle at a global level [104].

Along with the large data sets obtained from metabolomics platforms, there has been an increase in the availability of genomics data sets for different types of biofilms. Integration of the two can provide valuable information on the interaction between genes and metabolites. This would aid in establishing the direct relation between the cellular metabolic phenotypes and their gene expression levels. Multilevel integration of high-throughput omics data from various platforms such as genomics, transcriptomics and proteomics with metabolomics would be the next major stride in the field of biofilm metabolomics. This integrative 'omics' platform is capable of providing a comprehensive picture of changes occurring within any organism. This type of integration can associate the exact group of genes which are responsible for a particular phenotypic behaviour by comparison across proteome and metabolome levels. Numerous tools are now being developed to attain this perspective [105]. From a clinical point of view, this would further aid in the development of new strategies for overcoming drug resistance of biofilms, drug development, disease prevention, prediction and treatment, whereas from an environmental perspective, it would aid in unravelling the interactions within complex mixed species biofilm communities.

CORRESPONDING AUTHOR

Sanjay Swarup
Metabolites Biology Lab
Department of Biological Sciences (DBS)
Singapore Centre on Environmental Life Sciences Engineering (SCELSE)
NUS Environmental Research Institute (NERI)
Synthetic Biology for Clinical and Technological Innovation (SynCTI)
National University of Singapore
Singapore
sanjay@nus.edu.sg

REFERENCES

1. Battin TJ, Sloan WT, Kjelleberg S, Daims H, Head IM, Curtis TP et al. Microbial landscapes: New paths to biofilm research. *Nature Reviews Microbiology.* 2007;5(1):76–81.
2. Hall-Stoodley L, Costerton JW, Stoodley P. Bacterial biofilms: From the natural environment to infectious diseases. *Nature Reviews Microbiology.* 2004;2(2):95–108.
3. Sauer K. The genomics and proteomics of biofilm formation. *Genome Biology.* 2003;4(6):1.
4. Azevedo NF, Lopes SP, Keevil CW, Pereira MO, Vieira MJ. Time to "go large" on biofilm research: Advantages of an omics approach. *Biotechnology Letters.* 2009;31(4): 477–85.
5. Fiehn O. Metabolomics: The link between genotypes and phenotypes. *Plant Molecular Biology.* 2002;48(1–2):155–71.
6. Bino RJ, Hall RD, Fiehn O, Kopka J, Saito K, Draper J et al. Potential of metabolomics as a functional genomics tool. *Trends in Plant Science.* 2004;9(9):418–25.
7. Johnson CH, Gonzalez FJ. Challenges and opportunities of metabolomics. *Journal of Cellular Physiology.* 2012;227(8):2975–81.
8. Zhang B, Powers R. Analysis of bacterial biofilms using NMR-based metabolomics. *Future Medicinal Chemistry.* 2012;4(10):1273–306.
9. Beale D, Barratt R, Marlow D, Dunn M, Palombo E, Morrison P et al. Application of metabolomics to understanding biofilms in water distribution systems: A pilot study. *Biofouling.* 2013;29(3):283–94.
10. Lanni EJ, Masyuko RN, Driscoll CM, Aerts JT, Shrout JD, Bohn PW et al. MALDI-guided SIMS: Multiscale imaging of metabolites in bacterial biofilms. *Analytical Chemistry.* 2014;86(18):9139–45.
11. Masyuko RN, Lanni EJ, Driscoll CM, Shrout JD, Sweedler JV, Bohn PW. Spatial organization of *Pseudomonas aeruginosa* biofilms probed by combined matrix-assisted laser desorption ionization mass spectrometry and confocal Raman microscopy. *Analyst.* 2014;139(22):5700–8.
12. Stipetic LH, Dalby MJ, Davies RL, Morton FR, Ramage G, Burgess KE. A novel metabolomic approach used for the comparison of *Staphylococcus aureus* planktonic cells and biofilm samples. *Metabolomics.* 2016;12(4):1–11.
13. Agostini-Costa T, Vieira RF, Bizzo HR, Silveira D, Gimenes MA. Secondary metabolites. In Dhanarasu S (ed), *Chromatography and its applications. InTech.* 2012:131–64.
14. Peng B, Li H, Peng X-X. Functional metabolomics: From biomarker discovery to metabolome reprogramming. *Protein & Cell.* 2015;6(9):628–37.
15. Antti H, Fahlgren A, Näsström E, Kouremenos K, Sundén-Cullberg J, Guo Y et al. Metabolic profiling for detection of *Staphylococcus aureus* infection and antibiotic resistance. *PloS ONE.* 2013;8(2):e56971.
16. Yang Z, Marotta F. Pharmacometabolomics in drug discovery & development: Applications and challenges. *Metabolomics: Open Access.* 2012;2:5.
17. Wilson CM, Aggio RB, O'Toole PW, Villas-Boas S, Tannock GW. Transcriptional and metabolomic consequences of LuxS inactivation reveal a metabolic rather than quorum-sensing role for LuxS in *Lactobacillus reuteri* 100–23. *Journal of Bacteriology.* 2012;194(7):1743–6.
18. Patti GJ, Yanes O, Siuzdak G. Innovation: Metabolomics: The apogee of the omics trilogy. *Nature Reviews Molecular Cell Biology.* 2012;13(4):263–9.
19. Rai A, Umashankar S, Swarup S. Plant metabolomics: From experimental design to knowledge extraction. *Legume Genomics: Methods and Protocols.* 2013:279–312.
20. Baran R, Kochi H, Saito N, Suematsu M, Soga T, Nishioka T et al. MathDAMP: A package for differential analysis of metabolite profiles. *BMC Bioinformatics.* 2006;7(1):1.

21. Smith CA, Want EJ, O'Maille G, Abagyan R, Siuzdak G. XCMS: Processing mass spectrometry data for metabolite profiling using nonlinear peak alignment, matching, and identification. *Analytical Chemistry*. 2006;78(3):779–87.

22. Biswas A, Mynampati KC, Umashankar S, Reuben S, Parab G, Rao R et al. MetDAT: A modular and workflow-based free online pipeline for mass spectrometry data processing, analysis and interpretation. *Bioinformatics*. 2010;26(20):2639–40.

23. Pluskal T, Castillo S, Villar-Briones A, Orešič M. MZmine 2: Modular framework for processing, visualizing, and analyzing mass spectrometry-based molecular profile data. *BMC Bioinformatics*. 2010;11(1):1.

24. Biswas A, Rao R, Umashankar S, Mynampati KC, Reuben S, Parab G et al. datPAV: An online processing, analysis and visualization tool for exploratory investigation of experimental data. *Bioinformatics*. 2011;27(11):1585–6.

25. Xia J, Mandal R, Sinelnikov IV, Broadhurst D, Wishart DS. MetaboAnalyst 2.0: A comprehensive server for metabolomic data analysis. *Nucleic Acids Research*. 2012;40(W1):W127–W33.

26. Cottret L, Wildridge D, Vinson F, Barrett MP, Charles H, Sagot M-F et al. MetExplore: A web server to link metabolomic experiments and genome-scale metabolic networks. *Nucleic Acids Research*. 2010;38(Suppl 2):W132–W7.

27. Longnecker K, Futrelle J, Coburn E, Soule MCK, Kujawinski EB. Environmental metabolomics: Databases and tools for data analysis. *Marine Chemistry*. 2015;177:366–73.

28. Griffiths WJ, Koal T, Wang Y, Kohl M, Enot DP, Deigner HP. Targeted metabolomics for biomarker discovery. *Angewandte Chemie International Edition*. 2010;49(32):5426–45.

29. Vuckovic D. Current trends and challenges in sample preparation for global metabolomics using liquid chromatography–mass spectrometry. *Analytical and Bioanalytical Chemistry*. 2012;403(6):1523–48.

30. Putri SP, Nakayama Y, Matsuda F, Uchikata T, Kobayashi S, Matsubara A et al. Current metabolomics: Practical applications. *Journal of Bioscience and Bioengineering*. 2013;115(6):579–89.

31. Taymaz-Nikerel H, De Mey M, Ras C, ten Pierick A, Seifar RM, Van Dam JC et al. Development and application of a differential method for reliable metabolome analysis in *Escherichia coli*. *Analytical Biochemistry*. 2009;386(1):9–19.

32. Weibel KE, Mor J-R, Fiechter A. Rapid sampling of yeast cells and automated assays of adenylate, citrate, pyruvate and glucose-6–phosphate pools. *Analytical Biochemistry*. 1974;58(1):208–16.

33. de Koning W, van Dam K. A method for the determination of changes of glycolytic metabolites in yeast on a subsecond time scale using extraction at neutral pH. *Analytical Biochemistry*. 1992;204(1):118–23.

34. Putri SP, Fukusaki E. *Mass spectrometry-based metabolomics: A practical guide*. Boca Raton, FL: CRC Press; 2014.

35. de Jonge LP, Douma RD, Heijnen JJ, van Gulik WM. Optimization of cold methanol quenching for quantitative metabolomics of *Penicillium chrysogenum*. *Metabolomics*. 2012;8(4):727–35.

36. Spratlin JL, Serkova NJ, Eckhardt SG. Clinical applications of metabolomics in oncology: A review. *Clinical Cancer Research*. 2009;15(2):431–40.

37. Meyer H, Weidmann H, Lalk M. Methodological approaches to help unravel the intracellular metabolome of *Bacillus subtilis*. *Microbial Cell Factories*. 2013;12(1):1.

38. Wu XH, Yu HL, Ba ZY, Chen JY, Sun HG, Han BZ. Sampling methods for NMR-based metabolomics of *Staphylococcus aureus*. *Biotechnology Journal*. 2010;5(1):75–84.

39. Halouska S, Zhang B, Gaupp R, Lei S, Snell E, Fenton RJ et al. Revisiting protocols for the NMR analysis of bacterial metabolomes. *Journal of Integrated OMICS*. 2013;3(2):120.

40. Bligh EG, Dyer WJ. A rapid method of total lipid extraction and purification. *Canadian Journal of Biochemistry and Physiology.* 1959;37(8):911–7.
41. Maharjan RP, Ferenci T. Global metabolite analysis: The influence of extraction methodology on metabolome profiles of *Escherichia coli*. *Analytical Biochemistry.* 2003;313(1):145–54.
42. Tolker-Nielsen T, Sternberg C. Growing and analyzing biofilms in flow chambers. *Current Protocols in Microbiology.* 2011:1B. 2.1–B. 2.17.
43. Franklin MJ, Chang C, Akiyama T, Bothner B. New technologies for studying biofilms. *Microbiology Spectrum.* 2015;3(4), doi:10.1128/microbiolspec.MB-0016-2014.
44. Jonsson P, Wuolikainen A, Thysell E, Chorell E, Stattin P, Wikström P et al. Constrained randomization and multivariate effect projections improve information extraction and biomarker pattern discovery in metabolomics studies involving dependent samples. *Metabolomics.* 2015;11(6):1667–78.
45. Sysi-Aho M, Katajamaa M, Yetukuri L, Orešič M. Normalization method for metabolomics data using optimal selection of multiple internal standards. *BMC Bioinformatics.* 2007;8(1):1.
46. de Jong FA, Beecher C. Addressing the current bottlenecks of metabolomics: Isotopic Ratio Outlier Analysis™, an isotopic-labeling technique for accurate biochemical profiling. *Bioanalysis.* 2012;4(18):2303–14.
47. Ellis DI, Dunn WB, Griffin JL, Allwood JW, Goodacre R. Metabolic fingerprinting as a diagnostic tool. *Pharmacogenomics.* 2007;8(9):1243–66.
48. Sheridan H, Krenn L, Jiang R, Sutherland I, Ignatova S, Marmann A et al. The potential of metabolic fingerprinting as a tool for the modernisation of TCM preparations. *Journal of Ethnopharmacology.* 2012;140(3):482–91.
49. Inoue K, Tsutsui H, Akatsu H, Hashizume Y, Matsukawa N, Yamamoto T et al. Metabolic profiling of Alzheimer's disease brains. *Scientific Reports.* 2013;3. doi:10.1038/srep02364.
50. Williams HR, Willsmore JD, Cox IJ, Walker DG, Cobbold JF, Taylor-Robinson SD et al. Serum metabolic profiling in inflammatory bowel disease. *Digestive Diseases and Sciences.* 2012;57(8):2157–65.
51. Beale D, Morrison P, Key C, Palombo E. Metabolic profiling of biofilm bacteria known to cause microbial influenced corrosion. *Water Science and Technology.* 2014;69(1): 1–8.
52. Mugoni V, Medana C, Santoro MM. 13C-isotope-based protocol for prenyl lipid metabolic analysis in zebrafish embryos. *Nature Protocols.* 2013;8(12):2337–47.
53. Nakayama Y, Tamada Y, Tsugawa H, Bamba T, Fukusaki E. Novel strategy for nontargeted isotope-assisted metabolomics by means of metabolic turnover and multivariate analysis. *Metabolites.* 2014;4(3):722–39.
54. Hiller K, Wegner A, Weindl D, Cordes T, Metallo CM, Kelleher JK et al. NTFD: A stand-alone application for the non-targeted detection of stable isotope-labeled compounds in GC/MS data. *Bioinformatics.* 2013:btt119.
55. Trushina E, Mielke MM. Recent advances in the application of metabolomics to Alzheimer's disease. *Biochimica et Biophysica Acta (BBA): Molecular Basis of Disease.* 2014;1842(8):1232–9.
56. Ament Z, Masoodi M, Griffin JL. Applications of metabolomics for understanding the action of peroxisome proliferator-activated receptors (PPARs) in diabetes, obesity and cancer. *Genome Medicine.* 2012;4(4):1.
57. Junka AF, Deja S, Smutnicka D, Szymczyk P, Ziółkowski G, Bartoszewicz M et al. Differences in metabolic profiles of planktonic and biofilm cells in *Staphylococcus aureus*: (1) H Nuclear magnetic resonance search for candidate biomarkers. *Acta Biochimica Polonica.* 2013;60(4):701–6.

58. Zhang A, Sun H, Wang P, Han Y, Wang X. Modern analytical techniques in metabolomics analysis. *Analyst.* 2012;137(2):293–300.
59. Seger C, Sturm S, Stuppner H. Mass spectrometry and NMR spectroscopy: Modern high-end detectors for high resolution separation techniques–state of the art in natural product HPLC-MS, HPLC-NMR, and CE-MS hyphenations. *Natural Product Reports.* 2013;30(7):970–87.
60. Pitt JJ. Principles and applications of liquid chromatography-mass spectrometry in clinical biochemistry. *Clinical Biochemistry Review.* 2009;30(1):19–34.
61. Korfmacher WA. Foundation review: Principles and applications of LC-MS in new drug discovery. *Drug Discovery Today.* 2005;10(20):1357–67.
62. Theodoridis GA, Gika HG, Want EJ, Wilson ID. Liquid chromatography–mass spectrometry based global metabolite profiling: A review. *Analytica Chimica Acta.* 2012;711:7–16.
63. Gika HG, Theodoridis GA, Plumb RS, Wilson ID. Current practice of liquid chromatography–mass spectrometry in metabolomics and metabonomics. *Journal of Pharmaceutical and Biomedical Analysis.* 2014;87:12–25.
64. Fenn JB, Mann M, Meng CK, Wong SF, Whitehouse CM. Electrospray ionization–principles and practice. *Mass Spectrometry Reviews.* 1990;9(1):37–70.
65. Whitehouse CM, Dreyer R, Yamashita M, Fenn J. Electrospray ionization for mass-spectrometry of large biomolecules. *Science.* 1989;246(4926):64–71.
66. Leinonen A, Kuuranne T, Kostiainen R. Liquid chromatography/mass spectrometry in anabolic steroid analysis—Optimization and comparison of three ionization techniques: Electrospray ionization, atmospheric pressure chemical ionization and atmospheric pressure photoionization. *Journal of Mass Spectrometry.* 2002;37(7):693–8.
67. Raffaelli A, Saba A. Atmospheric pressure photoionization mass spectrometry. *Mass Spectrometry Reviews.* 2003;22(5):318–31.
68. Jansen R, Lachatre G, Marquet P. LC-MS/MS systematic toxicological analysis: Comparison of MS/MS spectra obtained with different instruments and settings. *Clinical Biochemistry.* 2005;38(4):362–72.
69. Forcisi S, Moritz F, Kanawati B, Tziotis D, Lehmann R, Schmitt-Kopplin P. Liquid chromatography–mass spectrometry in metabolomics research: Mass analyzers in ultra high pressure liquid chromatography coupling. *Journal of Chromatography A.* 2013;1292:51–65.
70. Byrdwell WC. Atmospheric pressure chemical ionization mass spectrometry for analysis of lipids. *Lipids.* 2001;36(4):327–46.
71. Thurman E, Ferrer I, Barcelo D. Choosing between atmospheric pressure chemical ionization and electrospray ionization interfaces for the HPLC/MS analysis of pesticides. *Analytical Chemistry.* 2001;73(22):5441–9.
72. Robb DB, Covey TR, Bruins AP. Atmospheric pressure photoionization: An ionization method for liquid chromatography-mass spectrometry. *Analytical Chemistry.* 2000;72(15):3653–9.
73. Politzer I, Dowty B, Laseter J. Use of gas chromatography and mass spectrometry to analyze underivatized volatile human or animal constituents of clinical interest. *Clinical Chemistry.* 1976;22(11):1775–88.
74. Akande WG. A review of experimental procedures of gas chromatography-mass spectrometry (GC-MS) and possible sources of analytical errors. *Earth Science.* 2012;1(1):1–9.
75. Chernushevich IV, Loboda AV, Thomson BA. An introduction to quadrupole–time-of-flight mass spectrometry. *Journal of Mass Spectrometry.* 2001;36(8):849–65.
76. Li B, An HJ, Hedrick JL, Lebrilla CB. Collision-induced dissociation tandem mass spectrometry for structural elucidation of glycans. *Glycomics: Methods and Protocols.* 2009:133–45.

77. Lange V, Picotti P, Domon B, Aebersold R. Selected reaction monitoring for quantitative proteomics: A tutorial. *Molecular Systems Biology.* 2008;4(1):222.
78. Freue GVC, Borchers CH. Multiple reaction monitoring (MRM) principles and application to coronary artery disease. *Circulation: Cardiovascular Genetics.* 2012;5(3):378.
79. Guilhaus M. Special feature: Tutorial. Principles and instrumentation in time-of-flight mass spectrometry. Physical and instrumental concepts. *Journal of Mass Spectrometry.* 1995;30(11):1519–32.
80. Dettmer K, Aronov PA, Hammock BD. Mass spectrometry-based metabolomics. *Mass Spectrometry Reviews.* 2007;26(1):51–78.
81. Stafford G. Ion trap mass spectrometry: A personal perspective. *Journal of the American Society for Mass Spectrometry.* 2002;13(6):589–96.
82. Perry RH, Cooks RG, Noll RJ. Orbitrap mass spectrometry: Instrumentation, ion motion and applications. *Mass Spectrometry Reviews.* 2008;27(6):661–99.
83. Glish GL, Burinsky DJ. Hybrid mass spectrometers for tandem mass spectrometry. *Journal of the American Society for Mass Spectrometry.* 2008;19(2):161–72.
84. Kivilompolo M, Obůrka V, Hyötyläinen T. Comparison of GC–MS and LC–MS methods for the analysis of antioxidant phenolic acids in herbs. *Analytical and Bioanalytical Chemistry.* 2007;388(4):881–7.
85. Garcia A, Barbas C. Gas chromatography-mass spectrometry (GC-MS)-based metabolomics. *Metabolic Profiling: Methods and Protocols.* 2011:191–204.
86. Smolinska A, Blanchet L, Buydens LM, Wijmenga SS. NMR and pattern recognition methods in metabolomics: From data acquisition to biomarker discovery: A review. *Analytica Chimica Acta.* 2012;750:82–97.
87. McPherson RA, Pincus MR, eds. *Henry's Clinical Diagnosis and Management by Laboratory Methods*, 22nd edition. 2011; Philadelphia, PA: Saunders/Elsevier.
88. Chandra Pati U, ed. *3-D Surface Geometry and Reconstruction: Developing Concepts and Applications.* 2012; Rourkela, India: National Institute of Technology.
89. Larive CK, Barding Jr GA, Dinges MM. NMR spectroscopy for metabolomics and metabolic profiling. *Analytical Chemistry.* 2014;87(1):133–46.
90. Zhang B, Halouska S, Schiaffo CE, Sadykov MR, Somerville GA, Powers R. NMR analysis of a stress response metabolic signaling network. *Journal of Proteome Research.* 2011;10(8):3743–54.
91. Veenstra TD. Metabolomics: The final frontier? *Genome Medicine.* 2012;4(4):1.
92. Lee JK, Williams PD, Cheon S. Data mining in genomics. *Clinics in Laboratory Medicine.* 2008;28(1):145–66.
93. Holmes E, Antti H. Chemometric contributions to the evolution of metabonomics: Mathematical solutions to characterising and interpreting complex biological NMR spectra. *Analyst.* 2002;127(12):1549–57.
94. Sugimoto M, Kawakami M, Robert M, Soga T, Tomita M. Bioinformatics tools for mass spectroscopy-based metabolomic data processing and analysis. *Current Bioinformatics.* 2012;7(1):96–108.
95. Flemming H-C, Neu TR, Wozniak DJ. The EPS matrix: The "house of biofilm cells". *Journal of Bacteriology.* 2007;189(22):7945–7.
96. Flemming H-C, Wingender J. The biofilm matrix. *Nature Reviews Microbiology.* 2010;8(9):623–33.
97. Lembre P, Lorentz C, Di Martino P, Di Martino P. Exopolysaccharides of the biofilm matrix: A complex biophysical world. In: Karunaratne DN (ed), *The complex world of polysaccharides.* Rijeka, Croatia: INTECH Open Access; 2012.
98. Nguyen T, Roddick FA, Fan L. Biofouling of water treatment membranes: A review of the underlying causes, monitoring techniques and control measures. *Membranes.* 2012;2(4):804–40.

99. D'Abzac P, Bordas F, Van Hullebusch E, Lens PN, Guibaud G. Extraction of extra-cellular polymeric substances (EPS) from anaerobic granular sludges: Comparison of chemical and physical extraction protocols. *Applied Microbiology and Biotechnology.* 2010;85(5):1589–99.
100. Subramaniam S, Yan S, Tyagi R, Surampalli R. Characterization of extracellular poly-meric substances (EPS) extracted from both sludge and pure bacterial strains isolated from wastewater sludge for sludge dewatering. *Water Research.* 2007;12:1–7.
101. Takahashi N, Washio J, Mayanagi G. Metabolomics of supragingival plaque and oral bacteria. *Journal of Dental Research.* 2010;89(12):1383–8.
102. Takahashi N, Washio J, Mayanagi G. Metabolomic approach to oral biofilm char-acterization: A future direction of biofilm research. *Journal of Oral Biosciences.* 2012;54(3):138–43.
103. Reuben S, Rai A, Pillai BV, Rodrigues A, Swarup S. A bacterial quercetin oxidoreduc-tase QuoA-mediated perturbation in the phenylpropanoid metabolic network increases lignification with a concomitant decrease in phenolamides in Arabidopsis. *Journal of Experimental Botany.* 2013;64(16):5183–94.
104. Hollywood K, Brison DR, Goodacre R. Metabolomics: Current technologies and future trends. *Proteomics.* 2006;6(17):4716–23.
105. Brink-Jensen K, Bak S, Jørgensen K, Ekstrøm CT. Integrative analysis of metabolomics and transcriptomics data: A unified model framework to identify underlying system path-ways. *PloS ONE.* 2013;8(9):e72116.

8 Biofilm Persisters
Formation, Molecular Mechanisms and Strategies for Tackling

Peng Li, Chaminda Jayampath Seneviratne and Lijian Jin

CONTENTS

INTRODUCTION

Microbial biofilms demonstrate an astounding ability to withstand stress, extremes of temperature, drug treatment and other harsh conditions imposed by the surrounding environment. Research into this aspect of microbial biofilms has generated various possibilities/theories/hypotheses regarding this phenomenon, and has also identified several genes or proteins that are associated with biofilm formation and drug resistance in different microorganisms. Currently, one of the more promising concepts that has the potential to explain this existential perseverance of microbial biofilms is that of persister cells. Persister cells are a metabolically quiescent subpopulation of microbial biofilms and planktonic cultures that can survive antimicrobial treatment at concentrations well above the minimal inhibitory concentration (MIC) [1]. Persisters differ from drug-resistant mutants in that they are phenotypic variants that have not acquired genetically heritable resistance. The occurrence of a subpopulation of resistant cells was first described in 1942 by Hobby et al., who found that approximately 1% of *Staphylococcus aureus* cells were not killed by penicillin. Similar observations on *S. pyogenes* was reported later in 1944 by Bigger and the concept of persisters was proposed [2]. The persister population of a culture can be quantified on addition of a lethal amount of antimicrobials. The resulting killing curve would be biphasic, with the bulk of the culture killed rapidly followed by a dramatic decrease of killing rate, giving rise to a small fraction of viable persister cells (Figure 8.1) [3–5]. Once antimicrobial treatment is interrupted/halted, persisters are capable of recovering from the challenges promptly, leading to the establishment of a new population. However, this newly formed population can be as sensitive as the original population to the antimicrobials and can produce a similar group of persisters [1].

Despite the discovery of persisters in the early 1940s, their importance was overlooked for a long time until the identification of persister cells in biofilms of predominant pathogens such as *Pseudomonas aeruginosa*, *Escherichia coli* and *Mycobacterium tuberculosis* [6–8]. In healthcare settings, the formation of biofilms accounts for at least 65% of infectious diseases, and is considered to be a critical cause of persistent infections and therapeutic failure [9,10]. In the recent literature, the persister populations are commonly referred to in association with the biofilm mode of growth of microorganisms. It is proposed that persisters are involved in the increased biofilm resistance to antimicrobials, and biofilm persisters are the underlying reason for recalcitrance and relapse of infectious diseases [11,12]. In this chapter, we discuss the general understanding of persister cells and the role of persister populations in biofilm-associated infections.

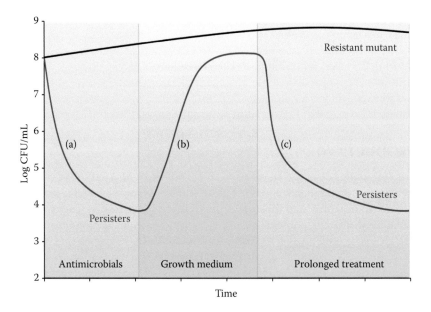

FIGURE 8.1 Schematic model for microbial persistence. A microbial population formed by a resistant mutant can grow in the presence of cidal antimicrobials and resist their treatments. The killing kinetics of a susceptible population by antimicrobials is characterised by a biphasic pattern, with the majority of cells killed and a small fraction of persisters remaining alive (a). When antimicrobial treatment ceases, persisters resume growth (b) and give rise to a population sensitive to the antimicrobial, as was the original population (c). Persisters are able to withstand prolonged antimicrobial therapy, leading to recurrent infections.

TYPE I AND TYPE II PERSISTERS

The presence of antimicrobial-tolerant persisters in a genetically clonal population reflects the adaptability of microorganisms in response to environmental challenges. To understand the formation of persisters, it is imperative to know whether this phenotype switch occurs before or after antimicrobial exposure. However, it is extremely challenging to study the state of persisters, as they constitute only a tiny part of the entire biofilm population. With the use of microfluidic devices and time-lapse fluorescent microscopy, an elegant study by Balaban et al. investigated high-persister (*hip*) mutants of *E. coli* at the single-cell level and demonstrated that persisters form before antibiotic (ampicillin) treatment [13]. These persisters are classified into two groups: type I persisters arise in response to an external trigger (e.g. starvation) and type II persisters are generated spontaneously and continuously during active population growth [13,14]. It is proposed that the number of type I persisters is proportional to the size of the inoculum from stationary-phase cells, whereas the number of type II persisters is determined by the total cell number of the culture [13]. It was shown that after inoculation of stationary-phase cells into fresh medium, the level of persisters remained stable at lag and early exponential phases (type I persisters) followed by a quick increase at mid- to late-exponential phases (type II persisters) [3]. Type I persisters vanished when a culture was maintained at the early exponential state by repeated cycles of inoculation, indicating that type I persisters are environmentally induced rather than spontaneously formed [3].

ENVIRONMENTAL TRIGGERS OF PERSISTER CELL FORMATION

A variety of environmental signals have been implicated in the occurrence of persisters among isogenic microbial populations, such as nutrient limitation, oxidative and nitrosative stress, cell envelope stress and antimicrobial exposure [15]. As mentioned previously, nutrient starvation and diauxic carbon-source transitions have been shown to stimulate formation of persisters in both planktonic and biofilm cells [16–19]. The microbial communication system, quorum sensing (QS) signalling, is involved in population growth and stationary phase response. A series of studies have demonstrated that microbial persistence can be positively influenced by QS molecules such as pyocyanin in *P. aeruginosa* [20], peptide pheromone in *Streptococcus mutans* [21] and indole in *E. coli* [22]. It should be noted that addition of spent medium to an early exponential culture induced elevated persister formation in *P. aeruginosa,* but not in *E. coli* and *S. aureus*, suggesting that the involvement of QS signalling in persistence is species specific [1,20]. In addition, oxidative stress induced by pretreatment with hydrogen peroxide or paraquat greatly increased the number of *E. coli* persisters tolerant to ofloxacin [22,23]. Heat shock was also identified to promote survival of persisters in the presence of antimicrobials [21,24]. Interestingly, exposure to subinhibitory concentrations of antibiotics can actually enhance the tolerance of microbes to the antibiotics per se [25,26]. Recent studies have also shown that host macrophages can induce antimicrobial tolerance of intracellular bacteria [27,28].

MECHANISMS BEHIND MICROBIAL PERSISTENCE

In an isogeneic microbial population, antimicrobials mainly target actively growing cells, thereby allowing non-growing cells to persist. Hence, it is generally assumed that growth arrest and dormancy account for microbial persistence [29]. The first direct evidence for this hypothesis comes from the observation of *E. coli* persisters that comprise non-growing or slowly growing cells, linking persistence to phenotypic switch from normal growth to reduced growth [13]. The phenomenon is viewed as a bet-hedging strategy, whereby persisters enter into a dormant state characterised by decreased cellular activities to withstand antimicrobial treatment. Gene loci known as toxin–antitoxin (TA) modules play a critical role in the induction of dormancy and persistence [30–34]. TA systems typically comprise two components: a stable toxin that inhibits cell growth by interfering with essential cellular processes (e.g. DNA replication and protein translation), and a labile antitoxin that regulates toxin activity [35]. Under normal growth conditions, an antitoxin neutralises the cognate toxin so that cell growth is unaffected. However, in stress circumstances, antitoxins are selectively degraded, which leaves active toxins to perform their functions.

Despite that dormancy has been a prevailing hypothesis accounting for persistence, increasing evidence suggests that growth arrest is not a universal mechanism for persistence [14]. For example, replicating persisters of mycobacteria have been identified in two independent studies [27,36]. Although reduced growth rate could increase the likelihood of a cell to become tolerant to antibiotic treatment, the majority of dormant cells are not persisters, and persisters can also arise from rapidly growing cells [37]. It is becoming clear that many active biological processes are engaged in microbial persistence along with dormancy, such as stringent response, SOS response and antioxidative response [15,18,38,39].

PERSISTERS IN BIOFILMS

When biofilms are exposed to antimicrobials, most of the cells can be killed, though leaving a subpopulation of biofilm persisters unaffected. It is generally believed that antimicrobials act in cooperation with host defenses to control infections, with the host cells eliminating pathogens surviving antimicrobial treatment. However, the three-dimensional structure of biofilms serves as a protective barrier against the immune system and prevents persisters within the biofilms from being eradicated by immune cells [40]. When the drug concentration decreases, persisters are able to resuscitate and repopulate the biofilms, leading to persistent infections. Interestingly, biofilms harbour higher proportions of persisters tolerant to lethal concentrations of antimicrobials as compared to planktonic cells, suggesting a protective role of biofilm for cellular survival [4,6,8,41]. The existence of biofilm persisters contributes to the recalcitrance of biofilm-related infections to antimicrobial therapy. It has been proposed that formation of persisters critically accounts for the increased antimicrobial resistance of biofilms [1,11,42].

Biofilms demonstrate extensive structural, chemical and biological heterogeneity, containing cells in various physiological states. In response to local environmental conditions, biofilms enrich differentiation of specific phenotypes with increased adaptability [43]. In biofilms, cells within the internal regions often encounter limited access to nutrients and enter into a dormant state [44]. In addition, bacteria trigger a stringent response that promotes cell survival under nutrient-limited conditions. This response is coordinated by RelA- and SpoT-mediated synthesis of the alarmone guanosine tetraphosphate (ppGpp) that massively reprogrammes gene expression via direct interaction with RNA polymerase or indirect σ-factor competition [45]. Indeed, antibiotic tolerance of bacterial biofilm persisters has been closely linked to TA operons, dormancy and stringent response. It has been reported that overexpression of the TA gene *yafQ* induces multidrug tolerance in *E. coli* biofilms, and disruption of *yafQ* reduces the level of persisters in the biofilms, but not in stationary-phase planktonic cells [46]. Inactivation of this stringent response by deletion of RelA and SpoT in *P. aeruginosa* resulted in a dramatic decrease of persistence in stationary phase and biofilms, and the reduced susceptibility was restored via complementation of the two genes [18]. The requirement of ppGpp for persistence has also been observed in *E. coli* biofilms, and it is demonstrated that ppGpp induces slow growth and antibiotic tolerance via activation of TA systems through inorganic polyphosphate- and Lon protease-dependent degradation of antitoxins [47].

In addition, the SOS response that mitigates DNA damage is required for hypertolerance of *E. coli* biofilm persisters to fluoroquinolone antibiotics on starvation to specific essential growth nutrients [17]. The starvation-induced biofilm tolerance is partially dependent on a stringent response and independent of the known SOS-related TA modules (TisAB, SymER, DinJ/YafQ and YafNO) [17]. Furthermore,

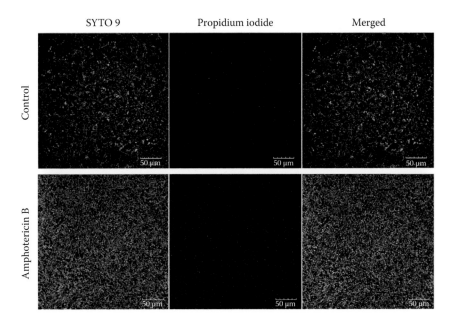

FIGURE 8.2 Persister of *Candida albicans* biofilms. *C. albicans* biofilms were treated with a lethal dose of antifungal amphotericin B and stained with viability indicators (SYTO 9 and propidium iodide). Live persister cells stain green and dead cells are red/yellow-coloured.

control of antibiotic-induced oxidative stress is a key element in ensuring the survival of bacterial biofilm persisters [18,41]. In *C. albicans* biofilms, the tolerance of persisters to miconazole is shown to be dependent on the protection against reactive oxygen species (ROS) mediated by superoxide dismutase (SOD) [48]. A recent high-throughput proteomic profiling of *Candida* biofilm persisters demonstrated that the antifungal tolerance of these survivors is determined by subtle metabolic regulation and activation of stress responses (Figure 8.2). In particular, the *Candida* biofilm persisters can withstand increased oxidative stress [42].

COMBATING PERSISTERS AND BIOFILM-RELATED INFECTIONS

Persister cells pose an important threat to healthcare because they are able to withstand the current therapeutic regimens. Novel approaches are of critical necessity to combat persister-based infections effectively. The currently evolving strategies for targeting persisters indicate that the capacity to kill persisters translates to the ability to manage biofilm-related infections [49,50].

As biofilm persisters are mainly slowly growing or dormant cells, strategies aiming to resuscitate persisters are of significant promise in restoring the susceptibility of persisters to antimicrobials. The combination of metabolites with gentamicin allowed appreciable reduction of biofilm viability both *in vitro* and in a mouse urinary tract infection model. However, the metabolite-enabled killing was limited to aminoglycosides and did not apply to β-lactams or fluoroquinolones. Interestingly, the potentiation was not based on growth resumption of the persisters, but on induction of a proton-motive force which in turn enhanced aminoglycoside uptake [51]. Recently, it was further demonstrated that the metabolic adjuvant L-arginine in combination with gentamicin could increase the killing of *in vitro* planktonic and biofilm persisters in *S. aureus*, *E. coli* and *P. aeruginosa* by affecting the pH gradient of the cell membrane. The effect was also confirmed in a mouse model of catheter-related infections showing a complete eradication of *S. aureus* and *E. coli* biofilms [49].

An alternative strategy to target persisters is to kill the biofilm persisters by inducing oxidative damage, as the survival of certain persister cells is linked to an antioxidative response. It was demonstrated that *Burkholderia cenocepacia* biofilm persisters avoided production of ROS via inhibition of the tricarboxylic acid cycle, while activating the alternative pathway glyoxylate shunt. Interestingly, the fraction of the biofilm persisters was reduced by itaconate, which inhibits the key enzyme of the glyoxylate shunt, isocitrate lyase [41]. Treatment of *C. albicans* biofilms with the SOD inhibitor diethyldithiocarbamate (DDTC) led to higher levels of endogenous ROS and an 18- to 200-fold reduction of the miconazole-tolerant persister fraction [48].

Other efforts have also been made to eradicate biofilm persisters. For example, BF8 is an inhibitor of QS and has been shown to sensitise both planktonic and biofilm persisters of *P. aeruginosa* and *E. coli* to antibiotics, though the exact mechanisms behind the action of BF8 remain unclear [52,53]. Acyldepsipeptides (ADEP) are a class of antibiotics that can activate a major protease ClpP, which leads to lethal degradation of proteins [54]. Kim Lewis's group found that the combination of ADEP4 and rifampicin could eradicate stationary-phase and biofilm cultures of *S. aureus* that otherwise contained antibiotic-tolerant cells. Importantly, combining ADEP4 with rifampicin cleared a deep-seated murine infection caused by *S. aureus* [50]. Most recently, it has been demonstrated that the U.S. Food and Drug Administration–approved anti-cancer drug mitomycin C (MMC) effectively kills planktonic and biofilm persisters of *E. coli*, *S. aureus* and *P. aeruginosa* by cross-linking DNA [55]. In addition, drugs interfering with pathways implicated in persistence, such as the stringent response and membrane stress response, may also contribute to the eradication of biofilm persisters [56,57].

CONCLUSIONS

The existence of persister cells in a wide variety of microbial subpopulations is becoming increasingly evident from recent studies. More and more treatment strategies end in failure because of the prevalence of persisters. Hence, this phenomenon of resistance can render therapeutic regimens ineffective unless they are effectively targeted. An expanding plethora of research in this direction is therefore warranted to necessitate both an understanding of the molecular mechanisms behind persister resistance and an efficient combative strategy against persisters. Altogether, persister cell biology has become one of the fascinating biofilm research areas of recent times, with a potential gold mine of understanding waiting to be uncovered.

CORRESPONDING AUTHOR

Lijian Jin
Faculty of Dentistry
The University of Hong Kong
Pok Fu Lam, Hong Kong
ljjin@hku.hk

REFERENCES

1. Lewis K. Persister cells. *Annual Review of Microbiology.* 2010;64:357–72.
2. Bigger JW. Treatment of staphylococcal infections with penicillin. *Lancet.* 1944: 497–500.
3. Keren I, Kaldalu N, Spoering A, Wang Y, Lewis K. Persister cells and tolerance to antimicrobials. *FEMS Microbiology Letters.* 2004;230(1):13–8.
4. Harrison JJ, Turner RJ, Ceri H. Persister cells, the biofilm matrix and tolerance to metal cations in biofilm and planktonic *Pseudomonas aeruginosa*. *Environmental microbiology.* 2005;7(7):981–94.
5. Sharma B, Brown AV, Matluck NE, Hu LT, Lewis K. *Borrelia burgdorferi*, the causative agent of Lyme disease, forms drug-tolerant persister cells. *Antimicrobial Agents and Chemotherapy.* 2015;59(8):4616–24.
6. Brooun A, Liu S, Lewis K. A dose-response study of antibiotic resistance in *Pseudomonas aeruginosa* biofilms. *Antimicrobial Agents and Chemotherapy.* 2000;44(3):640–6.
7. LaFleur MD, Kumamoto CA, Lewis K. *Candida albicans* biofilms produce antifungal-tolerant persister cells. *Antimicrobial Agents and Chemotherapy.* 2006;50(11):3839–46.
8. Ojha AK, Baughn AD, Sambandan D, Hsu T, Trivelli X, Guerardel Y et al. Growth of *Mycobacterium tuberculosis* biofilms containing free mycolic acids and harbouring drug-tolerant bacteria. *Molecular Microbiology.* 2008;69(1):164–74.

9. Hall-Stoodley L, Costerton JW, Stoodley P. Bacterial biofilms: From the natural environment to infectious diseases. *Nature Reviews Microbiology.* 2004;2(2):95–108.

10. Mah TF. Biofilm-specific antibiotic resistance. *Future Microbiology.* 2012;7(9):1061–72.

11. Van Acker H, Van Dijck P, Coenye T. Molecular mechanisms of antimicrobial tolerance and resistance in bacterial and fungal biofilms. *Trends in Microbiology.* 2014;22(6):326–33.

12. Fauvart M, De Groote VN, Michiels J. Role of persister cells in chronic infections: Clinical relevance and perspectives on anti-persister therapies. *Journal of Medical Microbiology.* 2011;60(Pt 6):699–709.

13. Balaban NQ, Merrin J, Chait R, Kowalik L, Leibler S. Bacterial persistence as a phenotypic switch. *Science.* 2004;305(5690):1622–5.

14. Balaban NQ, Gerdes K, Lewis K, McKinney JD. A problem of persistence: Still more questions than answers? *Nature Reviews Microbiology.* 2013;11(8):587–91.

15. Poole K. Stress responses as determinants of antimicrobial resistance in Gram-negative bacteria. *Trends in Microbiology.* 2012;20(5):227–34.

16. Amato SM, Orman MA, Brynildsen MP. Metabolic control of persister formation in *Escherichia coli. Molecular Cell.* 2013;50(4):475–87.

17. Bernier SP, Lebeaux D, DeFrancesco AS, Valomon A, Soubigou G, Coppee JY et al. Starvation, together with the SOS response, mediates high biofilm-specific tolerance to the fluoroquinolone ofloxacin. *PLoS Genetics.* 2013;9(1):e1003144.

18. Nguyen D, Joshi-Datar A, Lepine F, Bauerle E, Olakanmi O, Beer K et al. Active starvation responses mediate antibiotic tolerance in biofilms and nutrient-limited bacteria. *Science.* 2011;334(6058):982–6.

19. Fung DK, Chan EW, Chin ML, Chan RC. Delineation of a bacterial starvation stress response network which can mediate antibiotic tolerance development. *Antimicrobial Agents and Chemotherapy.* 2010;54(3):1082–93.

20. Moker N, Dean CR, Tao J. *Pseudomonas aeruginosa* increases formation of multidrug-tolerant persister cells in response to quorum-sensing signaling molecules. *Journal of Bacteriology.* 2010;192(7):1946–55.

21. Leung V, Levesque CM. A stress-inducible quorum-sensing peptide mediates the formation of persister cells with noninherited multidrug tolerance. *Journal of Bacteriology.* 2012;194(9):2265–74.

22. Vega NM, Allison KR, Khalil AS, Collins JJ. Signaling-mediated bacterial persister formation. *Nature Chemical Biology.* 2012;8(5):431–3.

23. Wu Y, Vulic M, Keren I, Lewis K. Role of oxidative stress in persister tolerance. *Antimicrobial Agents and Chemotherapy.* 2012;56(9):4922–6.

24. Cardoso K, Gandra RF, Wisniewski ES, Osaku CA, Kadowaki MK, Felipach-Neto V et al. DnaK and GroEL are induced in response to antibiotic and heat shock in *Acinetobacter baumannii. Journal of Medical Microbiology.* 2010;59(Pt 9):1061–8.

25. Dorr T, Lewis K, Vulic M. SOS response induces persistence to fluoroquinolones in *Escherichia coli. PLoS Genetics.* 2009;5(12):e1000760.

26. Johnson PJ, Levin BR. Pharmacodynamics, population dynamics, and the evolution of persistence in *Staphylococcus aureus. PLoS Genetics.* 2013;9(1):e1003123.

27. Adams KN, Takaki K, Connolly LE, Wiedenhoft H, Winglee K, Humbert O et al. Drug tolerance in replicating mycobacteria mediated by a macrophage-induced efflux mechanism. *Cell.* 2011;145(1):39–53.

28. Helaine S, Cheverton AM, Watson KG, Faure LM, Matthews SA, Holden DW. Internalization of *Salmonella* by macrophages induces formation of nonreplicating persisters. *Science.* 2014;343(6167):204–8.

29. Wood TK, Knabel SJ, Kwan BW. Bacterial persister cell formation and dormancy. *Applied and Environmental Microbiology.* 2013;79(23):7116–21.

30. Keren I, Shah D, Spoering A, Kaldalu N, Lewis K. Specialized persister cells and the mechanism of multidrug tolerance in *Escherichia coli*. *Journal of bacteriology*. 2004;186(24):8172–80.
31. Shah D, Zhang Z, Khodursky A, Kaldalu N, Kurg K, Lewis K. Persisters: A distinct physiological state of *E. coli*. *BMC Microbiology*. 2006;6:53.
32. Kim Y, Wood TK. Toxins Hha and CspD and small RNA regulator Hfq are involved in persister cell formation through MqsR in *Escherichia coli*. *Biochemical and Biophysical Research Communications*. 2010;391(1):209–13.
33. Maisonneuve E, Shakespeare LJ, Jorgensen MG, Gerdes K. Bacterial persistence by RNA endonucleases. *Proceedings of the National Academy of Sciences of the U S A*. 2011;108(32):13206–11.
34. Moyed HS, Bertrand KP. hipA, a newly recognized gene of *Escherichia coli* K-12 that affects frequency of persistence after inhibition of murein synthesis. *Journal of Bacteriology*. 1983;155(2):768–75.
35. Hayes F, Van Melderen L. Toxins-antitoxins: Diversity, evolution and function. *Critical Reviews in Biochemistry and Molecular Biology*. 2011;46(5):386–408.
36. Wakamoto Y, Dhar N, Chait R, Schneider K, Signorino-Gelo F, Leibler S et al. Dynamic persistence of antibiotic-stressed mycobacteria. *Science*. 2013;339(6115):91–5.
37. Orman MA, Brynildsen MP. Dormancy is not necessary or sufficient for bacterial persistence. *Antimicrobial Agents and Chemotherapy*. 2013;57(7):3230–9.
38. Germain E, Roghanian M, Gerdes K, Maisonneuve E. Stochastic induction of persister cells by HipA through (p)ppGpp-mediated activation of mRNA endonucleases. *Proceedings of the National Academy of Sciences of the U S A*. 2015;112(16):5171–6.
39. Cohen NR, Lobritz MA, Collins JJ. Microbial persistence and the road to drug resistance. *Cell Host & Microbe*. 2013;13(6):632–42.
40. Lewis K. Persister cells, dormancy and infectious disease. *Nature Reviews Microbiology*. 2007;5(1):48–56.
41. Van Acker H, Sass A, Bazzini S, De Roy K, Udine C, Messiaen T et al. Biofilm-grown *Burkholderia cepacia* complex cells survive antibiotic treatment by avoiding production of reactive oxygen species. *PloS ONE*. 2013;8(3):e58943.
42. Li P, Seneviratne CJ, Alpi E, Vizcaino JA, Jin LJ. Delicate metabolic control and coordinated stress response critically determine antifungal tolerance of *Candida albicans* biofilm persisters. *Antimicrobial Agents and Chemotherapy*. 2015;59(10):6101–12.
43. Stewart PS, Franklin MJ. Physiological heterogeneity in biofilms. *Nature Reviews Microbiology*. 2008;6(3):199–210.
44. Roberts ME, Stewart PS. Modelling protection from antimicrobial agents in biofilms through the formation of persister cells. *Microbiology*. 2005;151(Pt 1):75–80.
45. Dalebroux ZD, Swanson MS. ppGpp: Magic beyond RNA polymerase. *Nature Reviews Microbiology*. 2012;10(3):203–12.
46. Harrison JJ, Wade WD, Akierman S, Vacchi-Suzzi C, Stremick CA, Turner RJ et al. The chromosomal toxin gene yafQ is a determinant of multidrug tolerance for *Escherichia coli* growing in a biofilm. *Antimicrobial Agents and Chemotherapy*. 2009;53(6):2253–8.
47. Maisonneuve E, Castro-Camargo M, Gerdes K. (p)ppGpp controls bacterial persistence by stochastic induction of toxin-antitoxin activity. *Cell*. 2013;154(5):1140–50.
48. Bink A, Vandenbosch D, Coenye T, Nelis H, Cammue BP, Thevissen K. Superoxide dismutases are involved in *Candida albicans* biofilm persistence against miconazole. *Antimicrobial Agents and Chemotherapy*. 2011;55(9):4033–7.
49. Lebeaux D, Chauhan A, Letoffe S, Fischer F, de Reuse H, Beloin C et al. pH-mediated potentiation of aminoglycosides kills bacterial persisters and eradicates in vivo biofilms. *The Journal of Infectious Diseases*. 2014;20(9):1357–66.

50. Conlon BP, Nakayasu ES, Fleck LE, LaFleur MD, Isabella VM, Coleman K et al. Activated ClpP kills persisters and eradicates a chronic biofilm infection. *Nature.* 2013;503(7476):365–70.
51. Allison KR, Brynildsen MP, Collins JJ. Metabolite-enabled eradication of bacterial persisters by aminoglycosides. *Nature.* 2011;473(7346):216–20.
52. Pan J, Bahar AA, Syed H, Ren D. Reverting antibiotic tolerance of *Pseudomonas aeruginosa* PAO1 persister cells by (Z)-4-bromo-5-(bromomethylene)-3-methylfuran-2(5H)-one. *PloS ONE.* 2012;7(9):e45778.
53. Pan J, Xie X, Tian W, Bahar AA, Lin N, Song F et al. (Z)-4-Bromo-5-(bromomethylene)-3-methylfuran-2(5H)-one sensitizes *Escherichia coli* persister cells to antibiotics. *Applied Microbiology and Biotechnology.* 2013;97(20):9145–54.
54. Brotz-Oesterhelt H, Beyer D, Kroll HP, Endermann R, Ladel C, Schroeder W et al. Dysregulation of bacterial proteolytic machinery by a new class of antibiotics. *Nature Medicine.* 2005;11(10):1082–7.
55. Kwan BW, Chowdhury N, Wood TK. Combatting bacterial infections by killing persister cells with mitomycin C. *Environmental Microbiology.* 2015;17(11):4406–14.
56. Wexselblatt E, Oppenheimer-Shaanan Y, Kaspy I, London N, Schueler-Furman O, Yavin E et al. Relacin, a novel antibacterial agent targeting the stringent response. *PLoS Pathogens.* 2012;8(9):e1002925.
57. Lee S, Hinz A, Bauerle E, Angermeyer A, Juhaszova K, Kaneko Y et al. Targeting a bacterial stress response to enhance antibiotic action. *Proceedings of the National Academy of Sciences of the U S A.* 2009;106(34):14570–5.

9 Host–Biofilm Interactions at Mucosal Surfaces and Implications in Human Health

Nityasri Venkiteswaran, Kassapa Ellepola,
Chaminda Jayampath Seneviratne, Yuan Kun Lee,
Kia Joo Puan and Siew Cheng Wong

CONTENTS

INTRODUCTION

The ubiquitous occurrence of microbial biofilm communities on different surfaces was discussed briefly in the introductory chapter. Biofilms can exist on both abiotic and biotic surfaces under a wide spectrum of environmental and stress conditions [1]. This kind of adaptability and survivability of biofilms is extremely beneficial during their colonisation of the human host surfaces. For instance, all the exposed surfaces of the human body such as the oral cavity, skin, gastrointestinal tract and vagina are colonised with resident microbiota. The residing microbiota in each of these niches may be unique depending on the specific type and properties of the surfaces. The biofilm communities existing on teeth surfaces would be different from those on mucosal surfaces. In this chapter, we focus on the properties of mucosal biofilms and their interplay with host cells in affecting the overall health and disease condition of the host.

Mucosae are moist linings of the gastrointestinal, nasal and other orifices of the body in continuum with the skin at body openings. The term mucosa signifies a protective mucous membrane at these sites. The mucus thus secreted serves to prevent the invasion of the body by pathogenic microorganisms. In the past, therefore, host–microbial interactions at the mucosal surfaces were studied based on the notion that microorganisms exhibited a free-floating or 'planktonic' mode of growth. Hence, the precept of a 'mucosal biofilm' on mucosal surfaces remained unrecognised until recently. The advent of technology such as DNA sequencing has unravelled that even under healthy conditions, mucosal surfaces house a resident microbiota or mucosal microbiome comprising diverse bacteria and fungi [2]. It is therefore interesting to examine the circumstance under which the mucosal microbial community will develop into a pathogenic biofilm due to a disruption of the microbial balance (termed dysbiosis), compromised host defences or an invasion by a non-resident pathogenic organism capable of overcoming the host immune defences. Mucosal biofilm–associated infections can lead to serious health consequences and are linked with various human diseases including obesity and inflammatory bowel disease (IBD).

To gain a better understanding of the interplay between the host and mucosal biofilms, it is essential to examine some of the basic mechanisms involved in biofilms on mucosal surfaces and the resultant host immune response. The development, structure, composition and clinical implications of the microbial communities at the major mucosal surfaces of the human body are discussed in the first half of the chapter. The innate immune responses elicited by the host and the interactions at the host–mucosal biofilm interface are discussed in the latter part of the chapter. However, a detailed innate immune response of the mucosal surfaces is beyond the scope of this chapter. Readers can refer to some excellent reviews on this topic in the literature.

MUCOSAL BIOFILM FORMATION

The basic processes involved in biofilm development and maturation have been discussed in Chapter 1. Biofilm development on the mucosal surface follows a similar sequence. The attachment of microorganisms to the mucosa is guided by factors such as non-specific chemical bonds and specific microbial antigen–host receptor interactions [3]. Non-specific chemical bonds such as van der Waals forces, hydrophobic interactions, Brownian movement as well as electrostatic charges are important in determining the initial attachment of the microbes [4]. The energy released during such chemical bond formations can surmount 'long-distance' repulsive forces existing between the human cells and microbial cells [5]. The non-specific chemical bonding is followed by more specific interactions mediated through bacterial and fungal antigens with receptors expressed by host cells that promote a stronger attachment [6]. It is noteworthy that the microbial attachment to a mucosal surface is also governed by environmental factors such as temperature, pH, body fluids and the availability of nutrients.

HUMAN MUCOSAL MICROBIAL COMMUNITIES

All mucosal surfaces are always populated with either commensal or pathogenic microbiota depending on the health status of the host. However, the evidence of the biofilm mode of growth on the mucosal surfaces, such as respiratory and gastrointestinal system, is not distinctive enough. The initial attachment and colonisation of cells should be followed by subsequent cell divisions increasing the biomass and the production of an extracellular matrix (ECM) in which cells are encased. However, this classical picture seen in the mature *in vitro* biofilms may not be clearly evident in the *in vivo* situations. Although microorganisms are able to adhere to the mucosal surfaces and may develop into initial biofilm stages, this may not progress to a stage of maturation at the mucosal surfaces because many host factors as well as environmental factors *in vivo* may prevent the maturation phase of a mucosal biofilm. The mucosal cells are subjected to chronic wear and tear and are in a state of rapid turnover in an attempt to combat environmental stresses. As the mucosa is lined by a thin layer of mucus which is dynamic, it is also difficult for microorganisms to penetrate the mucus barrier and adhere to the mucosal epithelial cells to initiate biofilm formation.

Another problem in studying mucosal biofilms *in situ* is the poor accessibility of certain mucosal locations, such as the lower gastrointestinal tract, respiratory tract and the middle ear mucosa. Other factors that limit the study of mucosal biofilms include lack of suitable animal models and limited availability of human tissue samples. It is also important to use techniques that would preserve tissue samples in a manner that would avoid biofilm distortion. For example, the ECM is an essential component of the mucosal biofilm. The existing traditional microbial sampling techniques or histological processing can disrupt the spatial organisation of the mucosal biofilms. Aldehyde-based fixation and dehydration can damage the mucopolysaccharide-containing ECM. It has also been shown that it is impossible to observe biofilms on a formalin-fixed specimen, regardless of the visualisation technique employed [7]. Therefore, with this limitation is mind, we opted to select the term 'microbial community' on the mucosal surfaces to discuss the host–biofilm interactions at the mucosal surfaces.

MICROBIAL COMMUNITY OF THE ORAL MUCOSA

The oral cavity is a major entry route of microorganisms into the body and represents an ideal environment for the development of a mucosal microbial community. The epithelial lining in the oral cavity is keratinised on the tongue and hard palate and non-keratinised elsewhere. It is a primarily stratified squamous epithelium. The microbiota found on oral mucosa adapt to various challenges such as constantly changing environmental conditions including temperature, pH and salivary flow. This environment is always in contact with saliva, the presence of which has a paramount influence on the mucosal microbial communities. Saliva has a pH of 6.75–7.25 and has characteristic organic constituents such as amylase [8]. It acts as a main source of nutrients that favors the growth of resident microorganisms without a drop in pH. Salivary molecules such as lysozymes, lactoferrin and sIgA prevent attachment of extraneous organisms by playing a role in host defence against mucosal biofilm infections [8–10]. Salivary flow rate and viscosity also determine the microbial population in the mucosa. Hyposalivation has been shown to disrupt the microbial balance, leading to oral diseases such as dental caries and periodontitis [11].

A majority of bacteria in the oral mucosa belong to the phylum Firmicutes, followed by a lower population of Proteobacteria and Bacteroidetes (Figure 9.1a) [12].

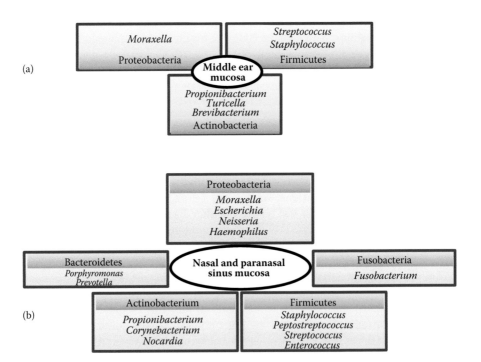

FIGURE 9.1 Common bacteria reported in the microbial community associated with the (a) middle ear mucosa and (b) the nasal and paranasal sinus mucosa.

The predominant genera in the buccal mucosa are *Streptococcus*, *Haemophilus*, *Prevotella* and *Veilonella* [13], of which *Streptococcus* is the most abundant [14,15]. The fungus *Candida albicans* can also be found in healthy mouths as a commensal. Resident bacteria are able to inhibit the overgrowth of the fungus by competitive inhibition of colonisation and modulation of the environment [16]. In certain oral mucosal pathologies such as recurrent aphthous stomatitis, the major bacteria may remain invariable although their proportions may vary. Bacteria such as *Veillonella parvula*, certain species of streptococci such as *Streptococcus salivarius* and *Prevotella intermedia* are seen in lesser abundance while certain species of the *Acinetobacter* genus which are not otherwise a part of the normal oral mucosal microbiota are seen in greater abundance [17].

MICROBIAL COMMUNITY OF THE MIDDLE EAR MUCOSA

The middle ear is another major port of external microbial entry into the host. Even though the middle ear is walled off from the external ear by means of the tympanic membrane, it is connected to the nasopharynx via the Eustachian tube, thereby maintaining its close proximity to the external environment. Most of the epithelium in the middle ear is pseudostratified ciliated columnar. It continues as simple cuboidal or columnar cells. Mucous secretory goblet cells usually lie parallel to the simple cuboidal cells such as in the Eustachian tube. Underlying the epithelium are lymphocytes and ceruminous glands, the secretions of which open through the mucosal surface [18].

Alpha-hemolytic streptococci inhabit the middle ear of healthy individuals and are believed to prevent infections by invaders [19]. Microbiota originating from the external ear such as *Staphylococcus aureus* and *Propionibacterium acnes* may be relocated into the middle ear through a perforated tympanic membrane and may develop into mucosal biofilms [20]. Middle ear mucosal biofilms in otitis media examined by 16S rDNA sequencing revealed the presence of bacterial species such as *S. aureus*, *Turicella otitidis*, *Brevibacterium mcbrellneri* and *Propionibacterium acnes* [21] (Figure 9.1a). Another study found the predominant sinus mucosal species originating from the nasopharynx of children affected with acute otitis media to be *Streptococcus pneumoniae*, non-typeable *Haemophilus influenzae* (NTHi) and *Moraxella catarrhalis* [22–24]. Microbiota of the upper respiratory tract can also be a source of middle ear infections such as otitis media via the Eustachian tube. It has been shown that removal of adenoids is a preventive therapy for otitis media, as it removes the source of microorganisms that might cause middle ear mucosal biofilm infections [25,26].

MICROBIAL COMMUNITY OF THE NASAL AND PARANASAL SINUS

The nasal cavity is lined by stratified squamous and respiratory pseudostratified ciliated columnar epithelium. Seromucinous glands are seen in the submucosa near the opening of the Eustachian tube. The sinuses are continuous with the nasal mucosa lined by pseudostratified ciliated columnar epithelium interspersed with fewer goblet cells and seromucinous glands. The mucus secreted in sinuses is slightly acidic (pH 5.5–6.5) [27]. The presence of villi increases the surface area of the sinuses, thereby helping to retain the moisture thus accounting for selection of the microbiota in this environment [28].

The commonly isolated bacteria in maxillary sinus of healthy individuals are *Corynebacterium diphtheriae* and *S. aureus* [29]. In addition, anaerobic bacteria such as *Porphyromonas gingivalis*, *P. intermedia*, *Fusobacterium nucleatum* and *Peptostreptococcus* spp. have also been isolated in this mucosal environment. Some studies have also reported the presence of *Staphylococcus pneumoniae* and *Streptococcus pyogenes*, coagulase-negative staphylococci, Corynebacteria and lactobacilli. Anaerobic bacteria including *Veillonella, Peptostreptococcus, Propionibacterium, Fusobacterium, Porphyromonas, Bacteroides, Prevotella* and *Bifidobacterium* have also been identified [30]. A recent study employing 16S rDNA sequencing has revealed that members of the phyla Actinobacteria, Firmicutes and Gammaproteobacteria predominated the nasal mucosa of healthy subjects, with the genera *Corynebacterium, Staphylococcus* and *Moraxella* being the most prominent [31]. Figure 9.1b shows the common bacteria associated with the nasal and paranasal sinus mucosa.

Bacterial communities residing in the middle meatus mucosa of healthy adults are reported to belong to coagulase-negative staphylococci, *Corynebacterium* spp. and *S. aureus* [32]. 16s rDNA sequencing revealed a rich diversity of bacteria in the middle meatus mucosa predominated by phyla Firmicutes, Proteobacteria and Actinobacteria [33]. The study also showed that *S. aureus, Staphylococcus epidermidis* and *P. acnes* were the most prominent and abundant organisms in healthy sinuses. Some potential pathogens such as *Escherichia coli, Enterococcus* spp. and *Fusobacterium* spp. have also been reported in the sinuses of healthy subjects [33].

A recent study on chronic rhinosinusitis (CRS) using 16S rDNA sequencing showed no unique bacterial signature in CRS patients *per se*, although the abundance of bacterial genera varied between healthy subjects and the subjects with disease. For instance, some bacterial genera such as *Corynebacterium* or *Moraxella* were higher in affected patients as compared to healthy subjects [31]. Similar findings were obtained in another study that employed sequencing for bacterial samples derived from sinuses [34]. Stressmann et al. reported that *S. aureus* was the most prevalent organism in CRS followed by *Staphylococcus epidermidis* and *P. acnes. S. aureus* was present in 10 times greater abundance as compared to the control healthy subjects. Moreover, it has been proposed that CRS patients may carry a unique microbiome at an individual level [35]. Foreman et al. demonstrated that *S. aureus* was identified in 50% of biofilms from patients with CRS followed by a lesser frequency of *H. influenzae* [36].

MICROBIAL COMMUNITY OF THE GASTROINTESTINAL MUCOSA

The gastrointestinal mucosa is colonised mainly by microorganisms belonging to the phyla Firmicutes and Bacteroidetes. Other phyla such as Actinobacteria, Proteobacteria and Verrucomicrobia are present in minor proportions. The bacterial diversity and abundance increases from the esophagus towards the distal gut and colon [37].

MICROBIAL COMMUNITY OF THE ESOPHAGEAL MUCOSA

Esophageal mucosa is composed of non-keratinised stratified squamous epithelium. Mucous glands are seen in the submucosa. The bacterial community merely passes through the esophagus, but some studies have shown the presence of certain microbiota in healthy subjects. Numerically, the esophagus has the least microbial population of the entire gastrointestinal tract [38]. Bacteria of oral origin such as streptococci and lactobacilli are dominant in the esophagus [38]. *Streptococcus mitis, Streptococcus sanguinis, Streptococcus mutans* and *S. salvarius* have been identified as the major streptococci [39]. In addition, bacteria from other genera such as *Fusobacterium, Neisseria* and *Haemophilus* are also present. rDNA sequencing of microbiota from Barrett's esophagus has shown a significant decrease in bacterial genera such as *Streptococcus, Staphyloccus, Rothia, Actinomyces* and *Bifidobacterium* compared to the healthy subjects. However, the difference in microbial composition was not directly associated with Barrett's esophagus [40]. One of the key findings of the foregoing study is that the distal esophagus displayed a greater bacterial diversity in subjects with Barrett's esophagus, including nitrate reducers such as *Campylobacter concisus* [40]. It was noteworthy to observe an association between the carcinogenic changes taking place in Barrett's esophagus and the presence of nitric oxide, a resultant product of nitrate reduction [40,41]. Whether this observation has a relationship with the esophageal microbiome is yet to be determined.

MICROBIAL COMMUNITY OF THE STOMACH MUCOSA

The epithelium lining the stomach is primarily of the simple columnar type. The lamina propria of the stomach, like in the oral cavity, consists of loose connective tissue. The lining is thrown into folds or rugae and contains mucous glands. The local pH in the stomach is about 2. Owing to its low pH, the stomach is thought to be uninhabitable for most microbes [42]. On the contrary, the resident microbial community on stomach mucosa is abundant. The predominant phyla observed are Proteobacteria, Firmicutes, Bacteroidetes, Actinobacteria and Fusobacteria [43]. *Streptococcus, Peptostreptococcus, Staphylococcus* and *Prevotella* have also been detected in the gastric mucosa apart from *Helicobacter*, which is known to colonise the gastric mucosal epithelium (Figure 9.2). Mucin of the stomach favours the planktonic life cycle of *Helicobacter pylori*. Situations that result in decreased mucin production lead to the biofilm lifestyle of these bacteria [44]. It has been found that *H. pylori* regulate the bacterial diversity in the stomach microenvironment. An absence of *H. pylori* accounts for greater numbers of transient microbiota in the stomach belonging to the genera *Streptococcus, Veillonella, Prevotella* and *Rothia* [45]. In conditions such as chronic atrophic gastritis, hyposecretion of acids leads to the specific colonisation by *Veillonella* and *Lactobacillus*.

MICROBIAL COMMUNITY OF THE INTESTINAL MUCOSA

The epithelial lining in the small and large intestine is similar to that of the stomach but with an additional feature of villi in the small intestine. The epithelial cells are interspersed with goblet cells in both the small and the large intestine. The gut mucosa is always covered by a layer of mucus secreted by goblet cells [46]. In addition, Paneth cells at the base of the crypts produce sIgA [47].

The human mucosa is fast growing, at an intriguing speed of four microns per minute [48]. This means the rate of mucosal proliferation is too high for any microorganism to even colonise, not to mention biofilm formation. Therefore, the small intestine is sparsely populated, and characterised by fast growing bacteria capable of overcoming host defences as well as competition from other bacteria. Another factor that accounts for less opportunity for the biofilm formation in the small intestine is the high flow rate of secretions such as bile acids and mucus [49]. The major genera in the small intestinal mucosal microbial community includes *Lactobacillus*, *Bacteroides*, *Clostridium*, *Mycobacterium* and *Enterococcus* [49] (Figure 9.2). Along the jejunal and illeal mucosa, the population of microorganisms may increase with the additional presence of *Bifidobacterium* spp. [50]. Nutrient resources are also instrumental in exerting a positive selection of certain species over others [47].

The colonic mucosa has certain restricted sites where colonisation and biofilm formation is easier owing to a lower rate of mucosal replication. This accounts for a greater microbial diversity in the colon as compared to the small intestine [51]. Unlike

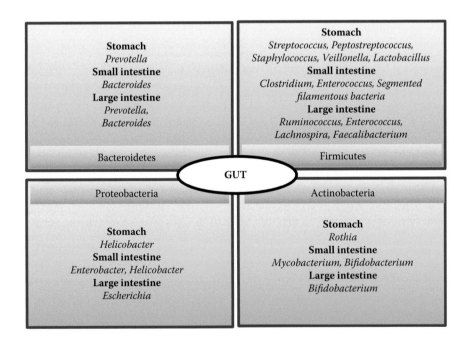

FIGURE 9.2 Common bacteria reported in the microbial community associated with the gut mucosa.

the small intestine, which has a single layer of tightly attached mucosa, the colonic mucus has two organised layers: a dense inner layer and a loose outer layer. The latter forms a favourable habitat for commensals such as *Bacteroides acidifaciens*, *Bacteroides fragilis*, *Akkermansia muciniphila* and those belonging to the family Bifidobacteriaceae. The dense inner mucus adjoining the crypts comprises a more restricted community of *Bacteroides* spp. and *Actinobacter* spp. [47]. The presence of the bacterial genera *Prevotella*, *Ruminococcus* and *Bacteroides* are indicative of a healthy microbiota in the intestine [52,53]. Microbiota belonging to the genera *Bacteroides* and *Bifidobacterium* are the prominent biofilm formers, which include *Bacteroides caccae*, *Bifidobacterium angulatum*, *Bifidobacterium adolescentis* and *Bifidobacterium bifidum*. *E. coli* and *Enterococcus faecalis* are the facultative anaerobes that frequently caused biofilm infections in the large intestine [54]. Owing to production of mucus in large quantities, the inner colonic mucus is relatively less populated. On the contrary, in conditions such as ulcerative colitis, the inner mucus barrier is defective, less dense and broken. This provides access to opportunistic pathogens such as *Bacteroides* and also to mucin degraders such as *A. muciniphila*, leading to inflammation in disease conditions such as Crohn's disease and ulcerative colitis [55]. Biofilms in the large intestine are associated with food residues, and therefore the microbial species and their biochemical activities are governed mainly by diet [56]. For instance, the infant gut demonstrates differences in microbiome based on the type of food to which it is introduced. Babies who are breast fed post-natally are predominated by organisms belonging to the Bacteroidetes and those fed with formula milk demonstrate higher amount of organisms belonging to the Firmicutes [57,58].

Fungal species such as *Candida* are normal inhabitants of the gut mucosa [59]. They have been detected in the gut microbiota of 30–70% of healthy adults [60]. *Candida* is capable of colonising and proliferating in the gut after it overcomes mechanical barriers composed of mucus, epithelial cells and the tight junctions between them, and chemical barriers such as the gastric secretions of acid, bile and digestive enzymes [61]. The indigenous commensal bacterial microbiota is antagonistic to *C. albicans*, thus making it further difficult for this fungus to establish pathogenicity. Bacteriocins, probiotics and other bacterial products prevent attachment of *Candida* to the gut mucosa [62]. However, if *Candida* manages to attach and colonise, it can create a hypoxic microenvironment in the human gut which favours the growth of strict anaerobes such as *B. fragilis* and *Clostridium perfringens* [63].

The resident microbiota in the host offer 'colonisation resistance' to the invasive microorganisms. Freter et al. proposed that the relative ability of a particular species to outcompete others depends entirely on its ability to devour specific limiting nutrients from the host. The limiting nutrients also govern the type of species that will predominate a certain area of the gut. Thus, the resident bacteria establish their own selective spatial niche based on these 'selective' nutrients that account for a positive selection of certain species over the others [47,64]. *E. coli* in gut mucosa typically exemplifies the phenomenon of colonisation resistance. Intestinal *E. coli* is unable to degrade polysaccharides derived from diet or the mucus layer for their nutritional requirements because of the lack of hydrolases [65]. It depends on other anaerobes present in the mucus for oligosaccharides needed for its growth. Thus, the existence of a mixed species of a microbial community feeds *E. coli*. This phenomenon has been described as the 'restaurant hypothesis' whereby *E. coli* resides in 'restaurants' and is exposed to a unique menu by means of its interaction with different anaerobic species. This accounts for a unique nutritional program per species of commensal *E. coli* [66]. Both commensal and pathogenic *E. coli* occupy distinct nutritional niches in the gut and are capable of utilising at least one nutritional component not utilised by the other. Their differing nutritional preferences allow both commensal and pathogenic *E. coli* to exist in unique niches of their own in the intestine [67].

Microbial Community of the Vaginal Mucosa

The vaginal mucosal epithelium is a non-keratinised stratified squamous epithelium. Vaginal epithelial cells lack a robust intercellular junction, thus making them permeable to microbial products and inflammatory mediators. The resident vaginal microbiota metabolise glycogen to glucose and subsequently ferment this glucose to lactic acid and hydrogen peroxide. Thus, a low pH of 3.8–4.2 is maintained. They also secrete bacteriocins and other organic products that have antibacterial properties against invading pathogens. However, these secretions also include certain biosurfactants that enable attachment to the epithelial cells and promote aggregation of different species of bacteria for the formation of mucosal biofilms [68–70].

Lactobacillus is the most common genus colonising the vagina of healthy women during their child-bearing age. The different species of lactobacilli seen are *Lactobacillus crispatus*, *Lactobacillus gasseri*, *Lactobacillus jensenii* and *Lactobacillus iners*. These originate primarily in the intestine and exhibit vaginotropism or pronounced affinity to attach to the vaginal mucosa. Other genera identified through DNA sequencing include *Atopobium*, *Prevotella*, and *Propionibacterium* [71,72]. Non-beneficial bacteria from genera such as *Streptococcus*, *Staphylococcus*, *Gardnerella* and *Enterococcus* may also be present in low concentrations in a healthy vagina but in insufficient numbers to cause disease [73,74]. The potentially pathogenic organisms that inhabit the vaginal mucosa are *Neisseria*, certain species of streptococci such as *S. pyogenes*, *S. pneumoniae*, *Haemophilus* and *Listeria* [75]. Figure 9.3 shows common bacteria associated with the vaginal mucosa.

The presence of *Lactobacillus* spp. in the vaginal microbiome decreases the risk of bacterial vaginosis and other sexually transmitted diseases caused by invading pathogens [76]. For instance, *Listeria monocytogenes* and *Chlamydia trachomatis* are inhibited by the lower vaginal pH [77,78]. Proliferation and colonisation of *Listeria* is favourable at around pH 6.5 [77]. The loss of beneficial bacteria such as *Lactobacilli* would favour simultaneous proliferation of pathogenic anaerobes responsible for bacterial vaginosis such as *Gardnerella vaginalis*, *Atopobium vaginae*, *Prevotella* spp. and those of the genus *Mobiluncus* and *Bacteroides* [79]. The most prevalent fungus *Candida* is also capable of thriving in the vaginal tract and forming biofilms. However, *Lactobacillus* can prevent hyphal growth in *Candida* and pathogenic transition of the fungus [80,81].

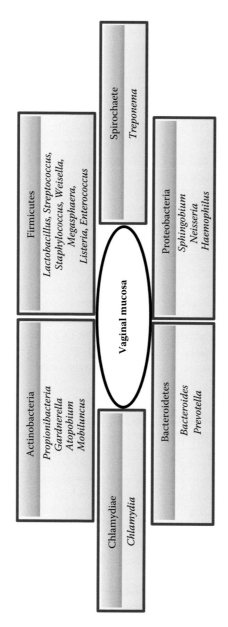

FIGURE 9.3 Common bacteria reported in the microbial community associated with the vaginal mucosa.

EXTRA CELLULAR MATRIX OF MUCOSAL BIOFILMS

Once firmly attached on the mucosal surface, the microorganisms undergo several rounds of cell division and form microcolonies. This is followed by the spatial-temporal arrangement of the microbes within a protective mesh of ECM. Microorganisms acquire nutrients from the surrounding epithelial cells and become embedded within the matrix. ECM is composed of self-secreted polymers including polysaccharides, proteins and DNA which produce a barrier to immune cells, opsonins and other host immune strategies [82]. Hence, microbes are 'hidden' in the ECM of the mucosal biofilm to protect themselves from the immune cells.

Generation of an ECM is a common trait in all biofilms, irrespective of abiotic or biotic surfaces. However, the dynamics behind this process may vary according to the surface characteristics and the flow conditions [83]. Compared to the abiotic surface biofilms, the composition of the ECM seen in the mucosal biofilm is inherently more complex owing to the fact that host proteins, mucopolysacccharides, nucleic acids and even host cells may participate in its development [82]. There is strong evidence that ECM components may play an important role in both structural and non-structural functions of the mucosal biofilms. Mutants defective in ECM generation lack the classical complex mucosal biofilm architecture [83,84]. The various components of the ECM perform specific functions within the biofilm microbial community and their secretion can be a function either of environmental factors or the genetic background of a specific strain. In microorganisms such as *Pseudomonas aeruginosa*, extracellular DNA (eDNA) in the ECM plays a pivotal role in guiding cellular migration within the biofilm structure. The ECM in the local vicinity of the pioneer cells directs the attachment of subsequent cells to establish the biofilm community [85]. ECM thus generates signals that help the colonies to expand in order to form larger territories.

INTERACTION OF MICROBES AND HOST AT THE MUCOSAL SURFACES

The various immune responses of the host and the constant evasion mechanisms of pathogens are part of the vicious cycle of mucosal infection. An understanding of the type of interactions occurring between the host and pathogen is of crucial importance in preventing the invasion and development of pathogenic biofilms on mucosal surfaces. However, studies on microbial and host interaction at mucosal surfaces are limited. Here, we provide a few examples of *in vitro* and *in vivo* models that have given some insight into this intriguing relationship between microbes and host surfaces.

Several studies have elucidated that the attachment and colonisation of the mucosal surfaces are mediated by defined surface molecules on the microorganisms that interact either with components of the mucosal intercellular matrix or with structures on the eukaryotic cell surface [86].

MICROBIAL-ASSOCIATED EXTRA CELLULAR MATRIX SENSORS

Molecules that specifically interact with ECM components such as fibronectin, collagen, laminin and elastin are commonly described as 'microbial surface components recognising adhesive matrix molecules (MSCRAMMs)' [87]. The expression of fibronectin-binding proteins could increase bacterial aggregation, suggesting that these proteins can promote the initiation of biofilm development. For example, mutant *S. aureus* lacking surface expression of fibronectin binding proteins (FnBPA and FnBPB) are defective in adhering to fibronectin-coated surfaces to form biofilms [88,89]. Similarly, two surface adhesins of *E. faecium*, SgrA and EcbA, showed binding to ECM components such as nidogen 1, nidogen 2, fibrinogen and collagen type V found in the basal lamina of mucosal surfaces [90]. In *H. influenzae*, an adhesin designated protein E was shown to bind vitronectin [91–93]. Mucin, a major glycoprotein component in mucus, could promote *P. aeruginosa* attachment and biofilm formation *in vitro* [94]. Glycoprotein-340 is another mucin-like protein found adsorbed to mucosal surfaces that could mediate the attachment of *S. mutans* and *Streptococcus gordonii* via surface adhesin SpaP [95,96] and SspA and SspB [97] respectively [98].

MICROBIAL-ASSOCIATED CELLULAR SENSORS

Other surface structures on microbes such as pili and flagella also serve as adhesins to facilitate early steps in biofilm formation and adhesion to mammalian cells. Specifically, *P. aeruginosa* type IV pili bind to glycosphingolipid receptors on epithelial cells [99–101]. *S. pyogenes* pili adhere and form microcolonies on human pharyngeal cells [102] and PilA of non-typeable *H. influenzae* (NTHi) strains mediates adherence to human respiratory epithelial cells both *in vitro* and *in vivo* [103]. Another interesting adhesin, FimH positioned on the tip of type I pili of several bacteria, including various species of *Salmonella*, specifically recognises mannose residues on epithelial cells and plays a significant role in biofilm formation *in vitro* [104–106]. Similarly, biofilm formation in *Neisseria meningitidis* is supported by pili-associated proteins such as PilQ [107] and PilX [108]. The binding of *P. aeruginosa* flagellar cap protein to Lewis^x oligosaccharides, a glycoprotein constituent of mucus, contributes to biofilm formation in cystic fibrosis patients [109]. Other specific cell surface adhesins such as CbpA and PsaA in *S. pneumoniae* and HrpA expressed on *N. meningitidis* have been shown to aid biofilm formation on mouse and human bronchial epithelial cells [110–113].

Similar to bacterial cell surface proteins, fungal cell wall proteins also have a major role in fungal biofilm formation on host surfaces. In *C. albicans,* Hwp1 is the first cell surface protein reported for biofilm formation *in vivo*, whereby the lack of Hwp1 results in poor adherence. It can also serve as a substrate for mammalian epithelial cell transglutaminase [114–116]. Other *C. albicans* adhesins such as Als3, a member of the agglutinin-like sequence (Als) family of proteins, and Eap1, a glycosylphosphatidylinositol-anchored cell wall protein, have also been shown to play a role in adhesion and biofilm formation both *in vitro* and *in vivo* [117,118].

The aforementioned studies clearly demonstrate the necessity of the microbe–host interaction at the mucosal surface for initial attachment and subsequent biofilm formation. However, our understanding of this cross-talk is still limited. Therefore, researchers should be encouraged to venture into this area of research to elucidate the fascinating aspects of host–microbial interactions at mucosal surfaces.

MICROBIAL-ASSOCIATED MOLECULAR PATTERN SENSORS

Besides the specific microbial adhesin interaction with ECM proteins and host surface molecules, there are additional interactions between the host and microorganisms that are based on the ability of the host to detect conserved ligands on microbes known as microbe-associated molecular patterns (MAMPs) [119,120]. Examples of MAMPs include lipoteichoic acid (LTA), lipopolysaccharides (LPS), nucleic acids, lipoproteins, surface glycoproteins and peptidoglycans (Table 9.1) [121]. MAMPs are recognised by pattern recognition receptors (PRRs) located on host epithelial and immune cells. PRRs can be either membrane bound or intracellular receptors [122]. Some of the common host PRRs include transmembrane receptors such as toll-like receptors (TLRs) and C-type lectin receptors (CLRs), and intracellular receptors such as nucleotide-binding oligomerisation domain (NOD-) like receptors (NLRs), AIM2-like receptor (ALR) and retinoic acid–inducible gene (RIG) I-like receptors (RLRs) [123]. Each receptor has unique recognition motifs for its binding to specific MAMPs.

Each of these PRR families consists of multiple members that display different patterns of expression on different cell types. For instance, TLR2 generally expressed on myeloid cells including dendritic cells, monocytes, macrophages and polymorphonuclear leukocytes is specific for recognising components of pathogens such as peptidoglycan and LTA of Gram-positive bacteria [124]. TLR3 is found primarily in dendritic cells and is involved in the recognition of dsRNA present in some viruses and implicated in immunity to viral infections [125].

TLR4, together with MD2 and CD14, mediates signal transduction by binding to a lipid component of the LPS [126] and is expressed mainly on monocytes, macrophages and also dendritic cells. LPS is a principal structural component present in the cell wall of all Gram-negative bacteria and some Gram-positive bacteria [127]. Other bacterial components such as flagellin, which is a structural protein of flagella present in all motile bacteria is recognised by TLR5 [128–136]. TLR9 senses unmethlyated CpG sequences in DNA found predominantly in bacteria [137]. In humans, TLR9 expression is restricted to B cells and plasmacytoid dendritic cells.

INNATE IMMUNE RESPONSE TO MUCOSAL BIOFILMS

On entry, pathogens do not directly establish contact with the host mucosa. Instead, they first encounter the complex community of commensal microorganisms and the mucosal immune defences. Whereas commensal organisms maintain a harmonious relationship with the mucosal surfaces, pathogens may either succumb to the immune defences or evade it. Successful adhesion and biofilm formation of invading microorganisms on the mucosal surface thus depends on their ability to overcome

TABLE 9.1
Microbial Adhesins Involved in Mucosal Attachment and Biofilm Formation

Category	Organism	Adhesin	Ligand	Type of Mucosa/Epithelial Cells	References
Gram-positive bacteria	S. mutans	SpaP	Glycoprotein 340	Oral mucosa	[96]
	S. gordonii	SspA and SspB	Glycoprotein 340	Oral mucosa	[97]
	S. pyogenes	Pili	—	Pharyngeal epithelial cells	[102]
	S. pneumoniae	CbpA	Choline	Nasopharyngeal mucosa	[112]
		PsaA	E-cadherin	Nasopharyngeal epithelial cells	[113]
	S. aureus	FnBPA/FnBPB	Fibronectin, elastin	Nasopharyngeal mucosa	[89]
	E. faecium	SgrA (Serine glutamate repeat A)	Fibrinogen and nidogen 1 and 2	Gastrointestinal mucosa	[90]
		EcbA	Collagen type V and fibrinogen	Gastrointestinal mucosa	[90]
Gram-negative bacteria	P. aeruginosa	Flagellin	TLR-5 receptors and cytosolic sensors at the cell surface	Respiratory mucosa	[135,136]
		Type IV pili	Glycosphingolipids (asialoGM1)	Lung epithelial cells	[100]
		Flagella cap protein	Lewisˣ oligosaccharides in mucin	Respiratory mucosa	[109]
	H. influenzae	Protein E (PE)	Vitronectin	Respiratory mucosa	[91,92]
		pilA	—	Respiratory epithelial cells	[103]
	Salmonella spp.	Std fimbrial adhesin	α(1,2)-Fucose	Cecal mucosa	[104–106]
		Type I fimbriae FimH	Mannose-containing glycoprotein	Epithelial cells	
	N. meningitidis	HrpA	—	Bronchial epithelial cells	[111]

(Continued)

TABLE 9.1 (CONTINUED)
Microbial Adhesins Involved in Mucosal Attachment and Biofilm Formation

Category	Organism	Adhesin	Ligand	Type of Mucosa/ Epithelial Cells	References
Fungi	C. albicans	Hwp1	Mammalian transglutaminases	Oral epithelial cells	[114–116,138]
		Als3	E-cadherin, N-cadherin, host cell ferritin	Oral mucosa	[117]
		Eap1	–	Oral mucosa	[118]

the host innate immune response, which acts as the first line of defence. The innate immune system encompasses a wide array of strategies ranging from expression of antimicrobial molecules, phagocytosis and proinflammatory mediators against the invading pathogens.

The secretions of the innate immune system prevent attachment of pathogens to mucosal sites and initiation of biofilm development. For example, lysozyme digests peptidoglycans in bacterial cell walls and the host plasma transferrin binds iron (Fe) with high affinity which otherwise is needed for microbial growth. Sodium chloride secreted from sweat glands interferes with ion transport and mucus, which contains mucin secreted by the mucosal epithelial cells, coats cell surfaces, rendering them unfavourable for microbial binding to mucosal surfaces.

HOST-DERIVED ANTIMICROBIAL PEPTIDES

In humans, a wide variety of proteins and peptides exhibit antimicrobial activity. Host-derived antimicrobial peptides (AMPs) form an essential part of the innate immune system. Defensins were the first natural antimicrobial peptides to be described in mammalian cells. Originally isolated from epithelial cells and neutrophils, they are small cationic peptides and function by binding to the bacterial plasma membrane. Defensins cause a disruption of the membrane integrity resulting in inhibition of DNA, RNA and protein synthesis. The nature of the interaction allows defensins to target both Gram-positive and Gram-negative bacteria, fungi and enveloped viruses. Two classes of defensins have been described in humans, alpha and beta. Both types consist of six conserved cysteine residues. Alpha-defensins are synthesised by polymorphonuclear leukocytes and Paneth cells. In contrast to alpha-defensins, beta-defensins are secreted by epithelial cells in the respiratory, gastrointestinal and urinary tracts. Defensins are secreted at low levels under normal physiological conditions but can be induced in response to microbial infections. Since their discovery, other functional roles have been ascribed to defensins [139]. For instance, alpha-defensins such as HNP1-3 have been demonstrated to function as chemoattractants for dendritic cells and naïve CD4 and CD8 T cells [140]. Alpha-defensins derived from human neutrophils have been shown to neutralise the anthrax lethal toxin [141], diphtheria toxin and *Pseudomonas* exotoxin A [141]. Recent investigations on human beta-defensin-3 have revealed its link to oral cancer [142].

Cathelicidins are a family of antimicrobial peptides derived from proteolysis. They consist of a conserved N-terminal domain and a C-terminal antibacterial domain. In humans, cleavage of hCAP-18 by proteinase 3 generates the active peptide LL-37, which possesses antibacterial activity (as extensively reviewed by Durr et al.) [143]. It is expressed in a wide variety of cell types including monocytes, NK cells, T cells and B cells as well as epithelial cells in the gastrointestinal tract, respiratory tract and the skin. Like defensins, it can exert antimicrobial activity on both Gram-positive and Gram-negative bacteria. Up-regulation of LL-37 expression has been implicated in a number of diseases including psoriasis, lupus, contact dermatitis, *Helicobacter pylori* infection and in tracheal aspirates of newborns during infection. Down-regulation of LL-37 is also reported in atopic dermatitis and Kostmann disease (an autosomal recessive disorder characterised by severe neutropenia). Patients with Kostmann disease are devoid of LL-37 in neutrophils and saliva [144]. Thus, patients with this disorder manifest with severe periodontal disease.

Histatins belong to a family of small histidine-rich peptides. They are produced by the salivary glands (submandibular, sublingual, parotid glands) and von Ebner's gland at the back of the tongue. Histatins exert antifungal and antibacterial activity, thereby playing a central role in maintaining good oral health. In humans, histatins 1, 3 and 5 have been described. Histatins 1 and 3 are encoded by two closely related genes. Among all the histatins, histatin 5 is a product processed from histatin 3 and demonstrates the most potent antifungal activity against pathogenic fungi including *Aspergillus fumigatus*, *Cryptococcus neoformans* and *C. albicans*. The exact mode of action of histatins in killing fungi is not clear. Earlier studies showed that histatin 5 interferes with *Candida* respiration by targeting the mitochondria [145,146]. Later studies have shown histatin 5 disrupts the *Candida* cell membrane by binding to the potassium ion transporter Trk1. This results in the loss of intracellular potassium and ATP leading to activation of cell death pathway [147].

HOST INNATE IMMUNE CELLS

Apart from secretions at mucosal sites, innate immune cells such as neutrophils, macrophages and dendritic cells also play a major role in mucosal defense [148]. These cells are capable of phagocytosis, one of the key processes in innate immunity during which the invading microbes are engulfed and destroyed by the aforementioned cells.

Neutrophils are the first cells to arrive at a site of bacterial infection [149]. Biofilms are not inherently protected from neutrophils. Numerous factors such as chemokines and cytokines released by host cells and bacteria-derived products such as *N*-acyl homoserine lactone (AHL) and formyl-Met-Leu-Phe (fMLP) at the infection site serve as chemoattractants, causing neutrophils to emigrate from blood vessels and actively migrate through the tissue to the site of infection. Several *in vitro* and *in vivo* studies have observed the localisation of neutrophils within, on and around biofilms. Once at the site of infection, neutrophils sense the microbes through their PRRs, phagocytose the microbes and release enzymes and reactive oxygen species (ROS). Neutrophils also produce neutrophil extracellular traps (NETs) [150,151] in a process known as NETosis. These NETs consist of nuclear and mitochondrial DNA filaments with high local concentrations of anti-microbial proteins and are able to immobilise vast amount of microbes to prevent further spread from occurring. NETosis is triggered by bacterial cell wall components activating receptors expressed on neutrophils [152]. This mechanism of killing has been demonstrated against microbes such as *C. albicans, S. aureus* and *S. flexneri* [153]. In addition, NETs from neutrophils also serve as opsonins on binding the microbes, promoting enhanced clearance by macrophages [154].

In the early stages of biofilm formation during which the bacterial aggregates are still small, they are predominantly cleared by neutrophil phagocytosis. When the biofilm is more established, phagocytosis becomes ineffective and neutrophils will promote microbe clearance through the release of enzymes and ROS, which can result in host tissue damage as well. In oral mucosa, periodontopathogenic bacterial species such as *P. gingivalis* could induce the expression of TREM-1, a proinflammatory receptor on neutrophils or interleukin-8 gene expression in gingival epithelial cells and fibroblasts [155]. Furthermore, the transition to biofilm development was shown to be dependent on cyclic dinucleotides (c-di-NMPs) such as c-di-GMP acting as a secondary messenger in a diverse array of microbes. These c-di-NMPs can act as pathogen-associated molecular patterns and specifically elicit a host type-I interferon innate immune response through their binding to STING and DDX41, both of which are cytoplasmic PRRs [156–158]. In fact, they have been tested as vaccine adjuvants in a mouse model of mastitis infection where administration of synthetic c-di-GMP could reduce bacterial colonisation by a strain of *S. aureus* that is capable of forming biofilm [159].

IMMUNE TOLERANCE TO COMMENSALS IN MUCOSAL BIOFILMS

Unlike abiotic surfaces, the mucosal surface composition is complex, with the presence of a host epithelial cell layer that secretes mucin, which forms a mucous membrane that is endowed with cells of the innate immune system. A biofilm consisting of commensal microorganisms is also present. Under physiological, non-inflammatory conditions, an immunological equilibrium exists between the commensal microorganisms of mucosal biofilms and the host mucosal defences owing to the constitutive presence of microorganisms. The commensals are capable of inducing specific signalling pathways through PRRs on epithelial cells, which elicit a tolerogenic immune response leading to immune homeostasis [160]. For instance in the gut, the MAMP–PRR signalling cascade helps maintain a symbiotic host–microbe relationship either by stabilising the gut barrier through mucus production or maintaining a tolerogenic immune response on MAMP recognition. In certain scenarios, the commensal organisms are capable of modifying the structure of their MAMPs such as pentacylation of lipid A in *Bacteroides* or exopolysaccharide expression on the surface of *Bifidobacterium*, which can evade PRR signalling by influencing components of the NF-κB pathway. This shapes the gut immune cells tolerogenically, thereby maintaining homeostasis [161,162]. Other means of immune tolerance are maintained through either a lack of T-cell activation in the context of anergy or suppression of effector T-cell activation by regulatory T cells [163,164]. Thus, the commensal organisms of the mucosal biofilms maintain a stable niche in the host mucosa through tight regulation of their interactions with the host, resulting in an equilibrium state whereby the host does not mount an overt immune response against them. It is when this equilibrium becomes disrupted that pathogenic organisms invade the mucosa.

EVASION OF HOST IMMUNE RESPONSE BY MUCOSAL BIOFILMS

The successful colonisation and biofilm development of pathogenic microorganisms on mucosal surfaces can lead to several serious consequences to the host. The compromised immunity of the host and the release of cytotoxic substances by the microbes are major factors in establishing the pathogenesis of mucosal biofilms. Here, we summarise some of the main evasion strategies and virulence factors associated with microbial pathogenesis caused by microbial biofilm.

For the host cationic antimicrobial peptides (AMPs) to work effectively, AMPs need to gain access to the cytoplasmic membrane of the microbes. In Gram-positive bacteria, the thick peptidoglycan cell wall is cross-linked with lipotechoic acids which serve as a barrier against AMPs, whereas in Gram-negative bacteria AMPs need to penetrate the cell wall, which is largely composed of negatively charged lipopolysacchride. AMP-resistant bacteria are known to increase their net positive surface charge through modifications resulting in electrostatic repulsion of AMP [165]. This prevents access of AMP to the cytoplasmic membrane.

Recent reports by Kang et al. have demonstrated that MSCRAMM of some Gram-positive bacteria can inhibit complement activation of the classical pathway by targeting C1q [166]. Biofilm bacteria of *P. aeruginosa* do not trigger oxidative bursts of polymorphonuclear leukocytes (PMNs) to the same degree as that of planktonic bacteria, thereby halting the activation of immune cells [167–169]. In addition, *P. aeruginosa* biofilms produce the exopolysaccharide alginate, which protects the bacteria from being killed by macrophages [170]. Alginate has also been shown to induce conformational changes to AMP and cause aggregation of the AMP, preventing access to the cytoplasmic membrane [171].

Elastase LasB is an important extracellular virulence factor that regulates the inflammatory response during biofilm formation. Bacterial elastase has been shown to inactivate and degrade LL-37 [172]. The lasB deletion mutant ($\Delta lasB$) displayed significantly decreased bacterial attachment, microcolony formation, extracellular matrix production and biofilm formation [173]. LasB cleaves host protease-activated receptors PAR2 in respiratory epithelial cells [174]. PAR2 signalling is known to regulate host inflammatory responses, particularly in the lung. Recent studies have demonstrated that the loss of PAR2 on neutrophils significantly decreased phagocytic uptake of *P. aeruginosa*, whereas activation of PAR2 caused recruitment of phagocytic machinery such as MAP kinases, Rho-Rac GTPases and actin, probably by acting as a direct phagocytic receptor [175,176]. Hence, the expression of elastase by virulent strains of *P. aeruginosa* could potentially modulate both inflammatory responses and phagocytosis through PAR2 inhibition during chronic biofilm formation.

Modification of neutrophil shape and function is another evasive strategy shown by mucosal biofilms. An interesting study demonstrated that on settling on *P. aeruginosa* biofilms, neutrophils become bloated in shape and partially degranulated. The cells become immobilised and phagocytically inert, showing little or no bactericidal activity [177]. The deposition of neutrophils also increased the oxygen consumption of the system by increasing bacterial respiration and the neutrophil respiratory burst, thereby decreasing the oxidative potential of the system. Overall, the study showed that the host defence becomes compromised as neutrophils remain immobilised with a diminished oxidative potential while biofilm bacteria escape.

Quorum sensing (QS) molecules are signalling molecules produced by bacteria that allow communication between bacteria, enabling them to control population density, regulate biofilm formation and produce virulence factors. As such, these QS molecules play a central role in host invasion and pathogenesis. QS molecules from *P. aeruginosa* infections are known to promote the production of rhamnolipids, which cause rapid cell death in neutrophils [178]. QS molecules such as

3-oxo-C12-homoserine lactone (3-oxo-C12-HSL) induce the transcription of virulence factors including elastase and proteases. Although 3-oxo-C12-HSL concentrations are recorded at submicromolar levels in planktonic culture supernatants of *P. aeruginosa*, they are as high as 600 μM in biofilms [179]. *In vitro* studies on immune modulation by 3-oxo-C12-HSL revealed that a 10 μM concentration is sufficient to reduce the LPS-induced production of the proinflammatory cytokine IL-12 by monocytes [180]. More recent studies demonstrated that a synthetic form of 3-oxo-C12-HSL can induce morphological changes to human macrophages by acting through the water channels, aquaporins [181]. Other studies showed that this compound induces apoptosis in neutrophils, monocytes [182] and fibroblasts [183], reducing the host immune response. The induction of apoptosis in inflammatory cells would also favour the spread of invading bacteria [184]. Studies have revealed that 3-oxo-C12-HSL could also inhibit cytokine production by T lymphocytes [185–187] and modulate antibody production by B lymphocytes [180,186]. Hence, QS molecules secreted by mucosal biofilms may weaken not only innate immunity, but also the adaptive immunity of the host which results in chronic mucosal biofilm infections. However, more research is warranted to obtain detailed information on the role of QS molecules in mucosal biofilms and immunity [188].

Although production of pro-inflammatory cytokines by immune cells is important to control mucosal biofilm, such locally released factors can also act as biofilm-specific growth factors, promoting their growth [189]. Furthermore, microbial aggregates causing an aberrant immune and inflammatory response can lead to mucosal tissue damage, as in the case of IBD [7]. Another example is the excessive secretion of ROS by neutrophils to combat *P. aeruginosa* infection in the lung, and in the process also resulted in destroying the host tissues [177].

ECM of microbial biofilms can also modify the sequence of events in pathogenesis through its effect on immune cell recognition of microbial cells and antimicrobial host responses. For example, *P. aeruginosa* ECM consists of alginate that is capable of inhibiting phagocytosis and mediating directed migration of neutrophils *in vitro* [170,190]. ECM components thereby act as a defence mechanism against immunocompetent cells. Other benefits conferred by the ECM include protection from environmental stresses, controlling host cell behaviour and biofilm resistance to antimicrobial agents. Certain ECM compounds can enhance nutrient availability for the mucosal biofilm community [191]. ECM can also control gene expression in microbial communities. For example, *V. Cholerae* regulates the expression of its virulent genes by mechano-sensing the viscosity of the gut mucosal environment imparted by ECM. Viscosity induced by ECM is detected by means of its flagellar activity, which in turn translates into the amount of sodium influx and thus gene regulation in *V. cholerae* [192]. Hence, further insight into the ECM of mucosal biofilms will be essential to develop novel therapeutic strategies against mucosal biofilm-associated infections.

FUTURE DIRECTIONS FOR MUCOSAL BIOFILM RESEARCH

Much of the existing information on mucosal biofilm physiology and their interactions with the host have been gleaned from *in vitro* models and genetic and molecular biology based approaches. However, biofilm pathogenesis is a complex dynamic process involving the host and the microbe, where the host component largely determines the fate of infection, which is difficult to model in an *in vitro* environment. This necessitates the use of *in vivo* models ranging from non-mammalian models including invertebrates such as *Caenorhabditis elegans* (nematode) and *Drosophila melanogaster* (fruit-fly) and vertebrates such as *Danio rerio* (zebra fish) to murine and higher mammalian models such as monkeys and pigs. Use of *in vivo* models for studying mucosal biofilm infections can be quite challenging owing to the differences in susceptibility among different models and the extent of correlation of the different models with the human host. The environmental differences of the human host versus other mammalian models are also to be accounted for. Animal welfare and ethical concerns impose further restrictions on the usage of these models. Development of *ex vivo* models allows for an ethical alternative to using *in vivo* models. But the difficulty of modelling polymicrobial infections and their cost ineffectiveness again make them non-ideal. Concentrated efforts are now being directed towards the development of better *in vivo* models and cost-effective *ex vivo* models. Attaining the gold standard platform for modelling host–microbial interactions would significantly advance our understanding of mucosal biofilm biology.

The next major leap in understanding host–mucosal biofilm interactions could come from proteomic or metabolomic investigations of these interactions. Biological hierarchy comprises the genome, proteome and the metabolome, with proteome and metabolome giving the final picture of events occurring within an organism. Understanding the protein or metabolic activity of mucosal biofilms is essential to understanding their pathogenicity. Until recently, technological limitations of both proteomics and metabolomics were impeding progress in this direction. With advanced technologies, large amounts of information are now being gathered and processed in a single attempt to provide the macro view of events. Mucosal biofilm research is now at the imminent juncture of integrative omics platforms, that is, genomics, transcriptomics, proteomics and metabolomics data collected simultaneously and integrated using bioinformatics tools. This type of an integrated platform can help in addressing unanswered queries regarding host–pathogen interactions. Biofilm infections are clinically important because most of them are resistant to conventional antimicrobial therapies. Therefore, research in this area needs to progress with increasingly sophisticated approaches, which would help in designing more potent and less toxic agents. The development of better infection models, assembling post genomic data and integration of multilevel omics data are capable of accelerating pharmacological research in biofilm infections by aiding both drug design and prediction of drug targets.

CORRESPONDING AUTHORS

Siew Cheng Wong
Singapore Immunology Network (SIgN)
Agency for Science, Technology and Research (A*STAR)
Singapore
wong_siew_cheng@immunol.a-star.edu.sg

Chaminda Jayampath Seneviratne
Discipline of Oral Sciences
Faculty of Dentistry
National University of Singapore
Singapore
jaya@nus.edu.sg

REFERENCES

1. Donlan RM, Costerton JW. Biofilms: Survival mechanisms of clinically relevant microorganisms. *Clinical Microbiology Reviews.* 2002;15(2):167–93.
2. Tannock GW. *Normal microflora: An introduction to microbes inhabiting the human body.* New York: Springer Science & Business Media; 1995.
3. Nobbs AH, Lamont RJ, Jenkinson HF. *Streptococcus* adherence and colonization. *Microbiology and Molecular Biology Reviews: MMBR.* 2009;73(3):407–50.
4. van Loosdrecht MC, Lyklema J, Norde W, Schraa G, Zehnder AJ. Electrophoretic mobility and hydrophobicity as a measure to predict the initial steps of bacterial adhesion. *Applied and Environmental Microbiology.* 1987;53(8):1898–901.
5. Heckels JE, Blackett B, Everson JS, Ward ME. The influence of surface charge on the attachment of *Neisseria gonorrhoeae* to human cells. *Journal of General Microbiology.* 1976;96(2):359–64.
6. Pizarro-Cerda J, Cossart P. Bacterial adhesion and entry into host cells. *Cell.* 2006;124(4):715–27.
7. Swidsinski A, Weber J, Loening-Baucke V, Hale LP, Lochs H. Spatial organization and composition of the mucosal flora in patients with inflammatory bowel disease. *Journal of Clinical Microbiology.* 2005;43(7):3380–9.
8. Marsh PD. Role of the oral microflora in health. *Microbial Ecology in Health and Disease.* 2000;12(3):130–7.
9. Van der Hoeven J, Busscher H, Evans L. The ecology of dental plaque: The role of nutrients in the control of the oral microflora. In: Busscher HJ, Evans LV (eds), *Oral biofilms and plaque control* (pp. 57–82). Amsterdam: Harwood; 1998.
10. Kolenbrander PE, Jakubovics NS, Chalmers NI, Palmer Jr RJ, Staffan Kjelleberg K, Givskov M et al. Human oral multi-species biofilms: Bacterial communities in health and disease. *The Biofilm Mode of Life: Mechanisms and Adaptations.* 2007:175–94.
11. Almstahl A, Wikstrom M. Oral microflora in subjects with reduced salivary secretion. *Journal of Dental Research.* 1999;78(8):1410–6.
12. Vanhoecke B, De Ryck T, Stringer A, Van de Wiele T, Keefe D. Microbiota and their role in the pathogenesis of oral mucositis. *Oral Diseases.* 2015;21(1):17–30.
13. Consortium HMP. Structure, function and diversity of the healthy human microbiome. *Nature.* 2012;486(7402):207–14.
14. Theilade E. Factors controlling the microflora of the healthy mouth. In: Hill MJ, Marsh PD (eds), *Human microbial ecology* (pp. 1–56). Boca Raton, FL: CRC Press; 1990.

15. Zheng W, Zhang Z, Liu C, Qiao Y, Zhou D, Qu J et al. Metagenomic sequencing reveals altered metabolic pathways in the oral microbiota of sailors during a long sea voyage. *Scientific Reports.* 2015;5:9131.
16. Oever JT, Netea MG. The bacteriome-mycobiome interaction and antifungal host defense. *European Journal of Immunology.* 2014;44(11):3182–91.
17. Kim Y-j, Choi YS, Baek KJ, Yoon S-H, Park HK, Choi Y. Mucosal and salivary microbiota associated with recurrent aphthous stomatitis. *BMC Microbiology.* 2016;16(1):1.
18. Michaels L, Hellquist HB. *Ear, nose and throat histopathology.* New York: Springer Science+Business Media; 2012.
19. Roos K, Håkansson EG, Holm S. Effect of recolonisation with 'interfering' α streptococci on recurrences of acute and secretory otitis media in children: Randomised placebo controlled trial. *BMJ.* 2001;322(7280):210.
20. Tano K, Grahn-Hakansson E, Holm SE, Hellstrom S. Inhibition of OM pathogens by alpha-hemolytic streptococci from healthy children, children with SOM and children with rAOM. *International Journal of Pediatric Otorhinolaryngology.* 2000;56(3):185–90.
21. Wessman M, Bjarnsholt T, Eickhardt-Sørensen SR, Johansen HK, Homøe P. Mucosal biofilm detection in chronic otitis media: A study of middle ear biopsies from Greenlandic patients. *European Archives of Oto-Rhino-Laryngology.* 2015;272(5):1079–85.
22. Gray BM, Converse GM, Dillon HC. Epidemiologic studies of *Streptococcus pneumoniae* in infants: Acquisition, carriage, and infection during the first 24 months of life. *Journal of Infectious Diseases.* 1980;142(6):923–33.
23. Trottier S, Stenberg K, Svanborg-Eden C. Turnover of nontypable *Haemophilus influenzae* in the nasopharynges of healthy children. *Journal of Clinical Microbiology.* 1989;27(10):2175–9.
24. Aniansson G, Alm B, Andersson B, Larsson P, Nylen O, Peterson H et al. Nasopharyngeal colonization during the first year of life. *The Journal of Infectious Diseases.* 1992;165(Suppl 1):S38–42.
25. Gates GA, Avery CA, Prihoda TJ, Cooper Jr J. Effectiveness of adenoidectomy and tympanostomy tubes in the treatment of chronic otitis media with effusion. *New England Journal of Medicine.* 1987;317(23):1444–51.
26. Maw R, Bawden R. Spontaneous resolution of severe chronic glue ear in children and the effect of adenoidectomy, tonsillectomy, and insertion of ventilation tubes (grommets). *BMJ.* 1993;306(6880):756–60.
27. Beule AG. Physiology and pathophysiology of respiratory mucosa of the nose and the paranasal sinuses. *GMS Current Topics in Otorhinolaryngology, Head and Neck Surgery.* 2010;9:Doc07.
28. Kumar G. *Orban's oral histology & embryology.* Philadelphia: Elsevier Health Sciences; 2014.
29. Sobin J, Engquist S, Nord CE. Bacteriology of the maxillary sinus in healthy volunteers. *Scandinavian Journal of Infectious Diseases.* 1992;24(5):633–5.
30. Glück U, Gebbers JO. The nose as bacterial reservoir: Important differences between the vestibule and cavity. *The Laryngoscope.* 2000;110(3):426–8.
31. Biswas K, Hoggard M, Jain R, Taylor MW, Douglas RG. The nasal microbiota in health and disease: Variation withi n and between subjects. *Frontiers in Microbiology.* 2015;6:134.
32. Gordts F, Halewyck S, Pierard D, Clement PA, Kaufman L. Microbiology of the middle meatus: A comparison between normal adults and children. *Journal of Laryngology & Otology.* 2000;114(03):184–8.
33. Ramakrishnan VR, Feazel LM, Gitomer SA, Ir D, Robertson CE, Frank DN. The microbiome of the middle meatus in healthy adults. *PloS ONE.* 2013;8(12):e85507.

34. Boase S, Foreman A, Cleland E, Tan L, Melton-Kreft R, Pant H et al. The microbiome of chronic rhinosinusitis: Culture, molecular diagnostics and biofilm detection. *BMC Infectious Diseases.* 2013;13(1):1.

35. Stressmann FA, Rogers GB, Chan SW, Howarth PH, Harries PG, Bruce KD et al. Characterization of bacterial community diversity in chronic rhinosinusitis infections using novel culture-independent techniques. *American Journal of Rhinology & Allergy.* 2011;25(4):e133–e40.

36. Foreman A, Boase S, Psaltis A, Wormald P-J. Role of bacterial and fungal biofilms in chronic rhinosinusitis. *Current Allergy and Asthma Reports.* 2012;12(2):127–35.

37. O'Hara AM, Shanahan F. The gut flora as a forgotten organ. *EMBO Reports.* 2006;7(7):688–93.

38. Macfarlane S, Dillon J. Microbial biofilms in the human gastrointestinal tract. *Journal of Applied Microbiology.* 2007;102(5):1187–96.

39. Norder Grusell E, Dahlen G, Ruth M, Ny L, Quiding-Jarbrink M, Bergquist H et al. Bacterial flora of the human oral cavity, and the upper and lower esophagus. *Diseases of the Esophagus.* 2013;26(1):84–90.

40. Blackett K, Siddhi S, Cleary S, Steed H, Miller M, Macfarlane S et al. Oesophageal bacterial biofilm changes in gastro-oesophageal reflux disease, Barrett's and oesophageal carcinoma: Association or causality? *Alimentary Pharmacology & Therapeutics.* 2013;37(11):1084–92.

41. Buttar NS, Wang KK. Mechanisms of disease: Carcinogenesis in Barrett's esophagus. *Nature Clinical Practice Gastroenterology & Hepatology.* 2004;1(2):106–12.

42. Yang I, Nell S, Suerbaum S. Survival in hostile territory: The microbiota of the stomach. *FEMS Microbiology Reviews.* 2013;37(5):736–61.

43. Bik EM, Eckburg PB, Gill SR, Nelson KE, Purdom EA, Francois F et al. Molecular analysis of the bacterial microbiota in the human stomach. *Proceedings of the National Academy of Sciences of the U S A.* 2006;103(3):732–7.

44. Corfield AP, Myerscough N, Longman R, Sylvester P, Arul S, Pignatelli M. Mucins and mucosal protection in the gastrointestinal tract: New prospects for mucins in the pathology of gastrointestinal disease. *Gut.* 2000;47(4):589–94.

45. Andersson AF, Lindberg M, Jakobsson H, Backhed F, Nyren P, Engstrand L. Comparative analysis of human gut microbiota by barcoded pyrosequencing. *PLoS ONE.* 2008;3(7):e2836.

46. Atuma C, Strugala V, Allen A, Holm L. The adherent gastrointestinal mucus gel layer: Thickness and physical state in vivo. *American Journal of Physiology-Gastrointestinal and Liver Physiology.* 2001;280(5):G922–G9.

47. Donaldson GP, Lee SM, Mazmanian SK. Gut biogeography of the bacterial microbiota. *Nature Reviews Microbiology.* 2016;14(1):20–32.

48. Gustafsson JK, Ermund A, Johansson ME, Schütte A, Hansson GC, Sjövall H. An ex vivo method for studying mucus formation, properties, and thickness in human colonic biopsies and mouse small and large intestinal explants. *American Journal of Physiology-Gastrointestinal and Liver Physiology.* 2012;302(4):G430–G8.

49. von Rosenvinge EC, O'May GA, Macfarlane S, Macfarlane GT, Shirtliff ME. Microbial biofilms and gastrointestinal diseases. *Pathogens and Disease.* 2013;67(1):25–38.

50. Salton MRJ, Kim KS. In: Baron S (ed). *SourceMedical microbiology.* 4th edition. Galveston, TX: University of Texas Medical Branch at Galveston; 1996. Chapter 2.

51. Zoetendal EG, Raes J, van den Bogert B, Arumugam M, Booijink CC, Troost FJ et al. The human small intestinal microbiota is driven by rapid uptake and conversion of simple carbohydrates. *The ISME Journal.* 2012;6(7):1415–26.

52. Arumugam M, Raes J, Pelletier E, Le Paslier D, Yamada T, Mende DR et al. Enterotypes of the human gut microbiome. *Nature.* 2011;473(7346):174–80.

53. Hollister EB, Gao C, Versalovic J. Compositional and functional features of the gastrointestinal microbiome and their effects on human health. *Gastroenterology.* 2014;146(6):1449–58.

54. Macfarlane S, Macfarlane GT. Composition and metabolic activities of bacterial biofilms colonizing food residues in the human gut. *Applied and Environ Microbiol.* 2006;72(9):6204–11.

55. Johansson ME, Gustafsson JK, Holmén-Larsson J, Jabbar KS, Xia L, Xu H et al. Bacteria penetrate the normally impenetrable inner colon mucus layer in both murine colitis models and patients with ulcerative colitis. *Gut.* 2013:gutjnl-2012-303207.

56. Macfarlane GT, Cummings J. *The colonic flora, fermentation, and large bowel digestive function.* New York: Raven Press; 1991.

57. Wang M, Li M, Chapkin RS, Ivanov I, Donovan SM. Fecal microbiome and metabolites differ between breast and formula-fed human infants. *The FASEB Journal.* 2013;27(1 Supplement):850.4.

58. John GK, Mullin GE. The gut microbiome and obesity. *Current Oncology Reports.* 2016;18(7):1–7.

59. Kleinegger CL, Lockhart SR, Vargas K, Soll DR. Frequency, intensity, species, and strains of oral *Candida* vary as a function of host age. *Journal of Clinical Microbiology.* 1996;34(9):2246–54.

60. Schulze J, Sonnenborn U. Yeasts in the gut: From commensals to infectious agents. *Deutsches Ärzteblatt International.* 2009;106(51–52):837–42.

61. Yan L, Yang C, Tang J. Disruption of the intestinal mucosal barrier in *Candida albicans* infections. *Microbiological Research.* 2013 8/25/;168(7):389–95.

62. De Repentigny L, Aumont F, Bernard K, Belhumeur P. Characterization of binding of *Candida albicans* to small intestinal mucin and its role in adherence to mucosal epithelial cells. *Infection and Immunity.* 2000;68(6):3172–9.

63. Fox EP, Cowley ES, Nobile CJ, Hartooni N, Newman DK, Johnson AD. Anaerobic bacteria grow within *Candida albicans* biofilms and induce biofilm formation in suspension cultures. *Current Biology.* 2014;24(20):2411–6.

64. Freter R, Brickner H, Botney M, Cleven D, Aranki A. Mechanisms that control bacterial populations in continuous-flow culture models of mouse large intestinal flora. *Infection and Immunity.* 1983;39(2):676–85.

65. Hoskins LC, Agustines M, McKee WB, Boulding ET, Kriaris M, Niedermeyer G. Mucin degradation in human colon ecosystems: Isolation and properties of fecal strains that degrade ABH blood group antigens and oligosaccharides from mucin glycoproteins. *Journal of Clinical Investigation.* 1985;75(3):944.

66. Conway T, Cohen PS. Commensal and pathogenic *Escherichia coli* metabolism in the gut. *Microbiology Spectrum.* 2015;3(3).

67. Leatham MP, Banerjee S, Autieri SM, Mercado-Lubo R, Conway T, Cohen PS. Precolonized human commensal *Escherichia coli* strains serve as a barrier to *E. coli* O157: H7 growth in the streptomycin-treated mouse intestine. *Infection and Immunity.* 2009;77(7):2876–86.

68. Ventolini G. Vaginal *Lactobacillus*: Biofilm formation in vivo – Clinical implications. *International Journal of Women's Health.* 2015;7:243–7.

69. Ventolini G. Progresses on biofilm formation by vaginal lactobacilli. *Journal of Nature and Science.* 2015;1(4):e70.

70. Eroschenko VP, Di Fiore MS. *DiFiore's Atlas of Histology with Functional Correlations.* Philadelphia: Lippincott Williams & Wilkins; 2013.

71. Huse SM, Ye Y, Zhou Y, Fodor AA. A core human microbiome as viewed through 16S rRNA sequence clusters. *PloS ONE.* 2012;7(6):e34242.

72. Albert AY, Chaban B, Wagner EC, Schellenberg JJ, Links MG, Van Schalkwyk J et al. A study of the vaginal microbiome in healthy Canadian women utilizing cpn 60-based

molecular profiling reveals distinct *Gardnerella* subgroup community state types. *PloS ONE*. 2015;10(8):e0135620.

73. Marrazzo JM, Koutsky LA, Eschenbach DA, Agnew K, Stine K, Hillier SL. Characterization of vaginal flora and bacterial vaginosis in women who have sex with women. *Journal of Infectious Diseases*. 2002;185(9):1307–13.

74. Strömbeck L. Vaginal commensal bacteria: Interactions with cervix epithelial and mono-cytic cells and influence on cytokines and secretory leukocyte protease inhibitor, SLPI. Gothenburg, Sweden: Department of Infectious Medicine, Institute of Biomedicine; 2008.

75. Larsen B, Monif GR. Understanding the bacterial flora of the female genital tract. *Clinical Infectious Diseases*. 2001;32(4):e69–77.

76. Mastromarino P, Hemalatha R, Barbonetti A, Cinque B, Cifone M, Tammaro F et al. Biological control of vaginosis to improve reproductive health. The Indian *Journal of Medical Research*. 2014;140(Suppl 1):S91–7.

77. Borges SF, Silva JG, Teixeira PC. Survival and biofilm formation of *Listeria monocyto-genes* in simulated vaginal fluid: Influence of pH and strain origin. *FEMS Immunology & Medical Microbiology*. 2011;62(3):315–20.

78. Mahmoud EA, Svensson L-O, Olsson S-E, Mårdh P-A. Antichlamydial activity of vagi-nal secretion. *American Journal of Obstetrics and Gynecology*. 1995;172(4):1268–72.

79. Machado D, Castro J, Palmeira-de-Oliveira A, Martinez-de-Oliveira J, Cerca N. Bacterial vaginosis biofilms: Challenges to current therapies and emerging solutions. *Frontiers in Microbiology*. 2015;6. doi:10.3389/fmicb.2015.01528.

80. Noverr MC, Huffnagle GB. Regulation of *Candida albicans* morphogenesis by fatty acid metabolites. *Infection and Immunity*. 2004;72(11):6206–10.

81. Strus M, Kucharska A, Kukla G, Brzychczy-Włoch M, Maresz K, Heczko PB. The in vitro activity of vaginal *Lactobacillus* with probiotic properties against *Candida*. *Infectious Diseases in Obstetrics and Gynecology*. 2005;13(2):69–75.

82. Branda SS, Vik Å, Friedman L, Kolter R. Biofilms: The matrix revisited. *Trends in Microbiology*. 2005;13(1):20–6.

83. Steinberg N, Kolodkin-Gal I. The matrix reloaded: How sensing the extracellular matrix synchronizes bacterial communities. *Journal of Bacteriology*. 2015;197(13):2092–103.

84. Serra DO, Richter AM, Klauck G, Mika F, Hengge R. Microanatomy at cellular reso-lution and spatial order of physiological differentiation in a bacterial biofilm. *mBio*. 2013;4(2):e00103–13.

85. Gloag ES, Turnbull L, Huang A, Vallotton P, Wang H, Nolan LM et al. Self-organization of bacterial biofilms is facilitated by extracellular DNA. *Proceedings of the National Academy of Sciences of the U S A*. 2013;110(28):11541–6.

86. Westerlund B, Korhonen TK. Bacterial proteins binding to the mammalian extracel-lular matrix. *Molecular Microbiology*. 1993;9(4):687–94.

87. Patti JM, Allen BL, McGavin MJ, Hook M. MSCRAMM-mediated adherence of microorganisms to host tissues. *Annual Review of Microbiology*. 1994;48:585–617.

88. McCourt J, O'Halloran DP, McCarthy H, O'Gara JP, Geoghegan JA. Fibronectin-binding proteins are required for biofilm formation by community-associated methicillin-resistant *Staphylococcus aureus* strain LAC. *FEMS Microbiology Letters*. 2014;353(2):157–64.

89. Foster TJ, Geoghegan JA, Ganesh VK, Höök M. Adhesion, invasion and evasion: The many functions of the surface proteins of *Staphylococcus aureus*. *Nature Reviews Microbiology*. 2014 Jan;12(1):49–62.

90. Hendrickx AP, van Luit-Asbroek M, Schapendonk CM, van Wamel WJ, Braat JC, Wijnands LM et al. SgrA, a nidogen-binding LPXTG surface adhesin impli-cated in biofilm formation, and EcbA, a collagen binding MSCRAMM, are two novel adhesins of hospital-acquired *Enterococcus faecium*. *Infection and Immunity*. 2009;77(11):5097–106.

91. Ronander E, Brant M, Janson H, Sheldon J, Forsgren A, Riesbeck K. Identification of a novel *Haemophilus influenzae* protein important for adhesion to epithelial cells. *Microbes and Infection.* 2008;10(1):87–96.

92. Ronander E, Brant M, Eriksson E, Morgelin M, Hallgren O, Westergren-Thorsson G et al. Nontypeable *Haemophilus influenzae* adhesin protein E: Characterization and biological activity. *The Journal of Infectious Diseases.* 2009;199(4):522–31.

93. Hallstrom T, Blom AM, Zipfel PF, Riesbeck K. Nontypeable *Haemophilus influenzae* protein E binds vitronectin and is important for serum resistance. *Journal of Immunology* (Baltimore). 2009;183(4):2593–601.

94. Landry RM, An D, Hupp JT, Singh PK, Parsek MR. Mucin-*Pseudomonas aeruginosa* interactions promote biofilm formation and antibiotic resistance. *Molecular Microbiology.* 2006;59(1):142–51.

95. Loimaranta V, Jakubovics NS, Hytonen J, Finne J, Jenkinson HF, Stromberg N. Fluid-or surface-phase human salivary scavenger protein gp340 exposes different bacterial recognition properties. *Infection and Immunity.* 2005;73(4):2245–52.

96. Bowen WH, Schilling K, Giertsen E, Pearson S, Lee SF, Bleiweis A et al. Role of a cell surface-associated protein in adherence and dental caries. *Infection and Immunity.* 1991;59(12):4606–9.

97. El-Sabaeny A, Demuth DR, Park Y, Lamont RJ. Environmental conditions modulate the expression of the sspA and sspB genes in *Streptococcus gordonii*. *Microbial Pathogenesis.* 2000 Aug;29(2):101–13.

98. Jakubovics NS, Stromberg N, van Dolleweerd CJ, Kelly CG, Jenkinson HF. Differential binding specificities of oral streptococcal antigen I/II family adhesins for human or bacterial ligands. *Molecular Microbiology.* 2005;55(5):1591–605.

99. Engel JN. Molecular Pathogenesis of acute *Pseudomonas aeruginosa* infections. In: Hauser AR, Rello J (eds), *Severe infections caused by Pseudomonas aeruginosa* (pp. 201–29). New York: Springer Science+Business Media; 2003.

100. Saiman L, Prince A. *Pseudomonas aeruginosa* pili bind to asialoGM1 which is increased on the surface of cystic fibrosis epithelial cells. *The Journal of Clinical Investigation.* 1993;92(4):1875–80.

101. Comolli JC, Waite LL, Mostov KE, Engel JN. Pili binding to asialo-GM1 on epithelial cells can mediate cytotoxicity or bacterial internalization by *Pseudomonas aeruginosa*. *Infection and Immunity.* 1999;67(7):3207–14.

102. Manetti AG, Zingaretti C, Falugi F, Capo S, Bombaci M, Bagnoli F et al. *Streptococcus pyogenes* pili promote pharyngeal cell adhesion and biofilm formation. *Molecular Microbiology.* 2007;64(4):968–83.

103. Jurcisek JA, Bookwalter JE, Baker BD, Fernandez S, Novotny LA, Munson RS et al. The PilA protein of non-typeable *Haemophilus influenzae* plays a role in biofilm formation, adherence to epithelial cells and colonization of the mammalian upper respiratory tract. *Molecular Microbiology.* 2007;65(5):1288–99.

104. Boddicker JD, Ledeboer NA, Jagnow J, Jones BD, Clegg S. Differential binding to and biofilm formation on, HEp-2 cells by *Salmonella enterica* serovar *Typhimurium* is dependent upon allelic variation in the *fimH* gene of the *fim* gene cluster. *Molecular Microbiology.* 2002;45(5):1255–65.

105. Chessa D, Winter MG, Jakomin M, Bäumler AJ. Salmonella enterica serotype Typhimurium Stdfimbriae bind terminal alpha(1,2)fucose residues in the cecal mucosa. *Molecular Microbiology.* 2009 Feb;71(4):864–75.

106. Hase K, Kawano K, Nochi T, Pontes GS, Fukuda S, Ebisawa M, Kadokura K, Tobe T, Fujimura Y, Kawano S, Yabashi A, Waguri S, Nakato G, Kimura S, Murakami T, Iimura M, Hamura K, Fukuoka S, Lowe AW, Itoh K, Kiyono H, Ohno H. Uptake through glycoprotein 2 of FimH(+) bacteria by M cells initiates mucosal immune response. *Nature.* 2009 Nov 12;462(7270):226–30.

107. Yi K, Rasmussen AW, Gudlavalleti SK, Stephens DS, Stojiljkovic I. Biofilm formation by *Neisseria meningitidis*. *Infection and Immunity.* 2004;72(10):6132–8.
108. Lappann M, Haagensen JA, Claus H, Vogel U, Molin S. Meningococcal biofilm formation: Structure, development and phenotypes in a standardized continuous flow system. *Molecular Microbiology.* 2006;62(5):1292–309.
109. Scharfman A, Arora SK, Delmotte P, Van Brussel E, Mazurier J, Ramphal R et al. Recognition of Lewis x derivatives present on mucins by flagellar components of *Pseudomonas aeruginosa. Infection and Immunity.* 2001;69(9):5243–8.
110. Orihuela CJ, Gao G, Francis KP, Yu J, Tuomanen EI. Tissue-specific contributions of pneumococcal virulence factors to pathogenesis. *The Journal of Infectious Diseases.* 2004;190(9):1661–9.
111. Neil RB, Apicella MA. Role of HrpA in biofilm formation of *Neisseria meningitidis* and regulation of the hrpBAS transcripts. *Infection and Immunity.* 2009;77(6):2285–93.
112. Rosenow C, Ryan P, Weiser JN, Johnson S, Fontan P, Ortqvist A, Masure HR. Contribution of novel choline-binding proteins to adherence, colonization and immunogenicity of *Streptococcus pneumoniae. Molecular Microbiology.* 1997 Sep;25(5): 819–29.
113. Anderton JM, Rajam G, Romero-Steiner S, Summer S, Kowalczyk AP, Carlone GM, Sampson JS, Ades EW. E-cadherin is a receptor for the common protein pneumococcal surface adhesin A (PsaA) of *Streptococcus pneumoniae. Microbial Pathogenesis.* 2007 May–Jun;42(5–6):225–36.
114. Staab JF, Bradway SD, Fidel PL, Sundstrom P. Adhesive and mammalian transglutaminase substrate properties of *Candida albicans* Hwp1. *Science.* 1999;283(5407):1535–8.
115. Sundstrom P, Balish E, Allen CM. Essential role of the *Candida albicans* transglutaminase substrate, hyphal wall protein 1, in lethal oroesophageal candidiasis in immunodeficient mice. *Journal of Infectious Diseases.* 2002 Feb 15;185(4):521–30.
116. Dongari-Bagtzoglou A. Pathogenesis of mucosal biofilm infections: Challenges and progress. *Expert Review of Anti-infective Therapy.* 2008 Apr;6(2):201–8.
117. Liu Y, Filler SG. *Candida albicans* Als3, a multifunctional adhesin and invasin. *Eukaryotic Cell.* 2011;10(2):168–73.
118. Li F, Svarovsky MJ, Karlsson AJ, Wagner JP, Marchillo K, Oshel P et al. Eap1p, an adhesin that mediates *Candida albicans*: Biofilm formation in vitro and in vivo. *Eukaryotic Cell.* 2007;6(6):931–9.
119. Chu H, Mazmanian SK. Innate immune recognition of the microbiota promotes host-microbial symbiosis. *Nature Immunology.* 2013;14(7):668–75.
120. Dethlefsen L, McFall-Ngai M, Relman DA. An ecological and evolutionary perspective on human-microbe mutualism and disease. *Nature.* 2007;449(7164):811–8.
121. Janeway CA, Jr., Medzhitov R. Innate immune recognition. *Annual Review of Immunology.* 2002;20:197–216.
122. Brubaker SW, Bonham KS, Zanoni I, Kagan JC. Innate immune pattern recognition: A cell biological perspective. *Annual Review of Immunology.* 2015;33:257–90.
123. Jang J-H, Shin HW, Lee JM, Lee H-W, Kim E-C, Park SH. An overview of pathogen recognition receptors for innate immunity in dental pulp. *Mediators of Inflammation.* 2015;794143.
124. Schwandner R, Dziarski R, Wesche H, Rothe M, Kirschning CJ. Peptidoglycan- and lipoteichoic acid-induced cell activation is mediated by toll-like receptor 2. *The Journal of Biological Chemistry.* 1999;274(25):17406–9.
125. Alexopoulou L, Holt AC, Medzhitov R, Flavell RA. Recognition of double-stranded RNA and activation of NF-kappaB by Toll-like receptor 3. *Nature.* 2001;413(6857): 732–8.
126. Kawai T, Akira S. The role of pattern-recognition receptors in innate immunity: Update on Toll-like receptors. *Nature Immunology.* 2010;11(5):373–84.

127. Chow JC, Young DW, Golenbock DT, Christ WJ, Gusovsky F. Toll-like receptor-4 mediates lipopolysaccharide-induced signal transduction. *The Journal of Biological Chemistry.* 1999;274(16):10689–92.
128. Medzhitov R. Toll-like receptors and innate immunity. *Nature Reviews Immunology.* 2001;1(2):135–45.
129. Alexopoulou L, Holt AC, Medzhitov R, Flavell RA. Recognition of double-stranded RNA and activation of NF-κB by Toll-like receptor 3. *Nature.* 2001;413(6857):732–8.
130. Qureshi ST, Larivière L, Leveque G, Clermont S, Moore KJ, Gros P et al. Endotoxin-tolerant mice have mutations in Toll-like receptor 4 (Tlr4). *The Journal of Experimental Medicine.* 1999;189(4):615–25.
131. Hayashi F, Smith KD, Ozinsky A, Hawn TR, Eugene CY, Goodlett DR et al. The innate immune response to bacterial flagellin is mediated by Toll-like receptor 5. *Nature.* 2001;410(6832):1099–103.
132. Hemmi H, Takeuchi O, Kawai T, Kaisho T, Sato S, Sanjo H et al. A Toll-like receptor recognizes bacterial DNA. *Nature.* 2000;408(6813):740–5.
133. Gay NJ, Gangloff M. Structure and function of Toll receptors and their ligands. *Annual Review of Biochemistry.* 2007;76:141–65.
134. Bauer S, Hartmann G. *Toll-like receptors (TLRs) and innate immunity*: New York: Springer Science+Business Media; 2007.
135. Feldman M, Bryan R, Rajan S, Scheffler L, Brunnert S, Tang H, Prince A. Role of flagella in pathogenesis of *Pseudomonas aeruginosa* pulmonary infection. *Infection and Immunity.* 1998 Jan;66(1):43–51.
136. Bucior I, Pielage JF, Engel JN. *Pseudomonas aeruginosa* pili and flagella mediate distinct binding and signaling events at the apical and basolateral surface of airway epithelium. *PLOS Pathogens.* 2012;8(4):e1002616.
137. Krieg AM. CpG motifs in bacterial DNA and their immune effects. *Annual Review of Immunology.* 2002;20:709–60.
138. Dwivedi P, Thompson A, Xie Z, Kashleva H, Ganguly S, Mitchell AP, Dongari-Bagtzoglou A. Role of Bcr1-activated genes Hwp1 and Hyr1 in *Candida albicans* oral mucosal biofilms and neutrophilevasion. *PLoS One.* 2011 Jan 25;6(1):e16218.
139. Kim C, Kaufmann SH. Defensin: A multifunctional molecule lives up to its versatile name. *Trends in Microbiology.* 2006;14(10):428–31.
140. Bowdish D, Davidson D, Hancock R. Immunomodulatory properties of defensins and cathelicidins. In: *Antimicrobial peptides and human disease* (pp. 27–66). New York: Springer Science+Business Media; 2006.
141. Kim C, Gajendran N, Mittrucker HW, Weiwad M, Song YH, Hurwitz R et al. Human alpha-defensins neutralize anthrax lethal toxin and protect against its fatal consequences. *Proceedings of the National Academy of Sciences of the U S A.* 2005;102(13):4830–5.
142. Kesting MR, Loeffelbein DJ, Hasler RJ, Wolff KD, Rittig A, Schulte M et al. Expression profile of human beta-defensin 3 in oral squamous cell carcinoma. *Cancer Investigation.* 2009;27(5):575–81.
143. Durr UH, Sudheendra US, Ramamoorthy A. LL-37, the only human member of the cathelicidin family of antimicrobial peptides. *Biochimica et Biophysica Acta.* 2006;1758(9):1408–25.
144. Putsep K, Carlsson G, Boman HG, Andersson M. Deficiency of antibacterial peptides in patients with morbus Kostmann: An observation study. *Lancet.* 2002;360(9340):1144–9.
145. Helmerhorst EJ, Breeuwer P, van't Hof W, Walgreen-Weterings E, Oomen LC, Veerman EC et al. The cellular target of histatin 5 on *Candida albicans* is the energized mitochondrion. *The Journal of Biological Chemistry.* 1999;274(11):7286–91.
146. Gyurko C, Lendenmann U, Troxler RF, Oppenheim FG. *Candida albicans* mutants deficient in respiration are resistant to the small cationic salivary antimicrobial peptide histatin 5. *Antimicrobial Agents and Chemotherapy.* 2000;44(2):348–54.

147. Baev D, Rivetta A, Vylkova S, Sun JN, Zeng GF, Slayman CL et al. The TRK1 potassium transporter is the critical effector for killing of *Candida albicans* by the cationic protein, Histatin 5. *The Journal of Biological Chemistry.* 2004;279(53):55060–72.

148. Mogensen TH. Pathogen recognition and inflammatory signaling in innate immune defenses. *Clinical Microbiology Reviews.* 2009;22(2):240–73.

149. Nikolaus S, Bauditz J, Gionchetti P, Witt C, Lochs H, Schreiber S. Increased secretion of pro-inflammatory cytokines by circulating polymorphonuclear neutrophils and regulation by interleukin 10 during intestinal inflammation. *Gut.* 1998;42(4):470–6.

150. Mantovani A, Cassatella MA, Costantini C, Jaillon S. Neutrophils in the activation and regulation of innate and adaptive immunity. *Nature Reviews Immunology.* 2011;11(8):519–31.

151. Ivanov, II, Frutos Rde L, Manel N, Yoshinaga K, Rifkin DB, Sartor RB et al. Specific microbiota direct the differentiation of IL-17-producing T-helper cells in the mucosa of the small intestine. *Cell Host Microbe.* 2008;4(4):337–49.

152. Hirschfeld J. Dynamic interactions of neutrophils and biofilms. *Journal of oral Microbiology.* 2014;6:26102.

153. Fuchs TA, Abed U, Goosmann C, Hurwitz R, Schulze I, Wahn V et al. Novel cell death program leads to neutrophil extracellular traps. *The Journal of Cell Biology.* 2007;176(2):231–41.

154. Palaniyar N, Clark H, Nadesalingam J, Shih MJ, Hawgood S, Reid KB. Innate immune collectin surfactant protein D enhances the clearance of DNA by macrophages and minimizes anti-DNA antibody generation. *Journal of Immunology* (Baltimore). 2005;174(11):7352–8.

155. Bostanci N, Thurnheer T, Aduse-Opoku J, Curtis MA, Zinkernagel AS, Belibasakis GN. *Porphyromonas gingivalis* regulates TREM-1 in human polymorphonuclear neutrophils via its gingipains. *PloS ONE.* 2013;8(10):e75784.

156. Woodward JJ, Iavarone AT, Portnoy DA. c-di-AMP secreted by intracellular *Listeria monocytogenes* activates a host type I interferon response. *Science.* 2010;328(5986): 1703–5.

157. Shaw N, Ouyang S, Liu ZJ. Binding of bacterial secondary messenger molecule c di-GMP is a STING operation. *Protein & Cell.* 2013;4(2):117–29.

158. McWhirter SM, Barbalat R, Monroe KM, Fontana MF, Hyodo M, Joncker NT et al. A host type I interferon response is induced by cytosolic sensing of the bacterial second messenger cyclic-di-GMP. *The Journal of Experimental Medicine.* 2009;206(9):1899–911.

159. Hu DL, Narita K, Hyodo M, Hayakawa Y, Nakane A, Karaolis DK. c-di-GMP as a vaccine adjuvant enhances protection against systemic methicillin-resistant *Staphylococcus aureus* (MRSA) infection. *Vaccine.* 2009;27(35):4867–73.

160. Feller L, Altini M, Khammissa RAG, Chandran R, Bouckaert M, Lemmer J. Oral mucosal immunity. *Oral Surgery, Oral Medicine, Oral Pathology and Oral Radiology.* 2013;116(5):576–83.

161. Sellge G, Kufer TA. PRR-signaling pathways: Learning from microbial tactics. *Seminars in Immunology.* 2015;27(2):75–84.

162. Fanning S, Hall LJ, van Sinderen D. Bifidobacterium breve UCC2003 surface exopolysaccharide production is a beneficial trait mediating commensal-host interaction through immune modulation and pathogen protection. *Gut Microbes.* 2012;3(5):420–5.

163. Dhodapkar MV, Steinman RM. Antigen-bearing immature dendritic cells induce peptide-specific CD8(+) regulatory T cells in vivo in humans. *Blood.* 2002;100(1):174–7.

164. Mahnke K, Qian Y, Knop J, Enk AH. Induction of CD4+/CD25+ regulatory T cells by targeting of antigens to immature dendritic cells. *Blood.* 2003;101(12):4862–9.

165. Cole JN, Nizet V. Bacterial evasion of host antimicrobial peptide defenses. *Microbiology Spectrum.* 2016;4(1).

166. Kang M, Ko YP, Liang X, Ross CL, Liu Q, Murray BE et al. Collagen-binding microbial surface components recognizing adhesive matrix molecule (MSCRAMM) of Gram-positive bacteria inhibit complement activation via the classical pathway. *The Journal of Biological Chemistry.* 2013;288(28):20520–31.

167. Jensen ET, Kharazmi A, Hoiby N, Costerton JW. Some bacterial parameters influencing the neutrophil oxidative burst response to *Pseudomonas aeruginosa* biofilms. APMIS: *Acta Pathologica, Microbiologica, et Immunologica Scandinavica.* 1992;100(8):727–33.

168. Kharazmi A. Mechanisms involved in the evasion of the host defence by *Pseudomonas aeruginosa. Immunology Letters.* 1991;30(2):201–5.

169. Kharazmi A, Nielsen H. Inhibition of human monocyte chemotaxis and chemiluminescence by *Pseudomonas aeruginosa* elastase. *APMIS: Acta Pathologica, Microbiologica, et Immunologica Scandinavica.* 1991;99(1):93–5.

170. Leid JG, Willson CJ, Shirtliff ME, Hassett DJ, Parsek MR, Jeffers AK. The exopolysaccharide alginate protects *Pseudomonas aeruginosa* biofilm bacteria from IFN-gamma-mediated macrophage killing. *Journal of Immunology* (Baltimore). 2005;175(11):7512–8.

171. Chan C, Burrows LL, Deber CM. Helix induction in antimicrobial peptides by alginate in biofilms. *The Journal of Biological Chemistry.* 2004;279(37):38749–54.

172. Schmidtchen A, Frick IM, Andersson E, Tapper H, Bjorck L. Proteinases of common pathogenic bacteria degrade and inactivate the antibacterial peptide LL-37. *Molecular Microbiology.* 2002;46(1):157–68.

173. Yu H, He X, Xie W, Xiong J, Sheng H, Guo S et al. Elastase LasB of *Pseudomonas aeruginosa* promotes biofilm formation partly through rhamnolipid-mediated regulation. *Canadian Journal of Microbiology.* 2014;60(4):227–35.

174. Dulon S, Leduc D, Cottrell GS, D'Alayer J, Hansen KK, Bunnett NW et al. *Pseudomonas aeruginosa* elastase disables proteinase-activated receptor 2 in respiratory epithelial cells. *American Journal of Respiratory Cell and Molecular Biology.* 2005;32(5):411–9.

175. Moraes TJ, Martin R, Plumb JD, Vachon E, Cameron CM, Danesh A et al. Role of PAR2 in murine pulmonary pseudomonal infection. *American Journal of Physiology: Lung Cellular and Molecular Physiology.* 2008;294(2):L368–77.

176. Steinhoff M, Buddenkotte J, Shpacovitch V, Rattenholl A, Moormann C, Vergnolle N et al. Proteinase-activated receptors: Transducers of proteinase-mediated signaling in inflammation and immune response. *Endocrine Reviews.* 2005;26(1):1–43.

177. Jesaitis AJ, Franklin MJ, Berglund D, Sasaki M, Lord CI, Bleazard JB et al. Compromised host defense on *Pseudomonas aeruginosa* biofilms: Characterization of neutrophil and biofilm interactions. *Journal of Immunology* (Baltimore). 2003;171(8):4329–39.

178. Jensen PO, Bjarnsholt T, Phipps R, Rasmussen TB, Calum H, Christoffersen L et al. Rapid necrotic killing of polymorphonuclear leukocytes is caused by quorum-sensing-controlled production of rhamnolipid by *Pseudomonas aeruginosa. Microbiology* (Reading, UK). 2007;153(Pt 5):1329–38.

179. Charlton TS, de Nys R, Netting A, Kumar N, Hentzer M, Givskov M et al. A novel and sensitive method for the quantification of *N*-3-oxoacyl homoserine lactones using gas chromatography-mass spectrometry: Application to a model bacterial biofilm. *Environmental Microbiology.* 2000;2(5):530–41.

180. Telford G, Wheeler D, Williams P, Tomkins PT, Appleby P, Sewell H et al. The *Pseudomonas aeruginosa* quorum-sensing signal molecule N-(3-oxododecanoyl)-L-homoserine lactone has immunomodulatory activity. *Infection and immunity.* 1998;66(1):36–42.

181. Holm A, Magnusson K-E, Vikström E. *Pseudomonas aeruginosa N*-3-oxo-dodecanoyl-homoserine lactone elicits changes in cell volume, morphology, and AQP9 characteristics in macrophages. *Frontiers in Cellular and Infection Microbiology.* 2016;6:32.

182. Tateda K, Ishii Y, Horikawa M, Matsumoto T, Miyairi S, Pechere JC et al. The *Pseudomonas aeruginosa* autoinducer *N*-3-oxododecanoyl homoserine lactone accelerates apoptosis in macrophages and neutrophils. *Infection and immunity.* 2003;71(10):5785–93.

183. Shiner EK, Terentyev D, Bryan A, Sennoune S, Martinez-Zaguilan R, Li G et al. *Pseudomonas aeruginosa* autoinducer modulates host cell responses through calcium signalling. *Cellular Microbiology.* 2006;8(10):1601–10.

184. Rumbaugh KP, Griswold JA, Hamood AN. The role of quorum sensing in the in vivo virulence of *Pseudomonas aeruginosa. Microbes and Infection.* 2000;2(14):1721–31.

185. Chhabra SR, Harty C, Hooi DS, Daykin M, Williams P, Telford G et al. Synthetic analogues of the bacterial signal (quorum sensing) molecule *N*-(3-oxododecanoyl)-L-homoserine lactone as immune modulators. *Journal of Medicinal Chemistry.* 2003; 46(1):97–104.

186. Ritchie AJ, Yam AO, Tanabe KM, Rice SA, Cooley MA. Modification of in vivo and in vitro T- and B-cell-mediated immune responses by the *Pseudomonas aeruginosa* quorum-sensing molecule *N*-(3-oxododecanoyl)-L-homoserine lactone. *Infection and Immunity.* 2003;71(8):4421–31.

187. Ritchie AJ, Jansson A, Stallberg J, Nilsson P, Lysaght P, Cooley MA. The *Pseudomonas aeruginosa* quorum-sensing molecule *N*-3-(oxododecanoyl)-L-homoserine lactone inhibits T-cell differentiation and cytokine production by a mechanism involving an early step in T-cell activation. *Infection and Immunity.* 2005;73(3):1648–55.

188. Cooley M, Chhabra SR, Williams P. N-Acylhomoserine lactone-mediated quorum sensing: A twist in the tail and a blow for host immunity. *Chemistry & Biology.* 2008;15(11):1141–7.

189. McLaughlin RA, Hoogewerf AJ. Interleukin-1beta-induced growth enhancement of *Staphylococcus aureus* occurs in biofilm but not planktonic cultures. *Microbial Pathogenesis.* 2006;41(2–3):67–79.

190. Hansch GM, Brenner-Weiss G, Prior B, Wagner C, Obst U. The extracellular polymer substance of *Pseudomonas aeruginosa*: Too slippery for neutrophils to migrate on? *The International Journal of Artificial Organs.* 2008;31(9):796–803.

191. Nadell CD, Drescher K, Wingreen NS, Bassler BL. Extracellular matrix structure governs invasion resistance in bacterial biofilms. *The ISME Journal.* 2015;9(8):1700–9.

192. Häse CC. Analysis of the role of flagellar activity in virulence gene expression in *Vibrio cholerae. Microbiology.* 2001;147(4):831–7.

10 Synbiotics, a Fusion of Probiotics and Prebiotics, and Biogenics against Oral Biofilm-Associated Diseases

Tomoko Ohshima, Tomomi Kawai,
Yukako Kojima, Nobuko Maeda and
Chaminda Jayampath Seneviratne

CONTENTS

ORAL BIOFILM AND ORAL DISEASES

Most oral infectious diseases such as dental caries, periodontitis and oral candidiasis are caused by oral biofilms of bacteria or fungi. Hence, biofilm formation is an important factor in oral infectious diseases. It is important to remove dental plaque mechanically by brushing teeth daily to maintain good oral health. However, mechanical control of a dental plaque biofilm may be difficult under certain circumstances and in populations such as the elderly. Therefore, alternative methods must be explored to ensure good oral health by controlling the pathogenic transformation of oral biofilms.

The indigenous microbiota in the oral cavity plays a role in preventing the invasion of extraneous pathogenic microorganisms. Hence, oral microbiota live in a symbiotic state under healthy conditions. They become pathogenic only under conditions favourable for their overgrowth and cause diseases such as dental caries, periodontitis and oral candidiasis [1]. When the healthy microbial balance collapses (i.e. dysbiosis), oral pathogens can proliferate and cause a typical opportunistic infection. Therefore, oral microbial symbiosis that suppresses the overgrowth of pathogens is important for maintaining a healthy oral ecosystem.

In this regard, probiotics, prebiotics and synbiotics can be considered a potential preventive strategy against oral diseases. Prebiotics have a direct effect on microbial growth as they stimulate the growth of beneficial bacteria and suppress the growth of pathogens in the gastrointestinal tract. Probiotics render a local protective effect against pathogens and a systemic indirect effect on immunological amelioration. Synbiotics are fusion products of prebiotics and probiotics. In this chapter, the potential use and associated limitations of probiotics, prebiotics and synbiotics with respect to the promotion of oral health are discussed. As most of those preventive functions are considered as direct suppression of oral pathogens within oral biofilm, the details of active mode are explained here against representative pathogens of dental caries, periodontitis and candidiasis. We also introduce biogenics, a recent concept derived from the work on probiotics. Biogenics advocates the use of beneficial bioactive substances produced by probiotic bacteria, whose activities are independent from the viability of probiotic bacteria in human bodies.

PROBIOTICS

DEFINITION AND HISTORY

The term *'probiotics'*, in contrast to antibiotics, was proposed by Lilly and Stillwell et al. in 1965 [2], from the original ecological term *'probiosis'* used by Kollath et al. in the 1950s [3], meaning a symbiotic relationship between organisms. In 1989, Fuller defined probiotics as 'a live microbial feed supplement which beneficially affects the host animal by improving its intestinal microbial balance' [4]. Hence, at that time, probiotics were intended to be used only for the 'intestinal microbiota'. Subsequent studies revealed the general health benefits of probiotics, such as an enhancement of the human immune system and preventive effects in urinary and respiratory tract infections and allergic or atopic conditions in infants [5]. Hence, probiotics were redefined by Salminen et al. [6] as 'a viable microbial food supplement which beneficially influences the health of the host'. According to the Food and Agriculture Organization/World Health Organization, probiotics are defined as 'live microorganisms when administered in adequate amounts confer a health benefit on the host' [7].

Clinical Trials of Probiotics on Oral Infectious Diseases

There has been a gradual increase in the number of studies that focus on the application of probiotics for oral health. A number of clinical studies have already reported promising findings focussed on dental caries and periodontitis [reviewed in 8–11]. For prevention of caries, there were several trials from 2001 to 2015 using lactobacilli or *Bifidobacterium*, and all achieved good results in reducing the number of *mutans* streptococci or Decayed–Missing–Filled (DMF) score (Table 10.1). Some clinical studies have shown the usefulness of probiotics for periodontal diseases (Table 10.2). Krasse et al. [12] reported the recovery effect of gingivitis by administration of *Lactobacillus reuteri*. The trial of Riccia et al. [13] showed the lozenge of *L. brevis* had anti-inflammatory effects on periodontitis. Vivekananda et al. [14] reported that *L. reuteri* DSM 17938 and *L. reuteri* ATCC PTA 5289 reduced the number of *Porphyromonas gingivalis* cells in the oral cavity of periodontitis patients. Ishikawa et al. [15] showed that levels of three of the major periodontal pathogens, *P. gingivalis*, *Prevotella intermedia* and *Prevotella nigrescens*, were significantly reduced by a four-week oral administration of *Lactobacillus salivarius* TI2711 (LS1).

Contrary to research on caries and periodontitis, studies on the use of probiotics for oral candidiasis are sparse (Table 10.3). Ahola et al. [16] and Hatakka et al. [17] conducted double-blinded, randomised clinical trials using probiotic cheese on young healthy adults (18–35 years of age) or elderly populations with some oral health problems such as dry mouth, mucosal lesions and oral pain. When oral carriage of *Candida* was compared with or without intervention of probiotics, there was an observed trend that the probiotics could decrease the quantity of *Candida*. However, the effect was not significant [16] or was small without an improvement in the mucosal symptoms of the aforementioned conditions [17]. On the other hand, studies conducted by Mendonça et al. [18], Ishikawa et al. [19] and Kraft-Bodi et al. [20] reported a slight or moderate improvement of oral candidiasis when patients were treated with probiotics. Dos Santos et al. [21] reported a significant improvement of oral candidiasis on probiotic treatment.

In Vivo Animal and In Vitro Studies of Probiotics for Oral Biofilm Infections

Animal and *in vitro* tests are necessary to select effective probiotic strains and subsequently elucidate the mechanisms of the probiotic effect. However, *in vitro* and animal tests for caries and periodontitis prevention were scarce compared to clinical trials (Tables 10.1 and 10.2). Most of the foregoing studies have only performed screening assays to select or confirm the effective strains, but have not examined the mechanism of action. On the other hand, several *in vivo* animal studies have been performed to examine the effect of probiotics on oral *Candida* infections. However, the results remain controversial. Some reports suggested a local as well as systemic beneficial effect of probiotics on candidiasis [22–24], while others have not observed a positive effect [25]. These diverse observations may result from differences in the administration technique employed. Kojima et al. [26] demonstrated that the key

TABLE 10.1

Summary of Studies That Examined the Anti-Cariogenic Activity of Probiotics against *Streptococcus mutans*

References	Test Strain	Test Design/ Feature Tested	Results
		Clinical Studies	
Nase, N. et al. (2001) *Caries Res.* 35, 412–420	*L. rhamnosus* GG, ATCC 53103 (LGG) (milk)	Double-blind, placebo-RCT, n = 594, 1–6 years old	Seven-month consumption of probiotic milk reduced caries risk and *S. mutans* counts.
Ahola, A. J. et al. (2002) *Arch Oral Biol.* 47, 799–804	*L. rhamnosus* ATCC 53103 (LGG), LC705 (cheese)	Double-blind, placebo-RCT, n = 74, 18–35 years old	Three-week consumption of probiotic cheese reduced *S. mutans* and *Candida* counts.
Caglar, E. et al. (2006) *Acta Odontol Scand.* 64, 314–318	*L. reuteri* ATCC 55730 (tablets)	Placebo-controlled, n = 120, 21–24 years old	Three-week consumption of probiotic tablets reduced *S. mutans* counts.
Stecksen-Blicks, C. et al. (2009) *Caries Res.* 43, 374–381	*L. rhamnosus* LB21 milk supplement (10^7 CFU/ml)	Double-blind, placebo-RCT, n = 248, 1–5 years old	Twenty-one-month consumption of probiotic milk reduced DMF.
Nikawa, H. et al. (2004) *Int J Food Microbiol.* 95, 219–223	*L. reuteri* SD2112 (ATCC55730) (yogurt)	Double-blind, placebo-RCT, n = 40, 20 years old	Two-week consumption of probiotic yogurt reduced *S. mutans* counts.
Lexner, M. O. et al. (2010) *Oral Health Prev Dent.* 8, 383–388	*L. rhamnosus* LB21 (milk)	Double-blind, placebo-RCT, n = 18, 14.5 years old	Two-week consumption of probiotic milk did not reduce *S. mutans* counts of caries in active adolescents.
Singh, R. et al. (2011) *Acta Odontol Scand.* 69, 389–394	*B. lactis* Bb-12 ATCC27536, *L. acidophilus* La-5 (ice-cream)	Double-blind, placebo-cross-over, CT, n = 40, 12–14 years old	Ten-day consumption of probiotic ice-cream reduced *S. mutans* counts.
Jindal, G. et al. (2011) *Eur Arch Paediatr Dent.* 12, 211–215	*L. rhamnosus*, *Bifidobacterium* spp., *Bacillus coagulans*	Double-blind, placebo-RCT, n = 150, 7–14 years old	Two-week consumption of probiotic bacterial suspension reduced *S. mutans* counts.
Taipale, T. et al. (2012) *Caries Res.* 46, 69–77	*B. animalis* subsp. *lactis* BB-12 (tablets)	Double-blind, placebo-RCT, n = 106 infants	Average 15-month consumption of probiotic tablets did not allow the colonization of probiotics in 1–2-month-old infants, but reduced the colonization of *S. mutans*.

(Continued)

TABLE 10.1 (CONTINUED)
Summary of Studies That Examined the Anti-Cariogenic Activity of Probiotics against *Streptococcus mutans*

References	Test Strain	Test Design/ Feature Tested	Results
Campus, G. et al. (2013) *Clin Oral Invest.* doi: 10.1007/s00784 -013-0980-9	*L. brevis* CD2 (lozenge)	Double-blind, placebo-RCT, $n =$ 191, 6–8 years old, dental caries in active children	Three- and six-week consumption of probiotic lozenge reduced *S. mutans* counts, acidity in plaque and breeding on proving (BOP).
Burton, J. P. et al. (2013) *J Med Microbiol.* 62, 875–884	*S. salivarius* M18 (lozenge)	Double-blind, placebo-RCT, $n =$ 100, dental caries in active children, 5–10 years old	Three-month consumption of probiotic reduced *S. mutans* counts.
Taipale, T. et al. (2013) *Caries Res.* 47, 364–372	*B. animalis* subsp. *lactis* BB-12 (tablets)	Double-blind, placebo-RCT, $n =$ 106, 1–2-months-old infants	Two-year consumption with a spoon or pacifier during period of eruption of primary teeth reduced *S. mutans* counts. Permanent colonization of probiotics in the oral cavity was not observed.
Ashwin, D. et al. (2015) *J Clin Diagn Res.* 9. doi: 10.7860/JCDR/2015 /10942.5532	*Bifidobacterium lactis* Bb-12, *L. acidophilus* La-5 (ice-cream)	Double-blind, placebo-RCT, $n =$ 60, 6–12 years old	Seven-day consumption of probiotic ice-cream reduced *S. mutans* counts for 30 days.
Animal Tests			
Tanzer, J. M. et al. (2010) *J Dent Res.* 89, 921–926	*L. paracasei* DSMZ16671	Evaluation in caries model rats, 21 days old. Toxicity and mutagenesis tests were carried out with heat-killed probiotics.	Caries score of rats after *S. mutans* inoculation for three and six weeks was reduced in the heat-killed probiotic consumption group, without toxicity nor mutagenicity.
***In Vitro* Tests**			
Nikawa, H. et al. (2004) *Int J Food Microbiol.* 95, 219–223	*L. reuteri* SD2112 (ATCC55730)	Growth inhibitory test of *S. mutans* and demineralizing test of probiotics on hydroxyapatite	Probiotics inhibited the viability and demineralizing activity of *S. mutans*.

(Continued)

TABLE 10.1 (CONTINUED)

Summary of Studies That Examined the Anti-Cariogenic Activity of Probiotics against *Streptococcus mutans*

References	Test Strain	Test Design/ Feature Tested	Results
Kang, M. S. et al. (2011) *J Microbiol.* 49, 193–199	*L. reuteri* strains (KCTC 3594 and KCTC 3678), rat-derived L. reuteri KCTC 3679		Probiotic strains produced H_2O_2 and a bacteriocin-like compound inhibited *S. mutans* biofolm formation.
Soderling, E. M. et al. (2011) *Curr Microbiol,* 62, 618–622	*L. rhamnosus* GG (ATCC 53103), *L. reuteri* SD2112 (ATCC 55730), *L. reuteri* ATCC PTA 5289, *L. plantarum* 299v (DSM 9843)		Probiotic strains inhibited *S. mutans* biofolm formation with low pH dependency.
Teanpaisan, R. et al. (2011) *Lett Appl Microbial.* 53, 452–459	Ten of lactobacilli species of oral isolates; *L. fermentum* [195], *L. salivarius* [53], *L. casei* [20], *L. gasseri* [18], *L. rhamnosus* [14], *L. paracasei* [12], *L. mucosae* [12], *L. oris* [12], *L. plantarum* [11], *L. vaginolis* [10], totally 357 strains		The highest inhibitory activity on *S. mutans* and *S. sobrinius* viability and biofilm formation activity was shown in five species of *L. paracasei, L. plantarum, L. rhamnosus, L. casei,* and *L. salivalius.*
Saha, S. et al. (2014) *Benef Microbes.* 5, 447–460	*L. fermentum* NCIMB 5221, NCIMB 2797, NCIMB 8829, *L. reuteri* NCIMB 701089, NCIMB 701359, NCIMB 702655, NCIMB 702656, NCIMB 11951, *L. acidophilus* ATCC 314		Four strains of *L. reuteri* reduced *S.mutans* below the detection limit (<10 CFUs/mL). One strain of *L. fermentum* was buffered by saliva and coaggregated with *S. mutans.*
Kojima, Y. et al. (2016) *J Oral Biosci.* 58, 27–32.	*L. fermentum, L. plantarum, L. casei, L. paracasei,* per 12 species (40 strains)	Inhibition assays of insoluble glucan production by *S. mutans* with lactobacilli culture supernatant	Five strains were selected as candidates for probiotics to reduce biofilm formation of *S. mutans.*

TABLE 10.2
Summary of Studies That Examined Probiotic Activity against Periodontal Pathogens

References	Test Strains	Test Design/ Feature Tested	Results
		Clinical Studies	
Ishikawa, H. et al. (2003). *J Jpn Soc Periodontol.* 45, 105–112.	*L. salivarius* TI2711 (LS1) (tablet: 2×10^7 CFUs, 1×10^8 CFUs)	RCT, $n = 78$, 22–62 years old	Probiotic tablet consumption for 8 weeks reduced black-pigmented anaerobic rods (BPAR), but not reduced salivary pH.
Vivekananda, M. R. et al. (2004) *Int J Food Microbiol.* 95, 219–223	*L. reuteri* Prodentis (1×10^8 CFUs DSM17938 + 1×10^8 CFUs ATCC PTA 5289)	Placebo-RCT, $n = 30$, 34–50–year-old periodontitis patients	Probiotics intervention for 3 weeks reduced plaque index, inflammation, and counts of periodontal pathogens.
Krasse, P. et al. (2005) *Swed Dent J.* 30, 55–60	*L. reuteri* (chewing gum: 1×10^8 CFUs LR-1 or LR-2)	Double-blind placebo-RCT, $n = 59$ of gingivitis patients	After 2 weeks of intervention, gingival inflammation of LR-1 group was reduced.
Riccia, D. N. et al. (2007) *Oral Dis.* 13, 376–385	*L. brevis* CD2 (lozenge)	Double-blind paired-comparison study, chronic periodontitis patient $n = 21$, 30–51 years old, age-matched healthy control, $n = 8$	The clinical parameters were ameliorated and inflammation parameter (metalloproteinase, nitric oxide synthase (NOS) activity, IgA, prostaglandin E_2 (PGE_2), γ-interferon (IFN-γ)) in saliva was decreased.
Twetman, S. et al. (2008) *Acta Odontol Scand.* 1–6	*L. reuteri* (ATCC55730, ATCC PTA5289) 1×10^8 CFUs/ (chewing gum)	Double-blind, placebo-RCT, $n = 42$, average 24 years old, moderate gingivitis patients	After 2-week consumption, the clinical parameters were ameliorated and TNF-α and IL-8 levels among inflammatory cytokines of gingival crevicular fluid (GCF) were decreased.
Mayanagi, G. et al. (2009) *J Clin Periodontol.* 36, 506–513	*L. salivarius* WB21 (tablets)	Double-blind, placebo-RCT, $n = 66$, average 44.9 years old, healthy volunteer	Counts of periodontal pathogen of *A. actinomycetemcomitans*, *P. intermedia*, *P. gingivalis*, *T. denticola*, *T. forsythia* were reduced by probiotic oral administration for 8 weeks.

(Continued)

TABLE 10.2 (CONTINUED)
Summary of Studies That Examined Probiotic Activity against Periodontal Pathogens

References	Test Strains	Test Design/ Feature Tested	Results
Staab, B. et al. (2009) *J Clin Periodontol.* 36, 850–856	*L. casei* Shirota (milk beverage)	Parallel-designed, non-blinded, $n = 50$, 24.4 years old, dental and medical students	After 8-week consumption, the clinical index was not changed, but estelase, MMP-3 and MPO activities of PML were reduced.
Slawik, S. et al. (2011) *Eur J Clin Nutr.* 65, 857–863	*L. casei* Shirota (milk beverage)	Single-blind CT, $n = 28$, healthy volunteer	After 4-week consumption, clinical parameters of BOP and GCF volume were reduced.
Teughels, W. et al. (2013) *J Clin Periodontol.* 40, 1025–1035	*L. reuteri* DSM17938, ATCC PTA5289 (lozenge)	Double-blind, placebo-controlled, parallel-arm CT, $n = 30$, chronic periodontitis patients	After 12-week consumption, clinical parameters were reduced including probing depth.
Animal Tests			
Hillman, J. D. et al. (1988) *Arch Oral Biol.* 33, 395–401	*S. sanguinis* KJ3sm	Gnotobiotic rat model, parallel, open-label, placebo-controlled	Administration of probiotics with H_2O_2 production ability reduced the *A. actinomycetemcomitans* level on rat teeth.
Teughels, W. et al. (2007) *J Dent Res.* 86, 1078–1082	*S. salivarius*, *S. mitis*, *S. sanginis*	Injection of mixed probiotics to gingival pockets of model beagle dogs, split-mouth, RT, $n = 8$	Administration of mixed probiotics for 4 weeks reduced the gingivitis level and amount of black pigmented anaerobes.
Nackaerts, O. et al. (2008) *J Clin Periodontol.* 35, 1048–1052	*S. salivarius*, *S. mitis*, *S. sanginis*	Split-mouth, double-blind RT, $n = 8$ male beagle dogs	Administration of mixed probiotics for 4 weeks improved bone density in 12 weeks.
Nagaoka S. et al. (2009) *J. Oral Biosci.* 54, 224–229	*Bifidobacterium adolescentis* OLB6398, OLB6410, KH96	Hamster periodontitis model by infection of *P. gingivalis* around ligatured molars, open-label, placebo-controlled	Probiotic *B. sdolescentis* reduced *P. gingivalis* colonisation but not significantly.

(Continued)

TABLE 10.2 (CONTINUED)
Summary of Studies That Examined Probiotic Activity against Periodontal Pathogens

References	Test Strains	Test Design/ Feature Tested	Results
		In Vitro Tests	
Ishikawa, H. et al. (2003). *J Jpn Soc Periodontol.* 45, 105–112	*L. salivarius* TI2711 (LS1)	Coculture test	The periodontal pathogens (*P. gingivalis, P. intermedia, P. nigrescens,* 10^8 CFUs) died within 24 h.
Koll-Klais, P. et al. (2005) *Oral Microbiol Immunol.* 20, 354–361	Ten species including *L. gasseri, L. fermentum, L. plantarum, L. paracasei, L. rhamnosus, L. salivarius*	Antibacterial activity against cariogenic and periodontal pathogen was determined.	A total of 238 strains of lactobacilli were isolated and 69% of them inhibited *S. mutans*, 88% inhibited *A. actinomycetemcomitans*, 82% inhibited *P. gingivalis* and 65% inhibited *P. intermendia.*
Jones, S. E. (2009) *BMC Microbiol.* 9. doi: 10.1186/1471–2180-9-35	*L. reuteri* ATCC PTA 6475, ATCC PTA 5289, ATCC 55730, CF48–3A	Leuterin producing level in *L. reuteri* was determined. TNF level of human monocyte stimulated by LPS was determined.	Producing activity of reuterin, an antibiotic factor of *L. reuteri*, and regulatory activity of TNF level of *L. reuteri* increased biofilm formation.
Teanpaisan, R. et al. (2011) *Lett Appl Microbiol.* 53, 452–459	Ten species, *L. fermentum* [195], *L. salivarius* [53], *L. casei* [20], *L. gasseri* [18], *L. rhamnosus* [14], *L. paracasei* [12], *L. mucosae* [12], *L. oris* [12], *L. plantarum* [11], *L. vaginolis* [10], totally 357 strains	Inhibitory zone formation assay on agar plates	Most strains of oral lactobacilli suppressed the growth of periodontal pathogens (*P. gingivalis, A. actinomycetemcomitans*), and cariogenic bacteria (*S. mutams, S. sobrinus*) in a biofilm model.
Riccia, D. N. et al. (2007) *Oral Dis.* 13, 376–385	*L. brevis* CD2 lozenge	Wistar rats macrophage stimulated by LPS was used in *in vitro* culture test.	With *L. brevis* culture supernatant, releasing levels of PGE_2 and MMP9 of macrophage were decreased.
Kawai, T. et al. (2016) *J Prob Health.* 4. 1000135	*L. plantarum* [122], *L. fermentum* ALAL020 out of 50 strains	MIC assay and active component was purified with HPLC/ LC-MS.	Antibacterial constituents against *P. gingivalis* were sodium lactate and a low molecular weight substance.

TABLE 10.3

Summary of Studies That Examined the Antifungal Activity of Probiotics against *Candida albicans*

References	Test Strains	Test Design/ Feature Tested	Results
		Clinical Studies	
Ahola, A. J. et al. (2002) *Arch. Oral Biol.* 47, 799–804	*L. rhamnosus* GG/ LS8 (cheese)	Intervention with cheese, double-blind placebo-RCT	Reduction in the risk of a high level of *Candida*
Hatakka, K. et al. (2007) *J Dent Res.* 86, 125–130	*L. lactis, L. helveticus, L. rhamnosus* GG, *P. freudenreichii* (cheese)	Intervention of an elderly group with cheese for 16 weeks, Double-blind randomised placebo trial (tested group, $n = 136$; control group, $n = 140$)	10% reduction of the high *Candida* count rate in the tested group (after 16-week intervention)
dos Santos, A. L. et al. (2009) *Braz J Microbiol.* 40, 960–964	*L. casei. B. breve* (commercial probiotic drink)	No control group, 26 individuals, intervention with a commercial probiotic drink for 20 days	Reduction of the *Candida* carrying rate, reduction of the sIgA level
Mendonça, F. H. et al. (2012) *Braz Dent J.* 23, 534–538	*L. casei, B. breve* (commercial probiotic drink)	No control group, 42 individuals older than 65 years of age Intervention with a commercial probiotic drink for 30 days	Decrement of *Candida* prevalence, increment of sIgA level
Sutula, J. et al. (2013) *Microb Ecol Health Dis.* 24, 21003	*L. casei* (commercial probiotic drink)	No control group, 22 healthy individuals approximately 32 years of age Intervention with a commercial probiotic drink for 4 weeks	No reduction of the *Candida* CFU, reduction of the halitosis score; did not detect *L. casei* after tests
Ishikawa, K. H. et al. (2015) *J. Prosthodont.* 24, 194–199	*L. rhamnosus, L. acidophilus,* B. bifidum	Double-blind randomised trial (tested group, $n = 30$, control group, $n = 29$) Intervention with trial probiotic products for 5 weeks	Reduction of the *Candida* carrying rate in the tested group
Kraft-Bodi, E. et al. (2015) *J Dent Res.* 94, 181–186	*L. reuteri* (lozenges)	Double-blind placebo-RCT, elderly individuals living in a nursing home (tested group, $n = 84$; control group, $n = 90$) Intervention with probiotic lozenges	Improved the *Candida* score

(*Continued*)

TABLE 10.3 (CONTINUED)
Summary of Studies That Examined the Antifungal Activity of Probiotics against *Candida albicans*

References	Test Strains	Test Design/ Feature Tested	Results
Animal Studies			
Wagner, R. D. et al. (1997) *Infect Immun.* 4165–4172	*L. acidophilus, L. reuteri, L. casei, B. animalis*	Oral candidiasis model in immunodeficient *bg/ bg-nu/nu* mice Estimated by the CFUs and pathological examinations	Increased the life expectancy in the tested group
Elahi, S. et al. (2005) *Clin Exp Immun.* 141, 29–36	*L. acidophilus, L. fermentum*	*Candida* infection model using male DBA/2 mice (H-2d), 6–8 weeks of age Oral administration of probiotics	Reduction in the duration of *Candida* colonisation in the tested group
Matsubara, V. H. et al. (2012) *Oral Dis.* 18, 260–264	*L. acidophilus, L. rhamnosus*	DBA/2 murine oral *Candida* infection model. Control group was treated with nystatin; tested group was treated with probiotics.	Reduction of the *Candida* level in the tested group compared with the control group
Zavisic, G. et al. (2012) *Braz J Microbiol.* 418–428	*L. plantarum, L. casei*	Wister rats and NMRI Ham laboratory mice	Did not show an inhibition in *C. albicans* growth
Ishijima, S.A. (2012) *Appl. Environm. Microbiol.* 78, 190–199	*S. salivarius*	ICR mice, oral candidiasis model	Probiotics were not fungicidal, but inhibited *Candida* adhesion
***In Vitro* Tests**			
Chung, T. C. et al. (1989) *Microbial Ecol Health Dis* 2, 137–144	*L. reuteri*	MIC assay using partially purified reuterin	Reuterin, an antimicrobial substance with broad-spectrum effects, led to the reduction of *C. albicans block*
Koll, P. et al. (2008) *Oral Microbiol Immunol.* 23, 139–147	*L. plantarum, L. paracasei, L. salivarius, L. rhamnosus*	Antimicrobial activity was detected using the antagonism method.	Did not show an inhibition in *C. albicans* growth

(Continued)

TABLE 10.3 (CONTINUED)

Summary of Studies That Examined the Antifungal Activity of Probiotics against *Candida albicans*

References	Test Strains	Test Design/ Feature Tested	Results
Kohler, G. A. et al. (2012) *Infect Dis. Obstet. Gynecol.* ID 636474	*L. rhamnosus, L. reuteri*	Antimicrobial activity was detected using an overlay plate or coculture assay. The genome-wide transcriptional profile of *C. albicans* was assayed with a cDNA microarray.	*C. albicans* was antisepticized by inhibition of the metabolic activity under low pH.
Hasslof, P. et al. (2010) *BMC Oral Health.* 10, 18	*L. plantarum, L. rhamnosus* GG, *L. paracasei, L. reuteri, L. acidophilus*	Agar overlay interference tests	*Candida* growth was reduced; however, the effect was generally weaker than for *mutans* streptococci.
Jiang, Q. et al. (2014) *Benef Microbes* 6, 361–368	*L. rhamnosus* GG, *L. casei* Shirota, *L. reuteri* SD2112, *L. brevis* CD2, *L. bulgaricus* LB86, *L. bulgaricus* LB Lact	Estimated the inhibition effect by coculture test under different pH conditions and the combination of saccharides using EIR.	Inhibition capacity differed in the probiotic strains, *L. rhamnosus* GG showed the strongest inhibition effects against *C. albicans*, followed by *L. casei* Block, *L. reuteri* SD2112 and *L. brevis* CD2.
Shokryazdan, P. et al. (2014) *BioMed Res Int.* ID 927268	*L. acidophilus, L. buchneri, L. casei, L. fermentum*	Coculture test with 12 pathogenic microorganisms	The active substance was organic acid.
Kheradmand, E. et al. (2014) *DARU J. Pharm Sci.* 22:48	*L. johnsonii, L. plantarum*	After selenium treatment, the antimicrobial effects improved.	The active substances were exometabolites or novel anti-*Candida* compounds.
Kojima, Y. et al. (2016) *J Oral Biosci.* 58, 27–32.	*L. fermentum, L. plantarum, L. paracasei* per 12 species (40 strains)	Coculture and growth inhibition assays of *C. albicans* with lactobacilli culture supernatant or saccharides	Three saccharides and five strains became candidates for pre- and probiotics, respectively.

(*Continued*)

TABLE 10.3 (CONTINUED)
Summary of Studies That Examined the Antifungal Activity of Probiotics against *Candida albicans*

References	Test Strains	Test Design/ Feature Tested	Results
Jiang, Q. et al. (2016) *BMC Microbiol.* 16, 149.	*L. rhamnosus* GG	Coculture test with five oral pathogens and scanned with confocal laser scanning microscopy using an *in vitro* biofilm model	*L. rhamnosus* GG slightly suppressed the growth of *C. albicans* in all groups.
James, K. M. et al. (2016) *J. Med Microbiol.* 65, 328–336	*L. plantarum* SD5870, *L. helveticus* CBS N116411, *S. salivarius* DSM 14685	Coculture test of probiotics and *C. albicans* and inhibitory test with *Lactobacillus* cell supernatants using an *in vitro* biofilm model	When live probiotics or their supernatants were overlaid on preformed *C. albicans* biofilms, biofilm size was reduced and expression of certain genes involved in the yeast–hyphae transition was disrupted.
Matsubara, V. H. et al. (2016) *Appl Microbiol Biotechnol.* 1–12.	*L. rhamnosus,* *L. casei,* *L. acidophilus*	Coculture test with probiotics on the *C. albicans* and inhibitory test with *Lactobacillus* cell culture supernatants. The morphology was visualised by CLSM and SEM.	Microscopic analyses revealed that *L. rhamnosus* suspensions reduced *Candida* hyphal differentiation, leading to a predominance of budding growth.

factor for the effectiveness of probiotics may be the selection of an appropriate strain that works against *Candida*.

Previous studies on probiotics have used a diverse set of *lactobacilli* spp. The genome size of the genus *Lactobacillus* ranges from 1.23 to 4.91 Mb and the GC content spans 31.9–57.0% among different species [27]. In addition, the properties of strains within the same species of *Lactobacillus* have been shown to vary [28,29]. Some of these studies have selected probiotic *Lactobacillus* strains that are known to confer intestinal health benefits and assumed a similar beneficial effect on oral infections. Therefore, it is important to demonstrate the *in vitro* activity of a probiotic strain against oral pathogens and subsequently select an efficient strain for *in vivo* and clinical studies. Such studies are few and shown in Tables 10.1 through 10.3.

ANTIMICROBIAL PROBIOTICS PRODUCTS AGAINST ORAL PATHOGENS

Studies of probiotics on intestinal health have revealed several antibacterial substances produced by lactic acid bacteria: (I) organic acids such as lactic and acetic acids, (II) hydrogen peroxide, (III) bacteriocins [30–32] and (IV) low molecular weight antimicrobial substances.

(I) Organic Acids

There have been several reports on the antibacterial effects of lactobacilli against *P. gingivalis* [33,34]. Matsuoka et al. [35] showed that *L. salivarius* TI2711 had antibacterial activity against *P. gingivalis* and suggested that the antibacterial substance of the strain was lactic acid. Kang et al. [36] also reported the antimicrobial activity of *L. reuteri* against oral pathogens such as *P. gingivalis*, *Tannerella forsythia*, *Aggregatibacter actinomycetemcomitans*, *Fusobacterium nucleatum* and *S. mutans* was attributable to lactic acid. Furthermore, Takahashi et al. [37] reported that *P. gingivalis* was acid sensitive and that *P. gingivalis* proliferation was inhibited at a pH $\leq$ 6.5. However, it is possible that low pH conditions in the oral cavity may induce caries or hypersensitivity. In our study [38], an antibacterial test of lactobacilli culture supernatants against *P. gingivalis* was performed after the pH was adjusted to 7 with sodium hydroxide to exclude the influence of pH. Despite the neutral pH of the *L. plantarum* 122 and *L. fermentum* ALAL020 culture supernatants, both strains strongly inhibited the growth of *P. gingivalis*. These results indicate that sodium lactate, a neutralised form of lactic acid, also has antibacterial properties. The minimum inhibitory concentration (MIC) of sodium lactate against type strain of *P. gingivalis* ATCC33277 was 2%. This result is in line with the findings of Matsuoka et al. [35]. Probiotic lactobacilli coaggregate with *Candida* and produce antimicrobial substances that have a direct growth inhibitory effect on *Candida*. Under aggregating situation, lactobacilli universally produce lactic acid that inhibits the metabolic activity of *Candida* spp. [39], which has a weak antifungal activity [40].

(II) Hydrogen Peroxide

Hydrogen peroxide (H_2O_2) is produced by most lactobacilli in the presence of oxygen. As lactobacilli do not produce catalase, H_2O_2 does not undergo auto-degradation. It has a broad-spectrum effect on planktonic bacteria, but the effect decreases drastically on biofilm [41]. It appears that lactobacilli do not produce effective concentrations of H_2O_2 against fungi [42], unlike other bacteria [31].

(III) Bacteriocins

Lactic acid bacteria produce bacteriocins, proteinaceous antimicrobial substances with molecular weights of several thousand daltons or more. Bacteriocins can be divided into five classes according to their primary structure, molecular composition and properties [43,44], but recently a simpler classification into three groups has been suggested [45]. However, reports of bacteriocins produced by lactic acid bacteria against *S. mutans* and *P. gingivalis* are scarce. The two-peptide lantibiotic lactin 3147 has a broad spectrum including *S. mutans* [45]. A 56-kDa novel bacteriocin produced by *L. paracasei* HL32 inhibits the growth of periodontal pathogens includ-ing *P. gingivalis* [46]. Bacteriocin L23 produced by *Lactobacillus fermentum* L23 [44], plantaricin produced by *L. plantarum* [47] and pentocin TV35b produced by *L. pentosus* [48] appear to be effective against the yeast form of *Candida*. Bacteriocins effective for hyphal forms of *Candida* have been identified infrequently [49,50]. For instance, brevicin SG1 produced by *L. brevis* [51] and nisin broduced by *Lactococcus lactis* [52] inhibited the hyphal growth of *C. albicans*.

(IV) Low Molecular Weight Antimicrobial Substances

Reuterin, an antibacterial substance (also known as 3-hydroxypropionaldehyde; molecular weight, 74 Da; composition formula, $C_3H_6O_2$), is a product of glycerol fermentation which has been seen in several probiotic bacteria. These probiotic bac-teria include *L. reuteri* [53], *L. brevis*, *L. buchneri* [54] and *L. collinoides* [55]. Under anaerobic conditions, *L. coryniformis* [56] also produces a low molecular weight antimicrobial substance that does not contain amino acids [57]. Reuterin was found to exert its antibacterial effects by causing oxidative stress within bacterial cells [58]. In addition to reuterin, low molecular substances produced by lactobacilli, reuteri-cyclin [59] and dyacetyl [60], have also been shown to be effective against the yeast forms of *Candida* [61].

PREBIOTICS

The term *prebiotics* was defined by G. R. Gibson and M. B. Roberfroid in 1995 [62] as 'a non-digestible food ingredient that beneficially affects the host by selectively stimulating the growth and/or activity of one or a limited number of bacteria in the colon, and thus improves host health'. Studies on oral prebiotics are limited. Sugars and dietary fiber have been considered to be prebiotics for intestinal lactic acid bac-teria [62]. However, this is not the case for the oral environment, as the presence of sugars is thought to increase the risk of dental caries. The *mutans* group of strepto-cocci, the major cariogenic pathogen associated with dental caries, metabolises car-iogenic sugars, such as glucose and sucrose, and produces organic acid and insoluble glucan substrate that contribute to dental caries.

On the contrary, sugar alcohols such as xylitol suppress the growth of *S. mutans*. Xylitol, a reduced derivative of xylose, converts to xylitol-5-phosphate inside *S. mutans* cells and inhibits glycolysis. Similarly, arabinose, a member of the same aldopentose group as xylose, is not assimilated by *S. mutans* [63] and likely has an effect similar to that of xylitol. We recently demonstrated that xylitol, xylose and arabinose inhibited the growth of *S. mutans*, but were utilised for the growth of sev-eral lactobacilli strains we tested [26]. Although xylitol is generally not assimilated by lactobacilli, a recent report showed that 36% of lactobacilli strains isolated from human oral cavities were able to metabolise xylitol [64].

Our previous data on *C. albicans* type strain ATCC18804 showed decreased growth in the presence of three saccharides (xylitol, xylose and arabinose) com-pared with glucose [26]. There are conflicting reports on the ability of *C. albicans* to assimilate xylitol and aldopentose. Makinen et al. [65] and Maleszka and Schneider [66] showed that *C. albicans* is not capable of proper growth in the presence of xylitol. Uittamo et al. [67] suggested that xylitol metabolism of *Candida* might compete for the nicotinamide adenine dinucleotide (NADH) coenzyme, leading to the down-regulation of alcohol dehydrogenase (ADH). Clinical trials in Turku sugar studies showed significantly decreased colony counts and detection frequency of oral *Candida* in the xylitol intake group [68,69]. On the other hand, yeast is known to possess a pentose assimilation pathway that produces ethanol from arabinose and xylose by an enzymatic reaction [70,71]. Even if *Candida* is capable of slowly assimilating those three candidate sugars, the slower growth compared to that of probiotic bacteria may have a competitive inhibition on *Candida*. The presence of xylitol inhibits the adhesion of *Candida* to mucosal surfaces [72,73]. In an experimental murine model of gastrointestinal candidiasis, the colonisation and invasion of *C. albicans* was significantly reduced in the group supplemented with xylitol compared to the group supplemented with glucose [74].

Most of periodontal pathogens gain nutrients from cervical fluids, which are a serum leaked through capillary vessels located in gingival tissue. The main constituent is a proteinaceous component rather than carbohydrates or sugar. Moreover, *P. gingivalis*, the centerpiece of periodontal bacteria, cannot live under low-pH conditions [37] in the presence of organic acids produced by sugar-assimilating bacteria such as lactobacilli. Therefore, prebiotics directly affecting periodontal pathogens metabolically may not be applicable, but activating the inhibitory effect of probiotics on periodontal pathogens will be applicable for periodontal disease.

SYNBIOTICS

NOTEWORTHY FEATURES OF SYNBIOTICS ASSOCIATED WITH ORAL APPLICATION

Gibson and Roberfroid [62] proposed the use of probiotic and prebiotic fusion products, or 'synbiotics', for the intestinal tract microbiota [75]. However, the use of synbiotics for the oral microbiota has not been well studied [26]. It is important to understand the limitations associated with the oral application of synbiotics. Probiotic bacteria are not able to colonise adult oral cavities easily [29,76]. Therefore, it appears that synbiotics are more effective for oral applications than probiotics alone. One must, however, consider the risk of dental caries while applying lactic acid bacteria in the oral cavity. Lactobacilli have long been considered to be one of the cariogenic bacteria present in dental plaque [77]. Currently, there are two concepts regarding the association of lactobacilli with dental caries. Lactobacilli comprise a very small proportion of normal oral microbiota and are present primarily on the tongue dorsum, rather than in dental plaque [78]. However, they are hardly detected in the oral cavity of caries-free individuals [79]. The lactobacilli count in the saliva is an indicator of the dental caries activity because lactobacilli penetrate porous tooth surfaces in early caries lesions or adhere to type I collagen of dentine exposed in the carious portion of the tooth [27]. As the salivary lactobacilli count correlates with the amount and frequency of carbohydrate (sugar) intake [80,81], the presence of lactobacilli is a reliable indicator for the dental caries activity [82]. Therefore, if one can maintain good oral hygiene, oral probiotic therapy with lactobacilli alone may not contribute to the development of dental caries. In addition, if appropriate prebiotics are administered simultaneously, then synbiotic therapy may suppress the development of oral candidiasis.

Another important consideration for synbiotic therapy is to recognise the difference in the host immune response of the intestine and the oral cavity. The host immune response is directly associated with the onset and severity of periodontitis and candidiasis. Whereas activation of a substantial host immune response can be expected in the intestine, a similar phenomenon is not expected in the oral cavity, as it is not an organ of mucosa-associated lymphoid tissues (MALT). In the intestine, probiotic bacteria are incorporated into M cells in Peyer's patches (PP), which are a major component of gut-associated lymphoid tissues (GALT), and digested to form active antigens. Macrophages and dendritic cells in PP phagocytise probiotic bacteria and are activated to produce several cytokines, which stimulate T-cell and B-cell functions [83]. Moreover, daily supplementation of lactobacilli as part of the normal diet increase the number and activity of natural killer cells in healthy elderly individuals [29]. Thus, synbiotics in the intestinal tract can be expected to activate both innate immunity and acquired immunity of cell-mediated and humoral immunity. Conversely, the oral cavity is not an immune organ and phenomena such as direct antigen presentation to adaptive immune cells does not occur. Nevertheless, some probiotic clinical trials and animal studies using oral disease models have reported the reduction of inflammatory response and allergic reaction in periodontitis (Table 10.2) or an increase of sIgA against *Candida,* leading to the suppression of *Candida* in the oral cavity [18,22,23]. It is well known that secretion of sIgA from the salivary gland is through differentiated plasma cells from B cells stimulated at MALT. According to the results of clinical and animal studies described earlier, oral synbiotics appear to transition into intestinal synbiotics, as the oral cavity is connected to the intestine. Children who were carriers of oral lactobacilli were found to have similar lactobacilli in their feces [27]. Hence, it appears that the intestinal colonisation of lactobacilli is transmitted through the oral cavity, which may provide simultaneous synbiotic activity at the oral cavity and the intestine.

BIOGENICS

Previous studies have highlighted the limitation of colonisation and fixation of nonnatural probiotic bacteria in the intestinal tract [84]. This phenomenon of transiency but not permanency in colonisation is also relevant for the probiotic application in oral cavities [85–87]. Even if we are able to address the restriction of colonisation of probiotic bacteria in the oral cavity, it comes with a risk of dental caries due to a potential acidic environment generated by probiotic bacteria. To address the aforementioned concerns, the concept of 'biogenics' has been suggested as a solution [88]. Biogenics is defined as 'food ingredients which beneficially affect the host by directly immunostimulating or suppressing mutagenesis, tumorigenesis, peroxidation, hypercholesterolemia or intestinal putrefaction' [88]. Hence, previous studies have suggested the administration of nonviable probiotic bacteria to obtain some 'probiotic' effects. It was reported that the consumption of pasteurised fermented milk increased the lifespan of mice [89,90]. A significant reduction of the Ehrlich ascites tumor growth in mice was also reported [90]. In addition, it was shown that heat-inactivated *Enterococcus faecalis* [91] or *L. gasseri* [92] retained a beneficial regulatory function in the gut. Moreover, Nakamura et al. [93] identified an angiotensin I–converting enzyme (ACE) inhibitor in a Japanese sterilised milk beverage fermented by *L. helveticus* and *Saccharomyces cerevisiae*. The active substance in those fermented beverages was lactotripeptides metabolically generated in the fermentation pathway. Follow-up studies were able to determine the bioactive metabolites of probiotic bacteria in addition to the antimicrobial substances, such as bacteriocin [94,95], and other beneficial active substances, such as conjugated linoleic acid (CLA) [94–96], protein or peptides [97,98] and polyphenols [99,100]. Taking all these observations into account, the new concept of biogenics, which makes use of the bioactive metabolites as foods or medicine, was recently advocated [88,101]. The biogenics effect is independent of the colonisation and viability of probiotic bacteria. Hence, biogenics is the direct delivery of an isolated and purified active ingredient of probiotics to the local environment. As shown in Figure 10.1, a certain active component secreted in culture supernatant by probiotic *L. plantarum* 108 inhibited hyphal growth of *C. albicans* but was not toxic to human oral keratinocytes. This strategy may also be useful for prevention of oral disease. Microorganisms including oral pathogens have the potential to grow in biofilm and express pathogenic properties compared to planktonic type. Biofilm formation is stimulated by an intercellular communication process harmonised with the bacterial population density known as quorum sensing (QS) systems, which are based on small molecules termed autoinducers (AI) [102]. Recently, a QS inhibitor (QSI) and QS signal quencher (QQ) molecule attracted attention in overcoming biofilm infections. Some reports exhibited the bacteriocins produced by probiotic lactobacilli such as *L. acidophilus*, *L. plantarum* and *L. reuteri* acted as QSI or QQ molecules [103]. It may be possible to purify the active ingredients of probiotic bacteria that demonstrate anti-oral pathogenic activity in biofilm for use in the biogenics process. However, this idea requires further study before clinical use.

Confocal imaging using live/dead fluorescent stains

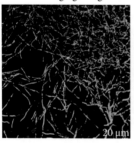 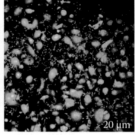 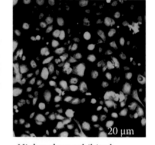

Control sample showing *Candida* infected cells

Lower dose inhibited hyphal formation and rescued the cells

Higher dose exhibited fungicidal activity without any damage to host cells

FIGURE 10.1 Effect of probiotic secretory products on *Candida albicans* biofilms formed on human oral keratinocytes. *Lactobacillus plantarum* 108 supernatants exhibited inhibitory properties on hyphal formation and fungicidal activity in a dose-dependent manner.

CONCLUSION

Taking the aforementioned studies into consideration, it is conceivable that an innovative combination of prebiotics, probiotics, synbiotics and biogenics will be instrumental in devising new therapies against oral biofilm infections such as dental caries, periodontitis and oral candidiasis. More comprehensive investigations on the mechanisms of synbiotics and biogenics are needed for this purpose. Hence, more studies are warranted to examine the bioactive metabolites of probiotic bacteria that induce favourable immunological outcomes and suppress oral pathogens residing in oral biofilms.

CORRESPONDING AUTHOR

Tomoko Ohshima
Department of Oral Microbiology
School of Dental Medicine
Tsurumi University
Kanagawa, Japan
ohshima-t@fs.tsurumi-u.ac.jp

REFERENCES

1. Sardi, J. C. O., Scorzoni, L., Bernardi, T., Fusco-Almeida, A. M. and Giannini, M. M. (2013). *Candida* species: Current epidemiology, pathogenicity, biofilm formation, natural antifungal products and new therapeutic options. *J Med Microbiol.* 62, 10–24.
2. Lilly, D. M. and Stillwell, R. H. (1965). Probiotics growth promoting factors produced by micro-organisms. *Science.* 147, 747–748.
3. Kollath, W. (1953). Ernahrung und Zahnsystem (Nutrition and the tooth system). *Dtsch Zahnarztl Z.* 8(11), 7–16.
4. Fuller, R. (1989). Probiotics in man and animals. *J Appl Bacteriol.* 66, 365–378.
5. Gourbeyre, P., Denery, S. and Bodinier, M. (2011). Probiotics, prebiotics, and synbiotics: Impact on the gut immune system and allergic reactions. *J Leukocyte Boil.* 89, 685–695.
6. Salminen, S., Bouley, C., Boutron-Ruault, M. C., Cummings, J. H., Franck, A., Gibson, G. R., Isolauri, E., Moreau, M. C., Roberfroid, M. and Rowland, I. (1998). Functional food science and gastrointestinal physiology and function. *Srit J Nutr.* 80, 147–171.
7. FAO/WHO. (2001). Evaluation of health and nutritional properties of probiotics in food including powder milk with live lactic acid bacteria. Report of a Joint FAO/WHO Expert Consultation. Available at: http://www.fao.org/es/ESN/food/foodandfoo_probio_en.stm.
8. Teughels, W., Loozen, G. and Quirynen, M. (2011). Do probiotics offer opportunities to manipulate the periodontal oral microbiota? *J Clin Periodontol.* 38(s11), 159–177.
9. Yanine, N., Araya, I., Brignardello-Petersen, R., Carrasco-Labra, A., González, A., Preciado, A., Villanueva, J., Sanz, M. and Martin, C. (2013). Effects of probiotics in periodontal diseases: a systematic review. *Clin Oral Invest.* 17, 1627–1634.
10. Saha, S., Tomaro-Duchesneau, C., Tabrizian, M. and Prakash, S. (2012). Probiotics as oral health biotherapeutics. *Expert Opin Biol Ther.* 12, 1207–1220.

11. Cagetti, M. G., Mastroberardino, S., Milia, E., Cocco, F., Lingström, P. and Campus, G. (2013). The use of probiotic strains in caries prevention: A systematic review. *Nutrients.* 5:7. 2530–2550.

12. Krasse, P., Carlsson, B., Dahl, C., Paulsson, A., Nilsson, A. and Sinkiewicz, G. (2006). Decreased gum bleeding and reduced gingivitis by the probiotic *Lactobacillus reuteri.* *Swedish Dent J.* 30, 55–60.

13. Riccia, D. N., Bizzini, F., Perilli, M. G., Polimeni, A., Trinchieri, V., Amicosante, G. and Cifone, M. G. (2007). Anti-inflammatory effects of *Lactobacillus brevis* (CD2) on periodontal disease. *Oral Dis.* 13: 376–385

14. Vivekananda, M. R., Vandana, K. L. and Bhat, K. G. (2010). Effect of the probiotic *Lactobacilli reuteri* (Prodentis) in the management of periodontal disease: A preliminary randomized clinical trial. *J Oral Microbiol.* 2, 5344: 2010.

15. Ishikawa, H., Aiba, Y., Nakanishi, M., Oh-hashi, Y. and Koga, Y. (2003). Suppression of periodontal pathogenic bacteria in the saliva of humans by the administration of *Lactobacillus salivarius* TI2711. *J Jpn Soc Periodontol.* 45, 105–112.

16. Ahola, A. J., Yli-Knuuttila, H., Suomalainen, T., Poussa, T., Ahlström, A., Meurman, J. H. and Korpela, R. (2002). Short-term consumption of probiotic-containing cheese and its effect on dental caries risk factor. *Arch Oral Biol.* 47, 799–804.

17. Hatakka, K., Ahola, A. J., Yli-Knuuttila, H., Richardson, M., Poussa, T., Meurman, J. H. and Korpela, R. (2007). Probiotics reduce the prevalence of oral candida in the elderly – A randomized controlled trial. *J Dent Res.* 86, 125–130.

18. Mendonça, F. H., dos Santos, S. S., de Faria, I. S., e Silva, C. R., Jorge, A. O. and Leão, M. V. (2012). Effects of probiotic bacteria on *Candida* presence and IgA anti-*Candida* in the oral cavity of elderly. *Braz Dent J.* 23, 534–538.

19. Ishikawa, K. H., Mayer, M. P., Miyazima, T. Y., Matsubara, V. H., Silva, E. G., Paula, C. R., Campos, T. T. and Nakamae, A. E. M. (2014). A multispecies probiotics reduces oral *Candida* colonization in denture wearers. *J Prosthodontics.* 24, 194–199.

20. Kraft-Bodi, E., Jørgensen, M. R., Keller, M. K., Kragelund, C. and Twetman, S. (2015). Effect of probiotic bacteria on oral candida in frail elderly. *J Dent Res.* 94, 181–186.

21. dos Santos, A. L., Jorge, A. O., dos Santos, S. S., e Silva, C. R. and Leão, M. V. (2009). Influence of probiotics on *Candida* presence and IgA anti-*Candida* in the oral cavity. *Braz J Microbiol.* 40, 960–964.

22. Wagner, R. D., Pierson, C., Warner, T., Dohnalek, M., Farmer, J., Roberts, L., Hilty, M. and Balish, E. (1997). Biotherapeutic effects of probiotic bacteria on candidiasis in immunodeficient mice. *Infect Immun.* 65, 4165–4172.

23. Elahi, S., Pang, G., Ashman, R. and Clancy, R. (2005). Enhanced clearance of *Candida albicans* from the oral cavities of mice following oral administration of *Lactobacillus acidophilus.* *Clin Exp Immunol.* 141, 29–36.

24. Matsubara, V. H., Silva, E. G., Paula, C. R., Ishikawa, K. H. and Nakamae, A. E. M. (2012). Treatment with probiotics in experimental oral colonization by *Candida albicans* in murine model (DBA/2). *Oral Dis.* 18, 260–264.

25. Zavisic, G., Petricevic, S., Radulovic, Z., Begovic, J., Golic, N., Topisirovic, L. and Strahinic, I. (2012). Probiotic features of two oral *Lactobacillus* isolates. *Braz J Microbiol.* 43, 418–428.

26. Kojima, Y., Ohshima, T., Seneviratne, C. J. and Maeda, N. (2016). Combining prebiotics and probiotics to develop novel synbiotics that suppress oral pathogens. *J Oral Biosci.* 58, 27–32.

27. Caufield, P. W., Schön, C. N., Saraithong, P., Li, Y. and Argimón, S. (2015) Oral lactobacilli and dental caries: A model for niche adaptation in humans. *J Dent Res.* 94, 110s–118s.

28. Koll, P., Mandar, R., Marcotte, H., Leibur, E. and Mikelsaar, M. (2008). Characterization of oral lactobacilli as potential probiotics for oral health. *Oral Microbiol Immunol.* 23, 139–147.

29. Tiihonen, K., Ouwehand, A. C. and Rautonen, N. (2010). Human intestinal microbiota and healthy ageing. *Ageing Res Rev.* 9, 107–116.
30. Taniguchi, M., Nakazawa, H., Takeda, O., Kaneko, T., Hoshino, K. and Tanaka, T. (1998). Production of a mixture of antimicrobial organic acids from lactose by co-culture of *Bifidobacterium longum* and *Propionibacterium freudenreichii*. *Biosci Biotechnol Biochem.* 62, 1522–1527.
31. Piard, J. C. and Desmazeaud, M. (1991). Inhibiting factors produced by lactic acid bacteria. 1. Oxygen metabolites and catabolism end-products. *Lait.* 71, 525–541.
32. Klaenhammer, T. R. (1988). Bacteriocins of lactic acid bacteria. *Biochime.* 70, 337–349.
33. Kõll-Klais, P., Mändar, R., Leibur, E., Marcotte, H., Hammarström, L. and Mikelsaar, M. (2005). Oral lactobacilli in chronic periodontitis and periodontal health: Species composition and antimicrobial activity. *Oral Microbiol Immunol.* 20, 354–361.
34. Teanpaisan, R., Piwat, S. and Dahlen, G. (2011). Inhibitory effect of oral *Lactobacillus* against oral pathogens. *Lett Appl Microbiol.* 53, 452–459.
35. Matsuoka, T., Nakanishi, M., Aiba, Y. and Koga Y. (2004). Mechanism of *Prophyromonas gingivalis* killing by *Lactobacillus salivalius* TI2711. *J Jpn Soc Periodontal.* 46, 118–126.
36. Kang, M. S., Oh, J. S., Lee, H. C., Lim, H. S., Lee, S. W., Yang, K. H., Choi, N. K. and Kim, S. M. (2011). Inhibitory effect of *Lactobacillus reuteri* on periodontopathic and cariogenic bacteria. *J Microbiol.* 49, 193–199.
37. Takahashi, N., Saito, K., Schachtele, C. F. and Yamada, T. (1997). Acid tolerance and acid-neutralizing activity of *Porphyromonas gingivalis*, *Prevotella intermedia* and *Fusobacterium nucleatum*. *Oral Microbiol Immunol.* 12, 323–328.
38. Kawai, T., Ohshima, T., Shin, R., Ikawa, S. and Maeda, N. (2016). Determination of the antibacterial constituents produced by lactobacilli against a periodontal pathogen: Sodium lactate and a low molecular weight substance. *J Prob Health.* 4. 1000135.
39. Köhler, G. A., Assefa, S. and Reid, G. (2012). Probiotic interference of *Lactobacillus rhamnosus* GR-1 and *Lactobacillus reuteri* RC-14 with the opportunistic fungal pathogen *Candidsa albicans*. *Infect Dis. Obstet Gynecol.* doi:10.1155/2012/636474.
40. Zalán, Z., Hudáček, J., Štětina, J., Chumchalová, J. and Halász, A. (2010). Production of organic acids by *Lactobacillus* strains in three different media. *Eur Food Res Technol.* 230, 395–404.
41. Perumal, P. K., Wand, M. E., Sutton, J. M. and Bock, L. J. (2014). Evaluation of the effectiveness of hydrogen-peroxide-based disinfectants on biofilms formed by Gram-negative pathogens. *J Hosp Infect.* 87, 227–233.
42. Shokryazdan, P., Sieo, C. C., Kalavathy, R., Liang, J. B., Alitheen, N. B., Jahromi, M. F. and Ho, Y. W. (2014). Probiotic potential of *Lactobacillus* strains with antimicrobial activity against some human pathogenic strains. *BioMed Res Int.* 2014 Article ID 927268, 16pp.
43. Chen, H. and Hoover, D. G. (2003). Bacteriocins and their food applications. *Compr Rev Food Sci Food Saf.* 2, 82–100.
44. Pascual, L. M., Daniele, M. B., Giordano, W., Pajaro, M. C. and Barberis, I. L. (2008) Purification and partial characterization of novel bacteriocin L23 produced by *Lactobacillus fermentum* L23. *Curr Microbiol.* 56, 397–402.
45. Cotter, P. D., Hill, C. and Ross, R. P. (2005). Bacteriocins: Developing innate immunity for food. *Nat Rev Microbiol.* 3, 777–788.
46. Hojo, K., Nagaoka, S., Ohshima, T. and Maeda, N. (2009). Bacterial interactions in dental biofilm development. *J Dent Res.* 88, 982–990.
47. Sharma, A. and Srivastava, S. (2014). Anti-*Candida* activity of two-peptide bacteriocins, plantaricins (Pln E/F and J/K) and their mode of action. *Fungal Biol.* 118, 264–275.

48. Okkers, D. J., Dicks, L. M. T., Silvester, M., Joubert, J. J. and Odendaal, H. J. (1999). Characterization of pentocin TV35b, a bacteriocin-like peptide isolated from *Lactobacillus* pentosus with a fungistatic effect on *Candida albicans*. *J Appl Microbiol*. 87, 726–734.

49. Calderone, R. A. and Fonzi, W. A. (2001). Virulence factors of *Candida albicans*. *Trends Microbiol*. 9, 327–335.

50. Douglas, L. J. (2003). *Candida* biofilm and their role in infection. *Trends Microbiol*. 11, 30–36.

51. Adebayo, C. O. and Aderiye, B. I. (2011). Suspected mode of antimycotic action of brevicin SG1 against *Candida albicans* and *Penicillium citrinum*. *Food Control*. 22, 1814–1820.

52. Le Lay, C., Akerey, B., Fliss, I., Subirade, M. and Rouabhia, M. (2008). Nisin Z inhibits the growth of *Candida albicans* and its transition from blastospore to hyphal form. *J Appl Microbiol*. 105, 1630–1639.

53. Talarico, T. L., Casas, I. A., Chung, T. C. and Dobrogosz, W. J. (1988). Production and isolation of reuterin, a growth inhibitor produced by *Lactobacillus reuteri*. *Antimicrob Agents Chemother*. 32, 1854–1858.

54. Schütz, H. and Radler, F. (1984). Anaerobic reduction of glycerol to propanediol-1.3 by *Lactobacillus brevis* and *Lactobacillus buchneri*. *Syst Appl Microbiol*. 5, 169–178.

55. Claisse, O. and Lonvaud-Funel, A. (2000). Assimilation of glycerol by a strain of *Lactobacillus collinoides* isolated from cider. *Food Microbiol*. 17, 513–519.

56. Magnusson, J., Ström, K., Roos, S., Sjögren, J. and Schnürer, J. (2003). Broad and complex antifungal activity among environmental isolates of lactic acid bacteria. *FEMS Microbiol. Lett*. 219, 129–135.

57. Talarico, T. L. and Dobrogosz, W. J. (1989). Chemical characterization of an antimicrobial substance produced by *Lactobacillus reuteri*. *Antimicrob Agents Chemother*. 33, 674–679.

58. Schaefer, L., Auchtung, T. A., Hermans, K. E., Whitehead, D., Borhan, B. and Britton, R. A. (2010). The antimicrobial compound reuterin (3–hydroxypropion-aldehyde) induces oxidative stress via interaction with thiol groups. *Microbiology*. 156, 1589–1599.

59. Ganzle, M. G. (2000). Characterization of reutericyclin produced by *Lactobacillus reuteri* LTH2584. *Appl Environ Microbiol*. 66, 4325–4333.

60. Jay, J. M. (1982). Antimicrobial properties of diacetyl. *Appl Environ Microbiol*. 44, 525–532.

61. Chung, T. C., Axelsson, L., Lindgren, S. E. and Dobrogosz, W. J. (1989). In vitro studies on reuterin synthesis by *Lactobacillus reuteri*. *Microb Ecol Health Dis*. 2, 137–144.

62. Gibson, G. R. and Roberfroid, M. B. (1995). Dietary modulation of the human colonic microbiota: Introducing the concept of prebiotics. *J Nutr*. 125, 1401–1412.

63. Coykendall, A. L. (1977). Proposal to elevate the subspecies of *Streptococcus mutans* to species status, based on their molecular composition. *Int J Syst Evol Microbiol*. 27(1), 26–30.

64. Almstahl, A., Lingstrom, P., Eliasson, L. and Carlen, A. (2013). Fermentation of sugars and sugar alcohols by plaque *Lactobacillus* strains. *Clin Oral Invest*. 17, 1465–1470.

65. Mäkinen, K. K., Ojanotko, A. and Vidgren, H. (1975). Effect of xylitol on the growth of three oral strains of *Candida albicans*. *J Dent. Res*. 54, 1239–1239.

66. Maleszka, R. and Schneider, H. (1982). Fermentation of D-xylose, xylitol, and D-xylulose by yeasts. *Can J Microbiol*. 28, 360–363.

67. Uittamo, J., Nieminen, M. T., Kaihovaara, P., Bowyer, P., Salaspuro, M. and Rautemaa, R. (2011). Xylitol inhibits carcinogenic acetaldehyde production by *Candida* species. *Int J Cancer*. 129, 2038–2041.

68. Larmas, M., Mäkinen, K. K. and Scheinin, A. (1974). Turku sugar studies III. An intermediate report on the effect of sucrose, fructose and xylitol diets on the numbers of salivary lactobacilli, *Candida* and streptococci. *Acta Odontol Scand.* 32, 423–433.
69. Larmas, M., Mäkinen, K. K. and Scheinin, A. (1976). Turku sugar studies VIII: Principal microbiological findings. *Acta Odontol Scand.* 34, 285–328.
70. Chiang, C. and Knight, S. G. (1960). A new pathway of pentose metabolism. *Biochem. Biophys Res Commun.* 3, 554–559.
71. Ōnishi, H. and Suzuki, T. (1966). The production of xylitol, L-arabinitol and ribitol by yeasts. *Agric Biol Chem.* 30, 1139–1144.
72. Pizzo, G., Giuliana, G., Milici, M. E. and Giangreco, R. (2000). Effect of dietary carbohydrates on the in vitro epithelial adhesion of *Candida albicans, Candida tropicalis,* and *Candida krusei. New Microbiol.* 23, 63–71.
73. Abu-Elteen, K. H. (2005). The influence of dietary carbohydrates on in vitro adherence of four *Candida* species to human buccal epithelial cells. *Microb Ecol Health Dis.* 17, 156–162.
74. Vargas, S. L., Patrick, C. C., Ayers, G. D. and Hughes, W. T. (1993). Modulating effect of dietary carbohydrate supplementation on *Candida albicans* colonization and invasion in a neutropenic mouse model. *Infect Immun.* 61, 619–626.
75. Panigrahi, P., Parida, S., Pradhan, L., Mohapatra, S. S., Misra, P. R., Johnson, J. A., Chaudhry, R., Taylor, S., Hansen, N. I. and Gewolb, I. H. (2008). Long-term colonization of a lactobacillus symbiotic preparation in the neonatal gut. *J Pediatr Gastroenterol Nutr.* 47, 45–53.
76. Lazarevic, V., Whiteson, K., Hernandez, D., François, P. and Schrenzel, J. (2009). Study of inter-and intra-individual variations in the salivary microbiota. *BMC Genom.* 11, 523–523.
77. Glass, R. L. (1952). The lack of relationship between salivary lactobacillus counts and dental caries activity. *Oral Surg Oral Med Oral Pathol.* 5, 210–213.
78. van Houte, J., Gibbons, R. J. and Pulkkinen, A. J. (1972). Ecology of human oral lactobacilli. *Infect Immun.* 6, 723–729.
79. Yang, R., Argimon, S., Li, Y., Gu, H., Zhou, X. and Caufield, P. W. (2010). Determining the genetic diversity of lactobacilli from the oral cavity. *J Microbiol Methods.* 82, 163–169.
80. Becks, H. (1950). Carbohydrate restriction in the prevention of dental caries using the LA count as one index. *J CA Dent Assoc.* 26, 53–58.
81. Jay, P. (1947). The reduction of oral *Lactobacillus acidophilus* counts by the periodic restriction of carbohydrate. *Am J Orthod.* 33(3), B162–184.
82. Crossner, C. G. (1981). Salivary lactobacillus counts in the prediction of caries activity. *Commun Dent Oral Epidemiol.* 9, 182–190.
83. Matsuzaki, T., Takagi, A., Ikemura, H., Matsuguchi, T., & Yokokura, T. (2007). Intestinal microflora: Probiotics and autoimmunity. *J Nutr.* 137, 798S–802S.
84. Mitsuoka, T. and Kaneuchi, C. (1977). Ecology of the bifidobacteria. *Am J Clin Nutr.* 30, 1799–1810.
85. Meurman, J. H., Antila, H. and Salminen, S. (1994). Recovery of *Lactobacillus* strain GG (ATCC 53103) from saliva of healthy volunteers after consumption of yoghurt prepared with the bacterium. *Microb Ecol Health Dis.* 7, 295–298.
86. Caglar, E., Topcuoglu, N., Cildir, S. K., Sandalli, N. and Kulekci, G. (2009). Oral colonization by *Lactobacillus reuteri* ATCC 55730 after exposure to probiotics. *Int J Paediatric Dent.* 19, 377–381.
87. Ravn, I., Dige, I., Meyer, R. L. and Nyvad, B. (2012). Colonization of the oral cavity by probiotic bacteria. *Caries Res.* 46, 107–112.

88. Mitsuoka, T. (2000). Significance of dietary modulation of intestinal flora and intestinal environment. *Biosci. Microflora.* 19, 15–25.
89. Arai, K., Murota, I., Hayakawa, K., Kataoka, M. and Mitsuoka, T. (1980). Effects of administration of pasteurized fermented milk to mice on the life-span and intestinal flora. *J Jpn Soc Nutr Food Sci.* 33, 219–223 [Japanese].
90. Takano, T., Arai, K., Murota, I., Hayakawa, K., Mizutani, T. and Mitsuoka, T. (1985). Effects of feeding sour milk on longevity and tumorigenesis in mice and rats. *Bifidobact Microflora.* 4, 31–37.
91. Terada, A., Bukawa, W., Kan, T. and Mitsuoka, T. (2004). Effects of the consumption of heat-killed *Enterococcus faecalis* EC-12 preparation on microbiota and metabolic activity of the faeces in healthy adults. *Microbial Ecol Health Dis.* 16, 188–194.
92. Sawada, D., Sugawara, T., Ishida, Y., Aihara, K., Aoki, Y., Takehara, I., Takano, K. and Fujiwara, S. (2016). Effect of continuous ingestion of a beverage prepared with *Lactobacillus gasseri* CP2305 inactivated by heat treatment on the regulation of intestinal function. *Food Res Int.* 79, 33–39.
93. Nakamura, Y., Yamamoto, N., Sakai, K., Okubo, A., Yamazaki, S. and Takano, T. (1995). Purification and characterization of angiotensin I-converting enzyme inhibitors from sour milk. *J Dairy Sci.* 78, 777–783.
94. Ross, R. P., Mills, S., Hill, C., Fitzgerald, G. F. and Stanton, C. (2010). Specific metabolite production by gut microbiota as a basis for probiotic function. *Int Dairy J.* 20, 269–276.
95. O'Shea, E. F., Cotter, P. D., Stanton, C., Ross, R. P. and Hill, C. (2012). Production of bioactive substances by intestinal bacteria as a basis for explaining probiotic mechanisms: Bacteriocins and conjugated linoleic acid. *Int J Food Microbiol.* 152, 189–205.
96. Hayes, M., Coakley, M., O'Sullivan, L. and Stanton, C. (2006). Cheese as a delivery vehicle for probiotics and biogenic substances. *Austral J Dairy Technol.* 61, 132.
97. Möller, N. P., Scholz-Ahrens, K. E., Roos, N. and Schrezenmeir, J. (2008). Bioactive peptides and proteins from foods: Indication for health effects. *Eur J Nutr.* 47, 171–182.
98. Bogsan, C. S., Florence, A. C. R., Perina, N., Hirota, C., Soares, F. A. S. M., Silva, R. C. and Oliveira, M. N. (2013). Survival of *Bifidobacterium lactis* HN019 and release of biogenic compounds in unfermented and fermented milk is affected by chilled storage at 4°C. *J Prob Health.* 4.114.
99. Monagas, M., Urpi-Sarda, M., Sánchez-Patán, F., Llorach, R., Garrido, I., Gómez-Cordovés, C., Andres-Lacueva, C. and Bartolomé, B. (2010). Insights into the metabolism and microbial biotransformation of dietary flavan-3-ols and the bioactivity of their metabolites. *Food Funct.* 1, 233–253.
100. Dharmaraj, S. (2010). Marine *Streptomyces* as a novel source of bioactive substances. *World J Microbiol Biotechnol.* 26, 2123–2139.
101. Mitsuoka, T. (2014). Development of functional foods. *Biosci Microbiot Food Health.* 33, 117–128.
102. Sperandio, V., Torres, A. G., Jarvis, B., Nataro, J. P. and Kaper, J. B. (2003). Bacteria–host communication: The language of hormones. *Proc Natl Acad Sci U S A.* 100, 8951–8956.
103. Liévin-Le Moal, V. and Servin, A. L. (2014). Anti-infective activities of *Lactobacillus* strains in the human intestinal microbiota: From probiotics to gastrointestinal anti-infectious biotherapeutic agents. *Clin Microbiol Rev.* 27, 167–199.

Index

Page numbers followed by f and t indicate figures and tables, respectively.